1998
YEAR BOOK OF
PLASTIC, RECONSTRUCTIVE, AND
AESTHETIC SURGERY®

Statement of Purpose

The YEAR BOOK Service

The YEAR BOOK series was devised in 1901 by practicing health professionals who observed that the literature of medicine and related disciplines had become so voluminous that no one individual could read and place in perspective every potential advance in a major specialty. In the final decade of the 20th century, this recognition is more acutely true than it was in 1901.

More than merely a series of books, YEAR BOOK volumes are the tangible results of a unique service designed to accomplish the following:

- to *survey* a wide range of journals of proven value
- to *select* from those journals papers representing significant advances and statements of important clinical principles
- to provide *abstracts* of those articles that are readable, convenient summaries of their key points
- to provide *commentary* about those articles to place them in perspective

These publications grow out of a unique process that calls on the talents of outstanding authorities in clinical and fundamental disciplines, trained literature specialists, and professional writers, all supported by the resources of Mosby, the world's preeminent publisher for the health professions.

The Literature Base

Mosby and its editors survey more than 1,000 journals published worldwide, covering the full range of the health professions. On an annual basis, the publisher examines usage patterns and polls its expert authorities to add new journals to the literature base and to delete journals that are no longer useful as potential YEAR BOOK sources.

The Literature Survey

The publisher's team of literature specialists, all of whom are trained and experienced health professionals, examines every original, peer-reviewed article in each journal issue. More than 250,000 articles per year are scanned systematically, including title, text, illustrations, tables, and references. Each scan is compared, article by article, to the search strategies that the publisher has developed in consultation with the 270 outside experts who form the pool of YEAR BOOK editors. A given article may be reviewed by any number of editors, from one to a dozen or more, regardless of the discipline for which the paper was originally published. In turn, each editor who receives the article reviews it to determine whether the article should be included in the YEAR BOOK. This decision is based on the article's inherent quality, its probable usefulness to readers of that YEAR BOOK, and the editor's goal to represent a balanced picture of a given field in each volume of the YEAR BOOK. In addition, the editor indicates when to include figures and tables from the article to help the YEAR BOOK reader better understand the information.

Of the quarter million articles scanned each year, only 5% are selected for detailed analysis within the YEAR BOOK series, thereby assuring readers of the high value of every selection.

The Abstract

The publisher's abstracting staff is headed by a seasoned medical professional and includes individuals with training in the life sciences, medicine, and other areas, plus extensive experience in writing for the health professions and related industries. Each selected article is assigned to a specific writer on this abstracting staff. The abstracter, guided in many cases by notations supplied by the expert editor, writes a structured, condensed summary designed so that the reader can rapidly acquire the essential information contained in the article.

The Commentary

The YEAR BOOK editorial boards, sometimes assisted by guest commentators, write comments that place each article in perspective for the reader. This provides the reader with the equivalent of a personal consultation with a leading international authority—an opportunity to better understand the value of the article and to benefit from the authority's thought processes in assessing the article.

Additional Editorial Features

The editorial boards of each YEAR BOOK organize the abstracts and comments to provide a logical and satisfying sequence of information. To enhance the organization, editors also provide introductions to sections or individual chapters, comments linking a number of abstracts, citations to additional literature, and other features.

The published YEAR BOOK contains enhanced bibliographic citations for each selected article, including extended listings of multiple authors and identification of author affiliations. Each YEAR BOOK contains a Table of Contents specific to that year's volume. From year to year, the Table of Contents for a given YEAR BOOK will vary depending on developments within the field.

Every YEAR BOOK contains a list of the journals from which papers have been selected. This list represents a subset of the more than 1,000 journals surveyed by the publisher and occasionally reflects a particularly pertinent article from a journal that is not surveyed on a routine basis.

Finally, each volume contains a comprehensive subject index and an index to authors of each selected paper.

The 1998 Year Book Series

Year Book of Allergy, Asthma, and Clinical Immunology: Drs. Rosenwasser, Boguniewicz, Borish, Nelson, Routes, and Spahn

Year Book of Anesthesiology and Pain Management®: Drs. Tinker, Abram, Chestnut, Roizen, Rothenberg, and Wood

Year Book of Cardiology®: Drs. Schlant, Collins, Gersh, Graham, Kaplan, and Waldo

Year Book of Chiropractic®: Dr. Lawrence

Year Book of Critical Care Medicine®: Drs. Parrillo, Balk, Calvin, Franklin, and Shapiro

Year Book of Dentistry®: Drs. Meskin, Berry, Jeffcoat, Leinfelder, Roser, Summitt, and Zakariasen

Year Book of Dermatologic Surgery®: Drs. Greenway, Papadopoulos, Whitaker, and Barrett

Year Book of Dermatology®: Dr. Thiers

Year Book of Diagnostic Radiology®: Drs. Osborn, Groskin, Dalinka, Maynard, Pentecost, Rebner, Ros, Smirniotopoulos, and Young

Year Book of Drug Therapy®: Drs. Lasagna and Weintraub

Year Book of Emergency Medicine®: Drs. Wagner, Dronen, Davidson, King, Niemann, and Roberts

Year Book of Endocrinology®: Drs. Bagdade, Braverman, Horton, Kannan, Landsberg, Molitch, Morley, Nathan, Odell, Poehlman, Rogol, and Ryan

Year Book of Family Practice®: Drs. Berg, Bowman, Davidson, Dexter, and Scherger

Year Book of Gastroenterology®: Drs. Aliperti and Fleshman

Year Book of Geriatrics and Gerontology®: Drs. Beck, Burton, Ostwald, Rabins, Reuben, Roth, Shapiro, and Whitehouse

Year Book of Hand Surgery®: Drs. Amadio and Hentz

Year Book of Hematology®: Drs. Spivak, Bell, Ness, Quesenberry, Wiernik, and Horowitz

Year Book of Infectious Diseases: Drs. Keusch, Barza, Bennish, Poutsiaka, Skolnik, and Snydman

Year Book of Medicine®: Drs. Klahr, Cline, McCallum, Frishman, Utiger, Malawista, Mandell, and Jett

Year Book of Neonatal and Perinatal Medicine®: Drs. Fanaroff, Maisels, and Stevenson

Year Book of Nephrology, Hypertension, and Mineral Metabolism: Drs. Schwab, Bennett, Emmett, Hostetter, Kumar, and Toto

Year Book of Neurology and Neurosurgery®: Drs. Bradley and Gibbs

1998

The Year Book of PLASTIC, RECONSTRUCTIVE, AND AESTHETIC SURGERY®

Editor

Stephen H. Miller, M.D., M.P.H., F.A.C.S.

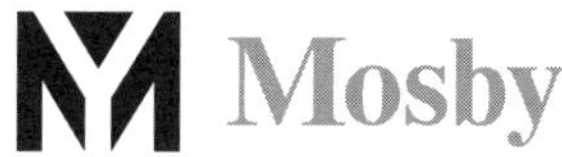

St. Louis   Baltimore   Boston   Carlsbad   Naples   New York   Philadelphia   Portland   London
Madrid   Mexico City   Singapore   Sydney   Tokyo   Toronto   Wiesbaden

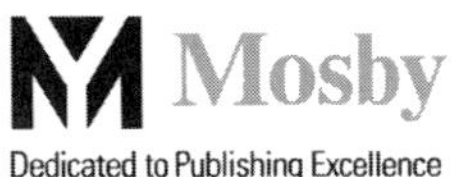

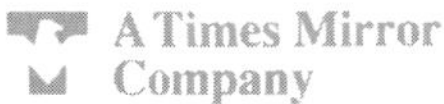

Publisher: Theresa Van Schaik
Director, Editorial Development: Gretchen C. Murphy
Developmental Editor: Marcy Reed
Manuscript Editor: Pat Costigan
Project Supervisor, Production: Joy Moore
Production Assistant: Laura Bayless
Manager, Literature Services: Idelle L. Winer
Illustrations and Permissions Coordinator: Phyllis K. Thompson

1998 EDITION
Copyright © 1998 by Mosby, Inc.

Printed in the United States of America
Composition by Reed Technology and Information Services, Inc.
Printing/binding by Maple–Vail

Editorial Office:
Mosby, Inc.
11830 Westline Industrial Drive
St. Louis, MO 63146
Customer Service: customer.support@mosby.com
        www.mosby.com/Mosby/CustomerSupport/index.html

International Standard Serial Number: 0140–175X
International Standard Book Number: 0–8151–9728–4

Associate Editors

Scott Bartlett, M.D.

Associate Professor of Surgery, University of Pennsylvania Medical Center and Children's Hospital of Philadelphia, Philadelphia, Pennsylvania

Warren Garner, M.D.

Associate Professor of Plastic and Reconstructive Surgery; Associate Professor of General Surgery, University of Michigan, Ann Arbor, Michigan

Peter W. McKinney, M.D., C.M., F.A.C.S.

Professor of Clinical Surgery (Plastic), Northwestern Medical School, Northwestern University, Chicago, Illinois

Robert L. Ruberg, M.D.

Professor and Director, Division of Plastic Surgery, Vice-Chair for Administrative Affairs, Department of Surgery, Ohio State University College of Medicine and Public Health, Columbus, Ohio

Roger Salisbury, M.D.

Professor of Surgery, Chief, Plastic and Reconstructive Surgery, New York Medical College Director, Burn Center, Westchester County Medical Center, Valhalla, New York

David J. Smith, Jr., M.D.

Professor and Section Head, Plastic and Reconstructive Surgery; Department of Surgery, University of Michigan, Ann Arbor, Michigan

Table of Contents

Associate Editors ix

Journals Represented xiii

Introduction xv

1. Congenital 1
   Experimental 1
   Craniofacial 4
   Maxillofacial 18
   Clefts 27
   Vascular and Lymphatic 34
   Other 36

2. Neoplastic, Inflammatory, and Degenerative Conditions 45
   Premalignant and Malignant Skin Tumors 45
   Head and Neck Reconstruction 51
   Degenerative and Inflammatory Conditions 56

3. Trauma 61
   Head and Neck 61
   Upper Extremity 67
   Burns 77

4. Aesthetic 97
   General 97
   Skin 100
   Skeletal 116
   Face, Neck, and Brow 125
   Eyelids 154
   Nose 167
   Extremities and Trunk 182
   Liposuction and Fat Grafting 184
   Additional Reading 197

5. Breast 199
   Silicone and Augmentation 199
   Reduction 213
   Cancer and Reconstruction 219

6. Flaps, Microsurgery, and Tissue Expansion 231

    Experimental 231

    Clinical 240

    Microsurgery 248

    Tissue Expansion 268

7. General 271

    Wound Healing and Scars 271

    Miscellaneous 292

    SUBJECT INDEX. 299

    AUTHOR INDEX 329

Journals Represented

Mosby and its editors survey more than 1,000 journals for its abstract and commentary publications. From these journals, the editors select the articles to be abstracted. Journals represented in this YEAR BOOK are listed below.

Acta Dermato-Venereologica
Aesthetic Plastic Surgery
American Journal of Clinical Nutrition
American Journal of Pathology
American Journal of Surgery
American Surgeon
Anesthesia and Plastic Surgery
Annales de Chirurgie Plastique et Esthetique
Annals of Plastic Surgery
Archives of Otolaryngology-Head and Neck Surgery
Archives of Surgery
Arthritis and Rheumatism
British Journal of Ophthalmology
British Journal of Plastic Surgery
British Medical Journal
Burns
Canadian Journal of Plastic Surgery
Childs Nervous System
Cleft Palate-Craniofacial Journal
Critical Care Medicine
Dermatologic Surgery
Diabetes Care
European Journal of Plastic Surgery
Journal of Bone and Joint Surgery (American Volume)
Journal of Burn Care and Rehabilitation
Journal of Clinical Investigation
Journal of Cranio-Maxillo-Facial Surgery
Journal of Hand Surgery (American)
Journal of Hand Surgery (British)
Journal of Laryngology and Otology
Journal of Neurosurgery
Journal of Oral and Maxillofacial Surgery
Journal of Pediatric Surgery
Journal of Reconstructive Microsurgery
Journal of Urology
Journal of Vascular Surgery
Journal of the American Academy of Dermatology
Journal of the American Medical Association
Lancet
Laryngoscope
Microsurgery
Neurosurgery
New England Journal of Medicine
Ophthalmic Plastic and Reconstructive Surgery
Pediatrics
Plastic and Reconstructive Surgery
Scandinavian Journal of Plastic and Reconstructive Hand Surgery

Southern Medical Journal
Transplantation
Wound Repair and Regeneration

STANDARD ABBREVIATIONS

The following terms are abbreviated in this edition: acquired immunodeficiency syndrome (AIDS), cardiopulmonary resuscitation (CPR), central nervous system (CNS), cerebrospinal fluid (CSF), computed tomography (CT), deoxyribonucleic acid (DNA), electrocardiography (ECG), health maintenance organization (HMO), human immunodeficiency virus (HIV), intensive care unit (ICU), intramuscular (IM), intravenous (IV), magnetic resonance (MR) imaging (MRI), and ribonucleic acid (RNA).

NOTE

The YEAR BOOK OF PLASTIC, RECONSTRUCTIVE, AND AESTHETIC SURGERY is a literature survey service providing abstracts of articles published in the professional literature. Every effort is made to assure the accuracy of the information presented in these pages. Neither the editors nor the publisher of the YEAR BOOK OF PLASTIC, RECONSTRUCTIVE, AND AESTHETIC SURGERY can be responsible for errors in the original materials. The editors' comments are their own opinions. Mention of specific products within this publication does not constitute endorsement.

To facilitate the use of the YEAR BOOK OF PLASTIC, RECONSTRUCTIVE, AND AESTHETIC SURGERY as a reference tool, all illustrations and tables included in this publication are now identified as they appear in the original article. This change is meant to help the reader recognize that any illustration or table appearing in the YEAR BOOK OF PLASTIC, RECONSTRUCTIVE, AND AESTHETIC SURGERY may be only one of many in the original article. For this reason, figure and table numbers will often appear to be out of sequence within the YEAR BOOK OF PLASTIC, RECONSTRUCTIVE, AND AESTHETIC SURGERY.

Introduction

We welcome Scott Bartlett, M.D., Warren Garner, M.D., and Roger Salisbury, M.D., to the editorial staff of the YEAR BOOK OF PLASTIC, RECONSTRUCTIVE, AND AESTHETIC SURGERY. Each of the new associated editors has enthusiastically joined with us to select and review cogent and timely articles pertinent to the modern-day practice of plastic, reconstructive, and aesthetic surgery. The quality of their selections and comments should prove beneficial for the edification of our audience. I believe that the YEAR BOOK, more than ever, provides each of its readers with a valuable and current resource for self-education.

I would like to thank the editorial staff of Mosby, Inc., Susan Fox, and Brenda Orf for their invaluable assistance during this transition year. Special thanks to the "old" hard-working associate editors, Peter McKinney, M.D., Robert Ruberg, M.D., and David Smith, M.D., for a great job and for adapting so well to the new system.

Stephen H. Miller, M.D., M.P.H., F.A.C.S.

1 Congenital

Experimental

Cranial Bone Graft to Reconstruct the Mandibular Condyle in *Macaca mulatta*

Dodson TB, Bays RA, Pfeffle RC, et al (Emory Univ, Atlanta, Ga)
J Oral Maxillofac Surg 55:260–267, 1997   1–1

Background.—Reconstructing the temporomandibular joint (TMJ) in adults is a surgical challenge. The efficacy of cranial bone grafts in the reconstruction of the mandibular condyle was investigated in a nonhuman primate model.

Methods.—Eight adult female monkeys were used. The right mandibular condyle was resected, and the mandible was reconstructed with autogenous, full-thickness cranial bone harvested from the frontal area of the skull and stabilized with rigid fixation. Assessments of joint function, facial symmetry, and occlusion were made before and for 1 year after surgery. Bone graft height was measured during surgery and 1 year later.

Findings.—Seven monkeys survived for 1 year with stable weights. No significant changes in maximal incisal opening or lateral excursion were observed. There were also no significant changes in facial symmetry or occlusion. The mean total reduction in graft height was 0.7 mm.

Conclusion.—In this primate model, full-thickness cranial bone grafts provided a functional joint that resisted resorption. Thus cranial bone may provide a suitable alternative to other autologous or alloplastic graft materials for reconstructing the human mandibular condyle in patients who are no longer growing.

▶ Reconstruction of the TMJ is fraught with problems. Not only is the conventional technique of costo-chondral grafting associated with a significant incidence of late ankylosis and either undergrowth or overgrowth, but the use of alloplastic joint replacements is problematic. In this article, the authors report on the use of cranial bone in a mature monkey model and show that, indeed, this material seems to be well tolerated. Not shown is a long-term analysis or any histologic data. One would be concerned that over the long term, progressive tightness and loss of junction of the joint apparatus would occur.

S.P. Bartlett, M.D.

Preliminary Report: A Ceramic Containing Crosslinked Collagen as a New Cranial Onlay and Inlay Material
Schendel S, Bresnick S, Cholon A (Stanford Univ, Calif)
Ann Plast Surg 38:158–162, 1997   1–2

Background.—Several different materials have been investigated for use in alloplastic bone grafting. The most frequently tested materials have been simple ceramics, but there are some important limitations to their use in craniomaxillary reconstruction. A new composite bone grafting material, consisting of particulate hydroxyapatite and cross-linked collagen, was tested in rabbits.

Methods.—The new material combined cross-linked collagen and hydroxyapatite into a pliable, carvable material designed to offer biocompatibility and structural integrity. In a time-sequence study, 5 rabbits had high- and low-loading composite only and inlay grafts placed in the parietal region of the skull. The animals were killed for histologic analysis of the parietal bones at 1, 2, 4, or 6 months after graft placement.

Results.—With both inlay and onlay grafts, there was tissue continuity and healing to the outer table of the skull. Both types of grafts showed bony ingrowth, with bone proliferation and vascularization. Ingrowth started as soon as 1 month after graft placement. The inlay grafts healed flush to the outer table. Both types of grafts still had at least 80% of graft volume at 6 months.

Conclusions.—This composite material may be very useful for craniomaxillary reconstruction. It is easy to handle and has good structural integrity and no brittleness. It maintains both its volume and shape, probably because of the combination of inorganic and organic components.

▶ This preliminary report demonstrates the utility of using a composite material containing both a ceramic and a collagen matrix. As the authors point out, this material may be more easy to handle and, in this preliminary report, is indeed biologically tolerated in the short term.

At the present time, new bioceramics are being reported almost daily. Each reportedly offers characteristics of bone growth incorporation similar to those of autogenous bone. With each of these, 6 questions will remain about the durability, safety, and capability for incorporation in the long term. As with this product, the answer will not be apparent for many years.

S.P. Bartlett, M.D.

The Viability of Cryopreserved Onlay Cranial Bone Allografts: A Comparative Experimental Study Versus Fresh Autografts
Sanz J, Elejabeitia J, Bazán A, et al (Univ of Navarra, Spain)
Ann Plast Surg 36:370–379, 1996   1–3

Introduction.—Calvarial bone grafts have some important advantages for use in craniofacial surgery, including ease of access and low reabsorption. There are some problems, however. Because of reabsorption, surgery must be repeated and new donor areas are needed. The amount of autogenous bone available is limited, and graft harvesting leads to increased surgical time and morbidity. Cryopreserved allografts are investigated as a possible alternative to calvarial bone autografts.

Methods.—The study examined the use of calvarial onlay bone grafts in sheep. After harvesting, the grafts were cryopreserved at −80°C. Their behavior was compared with that of fresh autografts implanted under identical conditions. After implantation, the 2 groups of grafts were compared for reabsorption rate over time. Light microscopic evaluation was performed to assess any histologic differences.

Results.—No evidence of infection or rejection was detected. Ninety-day reabsorption was 22% of the grafted volume with allografts vs. 20% with autografts; the difference was not significant. Loss of the diplöe led to reduced height in all onlay grafts. The allografts caused no inflammatory reaction, and the histologic findings were the same as those in fresh autografts. At sacrifice and throughout radiographic follow-up it was impossible to distinguish between the allografts and autografts.

Conclusions.—Cryopreserved calvarial bone allografts are a promising material for craniofacial surgery, as suggested by animal studies. This tissue undergoes creeping substitution and remains durable despite partial reabsorption. It is easy to work with and can be banked in virtually unlimited amounts.

▶ Allograft use in craniofacial reconstruction has prompted a great deal of research. These authors are the first to my knowledge to investigate the use of cranial bone allografts in an experimental model.

The early results are encouraging. At 90 days the authors found no statistical difference in volume retention between the 2 types of grafts and both graft types appeared to have similar histologic features. An obvious question remains, however: whether longer-term studies will bear this out. Early success with allografting of bones from other sources preserved by a variety of methods has been encouraging, only to see late resorption. Studies of this type on a long-term basis are needed.

The potential for this work is enormous. Although a great deal of experimental effort is now focused on the integration of complex bone substitutes with growth factors, it would be far simpler indeed and probably less costly if cranial allograft bone could be utilized.

S.P. Bartlett, M.D.

Craniofacial

The Differential Diagnosis of Posterior Plagiocephaly: True Lambdoid Synostosis Versus Positional Molding

Huang MHS, Gruss JS, Clarren SK, et al (Singapore Gen Hosp; Univ of Washington, Seattle)
Plast Reconstr Surg 98:765–774, 1996   1–4

Background.—Craniofacial surgery centers have noticed an increase in the number of patients referred for management of posterior plagiocephaly. There is ongoing debate about the diagnosis and treatment of this condition. There are insufficient data on the characteristics of true lambdoid synostosis, as opposed to deformational plagiocephaly related to positional molding. As a result, many infants with non-synostotic plagiocephaly have undergone major intracranial surgery. The findings of true lambdoid synostosis and positional plagiocephaly were compared and contrasted.

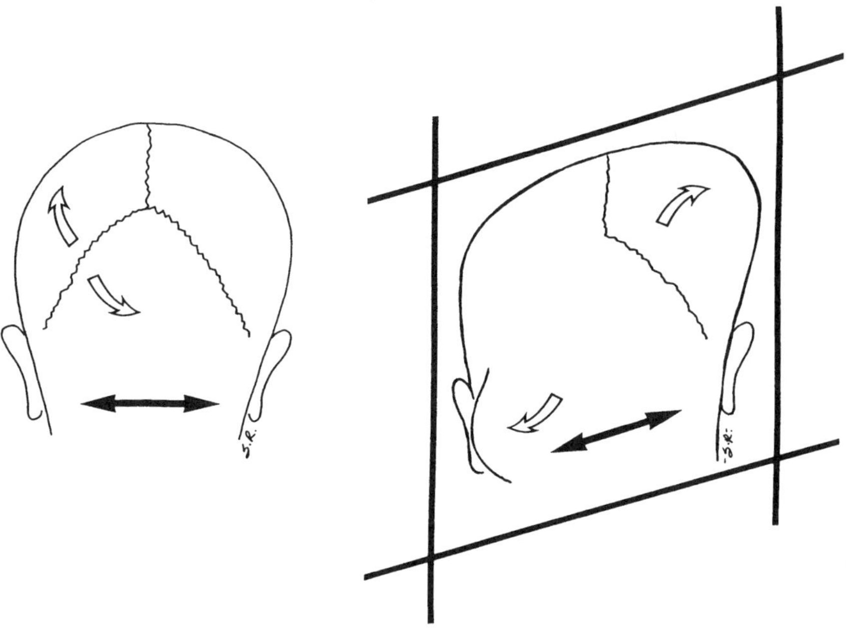

FIGURE 10.—Differences between deformational and synostotic posterior plagiocephaly from the posterior view (*clear arrows* indicate growth vectors; *solid arrows,* skull base axis). **Left,** positional molding. Growth occurs perpendicular to the suture, the skull base is horizontal, and the head shape is normal. **Right,** unilambdoid synostosis. Compensatory growth occurs parallel to the fused suture, resulting in contralateral parietal and ipsilateral occipitomastoid bossing, ipsilateral inferior tilt of the skull base, inferior displacement of the ipsilateral ear, and a parallelogram head shape. (Courtesy of Huang MHS, Gruss JS, Clarren SK, et al: The differential diagnosis of posterior plagiocephaly: True lambdoid synostosis versus positional molding. *Plast Reconstr Surg* 98:765–774, 1996.)

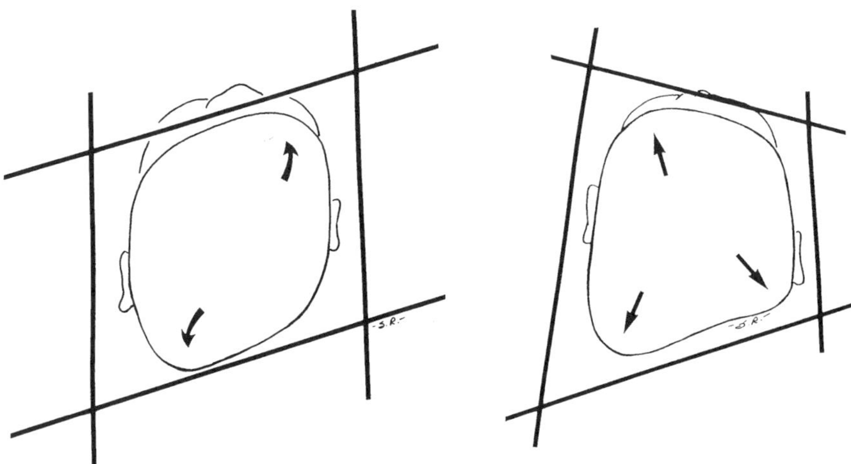

FIGURE 11.—Differences in head shape from the vertex view (*arrows* indicate directions of compensatory growth vectors). **Left,** positional molding produces a parallelogram-shaped head. **Right,** unilambdoid synostosis produces a trapezium-shaped head. (Courtesy of Huang MHS, Gruss JS, Clarren SK, et al: The differential diagnosis of posterior plagiocephaly: True lambdoid synostosis versus positional molding. *Plast Reconstr Surg* 98:765–774, 1996.)

Methods.—The study included 102 patients with posterior plagiocephaly evaluated at 1 craniofacial program from 1991 to 1994 and 130 patients undergoing surgery for craniosynostosis during the same period. The infants were evaluated by various specialists, including a pediatric dysmorphologist, a craniofacial surgeon, and a pediatric neurosurgeon. Appropriate diagnostic imaging studies were performed. Craniofacial surgery was performed in patients with lambdoid synostosis and those with severe, progressive positional molding. The clinical, imaging, and operative features of lambdoid synostosis and positional plagiocephaly were analyzed in detail and compared.

Results.—Just 3% of patients with craniosynostosis had the true clinical, imaging, and operative features of unilambdoid synostosis. Of the patients with positional molding, just 3% needed surgery. Unilambdoid synostosis was characterized by a thick ridge over the fused suture, just as is seen in other types of craniosynostosis when viewed from behind. These patients also had compensatory contralateral parietal and frontal bossing and an ipsilateral occipitomastoid bulge. There was an ipsilateral inferior tilt of the skull base, with accompanying inferior and posterior displacement of the ipsilateral ear. When viewed from above, these patients had a trapezoidal head shape. In contrast, patients with positional molding and open lambdoid sutures had the opposite clinical findings, corroborated by the diagnostic imaging findings. When viewed from posterior these patients had a normal head shape, but when viewed from above their heads resembled parallelogram.

Conclusions.—The differences between true lambdoid synostosis and positional molding are elucidated (Figs 10, 11, 12). True unilambdoid

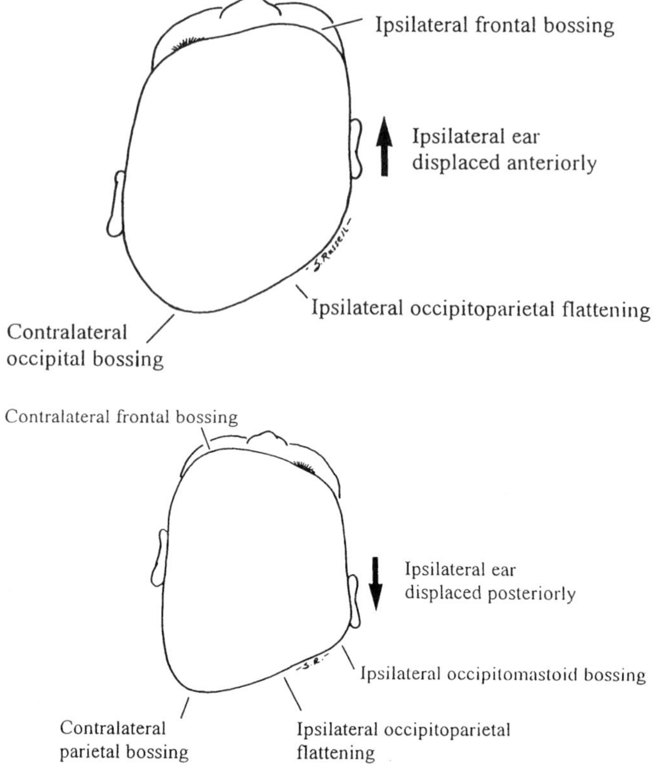

FIGURE 12.—Diagrammatic summary of some of the differences between positional molding (**left**) and unilambdoid synostosis (**right**). (Courtesy of Huang MHS, Gruss JS, Clarren SK, et al: The differential diagnosis of posterior plagiocephaly: True lambdoid synostosis versus positional molding. *Plast Reconstr Surg* 98:765–774, 1996.)

synostosis is a rare syndrome. Being aware of its specific features will permit more accurate diagnosis and treatment and prevent unnecessary surgery in patients with positional molding.

▶ This manuscript extends the original work of Mulliken, who categorized the differences in frontal plagiocephaly that can be caused by either unicoronal synostosis or molding. This information is of great interest to plastic surgeons, dysmorphologists, pediatricians, and geneticists.*

As the authors have emphasized, most patients with positional molding require no operative intervention. What is unknown is the incidence of problems such as elevated intracranial pressure and brain compression that are associated with true lambdoid synostosis, and the appropriate timing and type of intervention.

S.P. Bartlett, M.D.

---

*Experience at our center indicates that although these "classic" findings of lambdoid synostosis and positional molding may be seen and allow one to clearly differentiate these two entities, there remains an intermediary group which shares characteristics of each and in whom investigation with CT scans and close clinical follow-up is mandated.

Lambdoid Stenosis (Posterior Plagiocephaly) and Craniofacial Asymmetry: Long-term Outcomes

Goodrich JT, Argamaso R (Montefiore Med Ctr, Bronx, NY)
Childs Nerv Syst 12:720–726, 1996

1–5

Introduction.—As more and more infants are placed on their backs or sides to sleep, the number of cases of sudden infant death syndrome has decreased. At the same time, the number of positional cranial deformations has increased significantly. In their experience with lambdoid stenosis, or posterior plagiocephaly, the authors have noticed that rather severe craniofacial deformities can occur. Toward developing guidelines for selecting candidates for craniofacial reconstruction, the authors reviewed their experience with lambdoid stenosis.

Patients.—The analysis included 22 children who underwent surgery for lambdoid stenosis and were followed for 1 or more years. All had progressive deformation despite aggressive early positioning and helmet remodeling, with developing posterior plagiocephaly (severe deformation of the posterior occipital region). The authors developed criteria for selection of surgical candidates (Table 1). Most of the children in their series had "thumbprinting" and bone erosion over the posterior bone plates. Surgery consisted of a Marchac transposition or tiara reconstruction. Ideally, surgery was performed when the child was 6 to 12 months of age.

Outcomes.—There were no deaths and only minimal morbidity. None of the patients required revision surgery. The results were considered excellent in 77% of patients and good to very-good in the rest. Children undergoing early surgery had corrections of the "torquing" or "twisting" effect of lambdoidal sclerosis, leading to significantly fewer problems with facial scoliosis and temporomandibular joint malalignment.

Conclusions.—Most cases of lambdoid stenosis/positional deformation will respond to corrective positioning. Based on their experience, the authors outline selection criteria for surgical correction, when necessary.

TABLE 1.—Criteria Developed for Consideration for Surgery of a Child
With Lambdoid Stenosis

(a) Signs of increased intracranial pressure (digital markings on CT, papilledema, lack of head growth)
(b) Petrous ridge deformation (malpositioning of ear and axial shift of petrous ridge)
(c) Facial scolosis and/or orbital dystopia (similar to that in anteri- or plagiocephaly)
(d) Mandibular malalignment
(e) Forehead shifting secondary to compensatory bossing
(f) Failure of conservative regimes (e.g. positioning, helmet modeling) with further progression of asymmetry

(Courtesy of Goodrich JT, Argamaso R: Lambdoid stenosis (posterior plagiocephaly) and craniofacial asymmetry: Long-term outcomes. *Childs Nerv Sys* 12:720–726, 1996.)

With early recognition and surgical correction, the aesthetic results are highly satisfactory.

▶ The "hot topic" in craniofacial surgery today is posterior plagiocephaly. Numerous articles have been written, and a symposium dedicated almost completely to this topic has been completed. Questions remain, however, as to the definition and, more importantly, the management of this condition. I would call your attention to Table 1 which gives the criteria developed for the *consideration* of a child with lambdoid stenosis for surgery. The authors correctly state that these are criteria for considering an operation, not absolute indications for repair. It should be stressed, once again, that a period of observation is paramount, to see if these lesions are self-correcting.

It is becoming clear that true lambdoid synostosis and pure positional molding may represent just either end of a continuous spectrum. There remains a large group in the middle who tend to share some characteristics of the former and some characteristics of the latter. It is this intermediate group that deserves further investigation.

As an aside, these authors talk about "long-term outcomes." This is not a long-term outcome series. Further *true* long-term outcome studies of both surgically and nonsurgically treated treatment groups would be appropriate.

S.P. Bartlett, M.D.

Outcome Analysis of 85 Patients Undergoing the Pi Procedure for Correction of Sagittal Synostosis
Boop FA, Chadduck WM, Shewmake K, et al (Arkansas Children's Hosp, Little Rock; Children's Natl Med Ctr, Washington, DC)
J Neurosurg 85:50–55, 1996   1–6

Introduction.—For infants with sagittal synostosis, sagittal synostectomy can slow the progression of the deformity and, eventually, provide some improvement in skull contour. Some authorities recommend more complex procedures for cranial vault remodeling—such as the pi procedure—to improve the cosmetic results. Other authors criticize these procedures on the basis that they entail greater risk. To address these concerns, an experience with the pi procedure was reviewed.

Patients.—The review included 85 children with sagittal synostosis undergoing the pi procedure from 1986 to 1994. There were 69 boys and 16 girls, two thirds aged 6 months or younger. Sixty-five underwent preoperative CT, which always showed evidence of scaphocephaly; in 5% of patients, the scan also showed unsuspected intracranial pathology. Mean intraoperative blood loss was 115 mL, and was highest for children older than 1 year. All patients received blood transfusions, which were uncomplicated. Three patients experienced intraoperative dural lacerations. The average degree of foreshortening of the dolichocephalic skull was 13 mm.

Outcomes.—The cosmetic results were rated as excellent in 53% of children, good in 43%, and poor in 4%. Reoperation was required in 1 patient. All the poor outcomes occurred in infants younger than 8 weeks who had a reverse pi procedure. The best results were achieved in infants who were 3 to 6 months old at surgery.

Conclusions.—As an alternative for the treatment of sagittal synostosis, the pi procedure can be done with minimal morbidity. The cosmetic results are better than those achieved with strip craniectomy alone. The procedure is best done when the infant is 3 to 6 months old.

Synostectomy Versus Complex Cranioplasty for the Treatment of Sagittal Synostosis
Boop FA, Shewmake K, Chadduck WM (Arkansas Children's Hosp, Little Rock; Children's Natl Med Ctr, Washington, DC)
Childs Ncrv Syst 12:371–375, 1996   1–7

Background.—Strip craniectomy is the traditional therapy for infants with sagittal synostosis. This procedure is inadequate in many ways, however, as reflected by the large number of alternative procedures proposed. Arguments for and against the more complex cranioplasties for the treatment of sagittal synostosis were reviewed.

Discussion.—Sagittal synostectomy is effective in children treated within the first 8 weeks of life. However, there are several barriers to performing surgery at this time, including the fact that most children with craniosynostosis are not referred until 4 or 5 months of age. Further, infants treated with simple synostectomy during the first 8 weeks appear to have a high rate of re-stenosis. One argument against the use of more complex cranioplasties is that they carry higher rates of morbidity and mortality than strip craniectomy. However, experience with the pi procedure suggests that, with modern anesthetic and surgical techniques, morbidity is no higher than with strip or modified strip craniectomy. Opponents of complex cranioplasties also cite longer operative times and increased transfusion requirements. Intraoperative blood loss during the pi procedure can be limited to less than 125 mL, and it rarely is necessary to give more than 1 U of packed red blood cells. Thus, there is little increase in the risk of transmissible disease, compared with modified synostectomy. The argument that these operations lead to a longer hospital stay is irrelevant, considering that the goal of treatment is to give the child a normal appearance, not to provide a satisfactory appearance with a shorter hospital stay.

Recommendation.—Complex cranioplasties should be the treatment of choice for most infants with sagittal synostosis. The cosmetic results are better with the more complex procedures, and morbidity is little higher than that of synostectomy. It is safer to focus on careful blood screening rather than on avoiding or limiting blood transfusions during surgery. Strip craniectomy is best reserved for children referred during the first 2 months of life who have a rapidly progressive deformity with signs of increased intracranial pressure.

▶ These 2 papers (Abstracts 1–6 and 1–7) actually comment on the same group of patients who have undergone the more extensive pi procedure for the treatment of sagittal synostosis. Conventional treatment is an extended strip craniectomy done early in life (6 weeks to 3 months). The authors argue that these more extensive procedures done later improve results. Unfortunately, there is no group of patients who underwent craniectomy alone with which to compare these series, and until a prospective trial is performed to compare these techniques, this information will continue to be debated. At the present time, it seems prudent to recommend early extended strip craniectomies when possible and to perform more extreme cranioplasties (the type depending on and tailored to the deformity) when this is not possible or in those patients treated early who develop progressive deformity.

S.P. Bartlett, M.D.

Late Correction of Sagittal Synostosis in Children
Pensler JM, Ciletti SJ, Tomita T (Northwestern Univ, Chicago; Children's Mem Hosp, Chicago)
Plast Reconstr Surg 97:1362–1367, 1996   1–8

Introduction.—Surgery for correction of sagittal synostosis is best performed before the child is 2 months old. However, many children with scaphocephaly are not evaluated for reconstruction until they are more than 6 months old. These patients require the most extensive reconstructive surgery, which often yields disappointing results. A technique for late correction of scaphocephaly was described.

> *Technique.*—The operation is done with the child in the sphinx position to facilitate exposure from the supraorbital rim to the occipital prominence. A normal biparietal width is achieved by advancing the parietal tenons in tongue-in-groove fashion. This permits increases in parietal width of 2 cm per side, or 4 cm in total. An inverted triangle of bone is removed at the posterior border on the frontal bone; this facilitates posterior rotation of the frontal bone, reducing frontal bossing. Bipolar cautery is used to plicate the dura anteriorly, reducing the anteroposterior length of the skull. The frontal bone is scored to facilitate lateral expansion, and the occipital bone is treated in an analogous fashion. Microfixation plates and wires then are used to fix the cranial helmet to the cranial base. The remaining bony gaps are filled with hydroxyapatite and demineralized allograft bone gel.

Experience.—This technique has been used in 12 patients with late-diagnosed scaphocephaly. Intraoperative measurements suggested that anteroposterior length was reduced by a mean of 3 cm, whereas parietal width was increased by a mean of 4 cm. There were no problems with infection or bleeding, and no significant bone gaps after operation. The bone plates were palpable in 2 patients treated with 1.5–mm-thick plates.

Conclusions.—The procedure described is a safe and effective approach to the management of late-diagnosed sagittal synostosis. This technique provides controlled biparietal expansion of the cranial vault with a reduction in anteroposterior length and improvement in frontal and occipital bossing. Dual plication with bipolar ligation and suture ligation is used to ensure that the bone segments are placed in the optimal anatomical location during surgery.

▶ These authors add yet another technical modification for late correction of sagittal synostosis. In this manuscript, as in others that deal with this deformity, important points include the following: (1) a decrease in antero posterior dimension is essential and must be correlated with an increase in transverse dimension, and (2) osteotomies must be carried well into the cranial base, including the orbits, basiocciput, and sphenoparietal region.

S.P. Bartlett, M.D.

Classification of Previously Unclassified Cases of Craniosynostosis
Chumas PD, Cinalli G, Arnaud E, et al (Hôpital Necker Enfants–Malades, Paris; Gen Infirmary at Leeds, England)
J Neurosurg 86:177–181, 1997   1–9

Introduction.—A minority of patients with craniosynostosis are unable to be classified or are incorrectly classified. To determine whether there were any missed patterns of craniosynostosis, a 19-year retrospective review of a craniofacial data bank was done.

Methods.—Of 1,474 patients in the database, 53 (3.6%) were designated as nonsyndromic but unclassifiable. Patient records and radiographs were reviewed and compared with those of patients in the data bank who were classified as having simple craniosynostoses.

Results.—Patients previously considered unclassifiable were divided into 2 groups: group A—two-suture disease and group B—complex disease (more than 2 sutures involved).

Thirty-six group A patients showed clear evidence of simultaneous involvement of 2 sutures, but no progression over time, to suggest a more diffuse pansynostosis. Suture involvement was 17 patients with sagittal plus coronal; 7, sagittal and metopic; 6, sagittal and lambdoid; and 6, metopic and coronal.

Seventeen group B patients had severe morphologic changes and multiple suture involvement. Craniotomy was the only option in 6 group B patients because of large areas of lacunae within the cranial vault. Ten

TABLE 1.—Rates of Surgical Intervention in 53 Patients With Two-Suture or Complex Disease vs. Patients With Simple Craniosynostosis

	Type of Disease		
Factor	Two-Suture	Complex	Grouped Non-syndromic
no. of cases	36	17	1189
age at presentation (yrs)	1.2 ± 1.3	1 ± 1.9	1.3 ± 1.9
preop DQ (no. of pts)	93 ± 13 (18)	94 ± 12 (5)	99 ± 14 (701)
preop ICP (no. of pts)	13.9 (9)	10 (2)	10.6 (428)
no. treated surgically (%)	33 (92)	16 (94)	903 (76)
follow-up period (yrs)	4.1 ± 3.1	5.5 ± 5.1	4 ± 3.5
no. of operations			
one	25 pts (76%)	10 pts (62%)	858 pts (95%)
two	7 pts	6 pts	42 pts
three	1 pt		3 pts
final IQ (no. of pts)	99 ± 24 (25)	90 ± 20 (13)	101 ± 17 (737)
final morphological grade	1.6 ± 0.6	1.9 ± 0.6	1.3 ± 0.6

Abbreviations: DQ, development quotient; *pts,* patients.
(Courtesy of Chumas PD, Cinalli G, Arnaud E, et al: Classification of previously unclassified cases of craniosynostosis. *J Neurosurg* 86:177–181, 1997.)

group B patients had bilateral lambdoid plus sagittal suture involvement that resulted in marked occipital recession posteriorly. Six patients had a massive frontal bone that was associated with posteriorly located coronal sutures. Four patients with bilateral coronal plus metopic involvement had small frontal bones. Group B patients tended to have a lower intelligence quotient and worse morphologic outcome than patients with simple craniosynostoses. The incidence of second operations in group A patients, group B patients, and patients with simple craniosynostoses, respectively, was 24%, 37.5%, and 5% (Table 1).

Conclusions.—Patients with "two-suture synostosis" can be treated with standard craniosynostosis but have a higher rate of re-operation, compared with patients with simple craniosynostoses. Patients with "complex" disease have severe multisuture involvement and require a tailor-made approach to management that often necessitates a second operative procedure.

► Unclassified craniosynostosis, those not believed to be simple nonsyndromic or complex syndromic, are seen in any large-volume craniosynostosis practice. Each of us has anecdotal experience with these deformities and generally agrees with that of the authors: the more sutures involved and the more complex the deformity, the greater the number of operative interventions required to effect a satisfactory outcome.

Exciting changes in molecular genetics should shed light on this subject. The work of Muenke and coworkers[1] in defining growth factor receptor deficiencies should be helpful. It is likely that in the very near future, previously unclassified cases of craniosynostosis can be placed into more broad diagnostic groups, which will then allow for a more detailed analysis of specific deformities, their treatment, and outcome.

S.P. Bartlett, M.D.

Reference

1. Schell U, Hehr A, Feldman GJ, et al: Mutations in FGFR1 and FGFR2 cause familial and sporadic Pfeiffer syndrome. *Hum Mol Genet* 4:323–328, 1995.

Prognosis for Mental Function in Apert's Syndrome

Renier D, Arnaud E, Cinalli G, et al (Hôpital Necker Enfants-Malades, Paris)
J Neurosurg 85:66–72, 1996   1–10

Introduction.—Reports vary regarding the universality of mental retardation and the effectiveness of early surgery on improvement of intellectual development in children with Apert's syndrome. The mental development, the influence of surgical treatment, associated brain malformations, and the quality of the family environment were evaluated in children with Apert's syndrome.

Methods.—Of 70 children with Apert's syndrome, 60 underwent MRI of the head. There were 32 boys and 28 girls who underwent a mean initial examination at 20 months. The mean age of 53 patients who underwent surgery was 22 months. Thirty-seven patients underwent surgery before the age of 1 year. The initial procedure was forehead advancement in 49 patients, skull decompression by free flaps in 1, and the Le Fort III procedure in 3. Reoperation was performed for increased intracranial pressure in 6 patients, facial advancement of the Le Fort III type in 25, and cranioplasty for lack of re-ossification in 3. Seven children did not undergo surgery because of mild deformity or parental refusal. Ten children were institutionalized soon after birth. Forty-three children lived in a normal family environment and the family situation was not known in 7 children.

Results.—The mean IQ of 38 patients with an available final IQ assessment was 62 (range, 10 to 114). In 12 patients (32%), it was higher than 70. The major factor associated with changes in mental development was age at time of operation. The final IQ was higher than 70 in 50% of children who underwent surgery before the age of 1 year, compared to 7.1% of children who had surgery after the age of 1 year. There was no correlation between final IQ and malformations of the corpus callosum and size of the ventricles. Anomalies of the septum pellucidum had a significant effect. More than twice as many children with an IQ greater than 70 had a normal septum, compared to children with septal anomalies. Only 12.5% of institutionalized children had a normal IQ level, compared to 39.3% of children raised in a normal family environment.

Conclusion.—Time of operation, septal anomalies, and environment were the most important determinants of IQ in this series of patients with Apert's syndrome.

▶ Two important observations are made in this manuscript. The first is that children operated on before the age of 1 year had a significantly better IQ score than those operated on later in life. Second, the quality of the family environment contributed to intellectual development. One could argue that the exception to the former is the child with widely patent fontanels who has a decompressed neurocranium. This points out once again that, although general guidelines can be made in the treatment of these disorders, individualization is the rule. A series which more closely matches deformity types would be helpful. The quality of the child's environment cannot be overestimated.

S.P. Bartlett, M.D.

Extradural Deadspace After Infant Fronto-Orbital Advancement in Apert Syndrome

Moore MH, Abbott AH (Women's and Children's Hosp, North Adelaide, Australia)
Cleft Palate Craniofac J 33:202–205, 1996   1–11

Background.—Infant fronto-orbital advancement is currently a cornerstone of the treatment of craniosynostosis in Apert syndrome. It is assumed that the expanding brain rapidly advances in support of, and to remodel, the new frontal facade. However, no detailed analysis of the early intracranial changes after fronto-orbital advancement in infants with Apert syndrome had been published.

Methods.—Twenty-two infants with Apert syndrome underwent initial treatment of craniosynostosis between 1988 and 1993. All were younger than 15 months of age. Twelve infants in this group had enough early postoperative CT data available for assessing the intracranial dead space after fronto-orbital advancement. In all patients, fronto-orbital advancement of 10–20 mm was performed.

Findings.—Computed tomography in these infants showed a large extradural dead space persisting through the first week after surgery and not consistently obliterated until the fourth week. Early dead space effacement resulted from expansion of the prefrontal subarachnoid space, with no significant changes in frontal brain substance or ventricle size or shape. Brain growth or expansion was especially slow, and brain shape distortions were still apparent at late follow-up.

Conclusions.—A large extradural dead space seen in this series persisted through the first postoperative week, with consistent obliteration occurring only in the fourth week. Insignificant brain expansion and ventricular dilation occurred in the early postoperative period, as seen on qualitative CT scans. Early dead space obliteration was a result of the prefrontal subarachnoid space in all the patients.

▶ Early surgery in the treatment of Apert's craniosynostosis is frustrating indeed. Unlike many simple non-syndromic and syndromic synostosis cases, a high rate of "recurrence" of the deformity is seen. As Posnick[1] and co-workers pointed out, intracranial volume in these patients is frequently above normal. Hence, it comes as no surprise that fronto-orbital advancement is not associated with rapid filling of the fronto-orbital extradural dead space. Rather, this is a slow process, primarily associated with expansion of the prefrontal subarachnoid space.

Given these considerations, perhaps the most salient feature of this article can be found in the last paragraph. A delay in brain expansion and support for the advanced forehead may be a primary reason for the inconsistency in achieving good frontal contour. This necessarily leads to a higher rate of repeat surgery. Hence, delaying intervention in these patients may, indeed, be most appropriate, especially in cases in which there is no sign of elevated intracranial pressure or other compressive problems.

S.P. Bartlett, M.D.

Reference

1. Posnick JC, Bite U, Nakano P, et al: Indirect intracranial volume measurements using CT scans: Clinical applications for craniosynostosis. *Plast Reconstr Surg* 89:34–45, 1992.

Posterior Skull Surgery in Craniosynostosis
Sgouros S, Goldin JH, Hockley AD, et al (Queen Elizabeth and Children's Hosps, Birmingham, England)
Childs Nerv Syst 12:727–733, 1996
1–12

Purpose.—Historically, in the management of craniosynostosis, most attention has focused on the anterior portion of the skull. The authors performed posterior skull release in 2 patients with an unusual "cloverleaf" skull deformity. The resulting improvement in skull shape was such that no further surgery was needed. They review their experience with posterior skull surgery, emphasizing its role in the management of patients with complex craniosynostosis.

Methods.—From 1978 to 1994, 275 children underwent surgery for craniosynostosis. Of these, 22 had posterior skull release at some point. The patients were 13 boys and 9 girls with a mean age of 5 months at their first operation. Sixteen had complex syndromes with multiple suture involvement, 3 had coronal and lambdoid suture involvement, and 3 had isolated lambdoid synostosis. Posterior skull release was performed by circumferential occipital craniectomy and bilateral bone flap craniotomy. The patients were followed for a mean of 5 years.

Findings.—In the overall experience, 5% of patients had recurrent craniosynostosis requiring reoperation. This complication occurred when increased intracranial pressure required surgery before 6 months of age. Beginning in 1986, the authors performed initial posterior skull release or decompression in patients with significantly increased intracranial pressure. The procedure removed the pressure of the growing brain from the orbits, permitting deferral of fronto-orbital advancement to 1 year of age or older. Early posterior skull release completely avoided the need for anterior skull surgery in 3 patients. An additional 9 patients did not need repeat surgery for recurrent anterior skull deformity. Early posterior skull surgery was not performed in patients with severe, vision-threatening exorbitism. This group needed early fronto-orbital advancement, sometimes supplemented by later posterior skull release. Satisfactory results were achieved with posterior skull release for children with deformity related to isolated lambdoid synostosis or for children with nonsyndromic lambdoid and coronal synostosis who had pronounced "copper beating" of the posterior skull.

Conclusion.—Posterior skull surgery can play an important role in the management of craniosynostosis. It can reduce high intracranial pressure in patients with complex craniosynostosis, sometimes correcting skull deformity to the point where fronto-orbital advancement can be avoided completely. Early posterior skull release allows anterior skull surgery to be delayed until after 1 year of age, making surgery easier and reducing the risk of recurrent craniosynostosis.

▶ This review addresses the small subgroup of the total patient population with craniosynostosis, but in whom the ramifications of the disease are severe. It is agreed that there has been a tendency to give less emphasis to the posterior vault, as it is frequently "covered by hair." However, as these authors point out, there may, indeed, be a role for early posterior skull release in these patients to bide time and reduce the total number of interventions on the anterior vault. This may also give one time for the anterior bone to mature and permit more accurate osteotomies, advancement, and fixation. This technique may also be of value in the young patient with severe progressive turribrachycephaly; releasing the posterior vault may permit less progression of the deformity.

S.P. Bartlett, M.D.

Treatment of Obstructive Sleep Apnoea Using Nasal CPAP in Children With Craniofacial Dysostoses
Gonsalez S, Thompson D, Hayward R, et al (Great Ormond Street Hosp for Children, London)
Childs Nerv Syst 12:713–719, 1996   1–13

Background.—Upper airway function can be adversely affected in patients with craniofacial dysostoses. Obstructive sleep apnea is a common problem for these patients, and surgery is best delayed until facial growth is complete. Adults with obstructive sleep apnea may be treated with nasal continuous positive airway pressure (n-CPAP). This approach to the palliation of obstructive sleep apnea was tested in children with craniofacial dysostosis.

Methods.—The study included 8 consecutive children with craniofacial dysostosis and obstructive sleep apnea confirmed by sleep studies. The children ranged from 2 to 15 years of age. They were studied at baseline and during follow-up with nighttime respiratory sleep studies. After an

TABLE 1.—Summary of Clinical Characteristics, Time Taken to Acclimatize to Nasal Continuous Positive Airway Pressure, Results of the First Trial, and Outcome

Patient	Age (years)	Syndrome	Previous treatment for upper airway problems	Time taken to acclimatise to n-CPAP	Result of first n-CPAP trial	Outcome
1	15.0	Pfeiffer	None	1 night	Good	On n-CPAP for 14 months, awaiting midface surgery
2	2.2	Crouzon	Midface advancement	2 months	Good	On n-CPAP for 12 months
3	3.2	Crouzon	None	1 month	Good	On n-CPAP for 12 months
4	13.0	Apert	None	1 night	Partial improvement	On n-CPAP for 3 months, awaiting nasal + pharyngeal endoscopy
5	13.8	Pfeiffer	Adenotonsillectomy	1 night	Good	On n-CPAP for 2 months
6	3.0	Apert	None	Not tolerated after 1 month	Not assessed	On home acclimatisation to n-CPAP
7	2.5	Apert	Nasopharyngeal airway	3 nights	Poor	Well, with nasopharyngeal airway
8	5.5	Crouzon	Tracheostomy	Not tolerated	Not assessed	Well, with tracheostomy

Abbreviation: n-CPAP, nasal continuous positive airway pressure.
(Courtesy of Gonsalez S, Thompson D, Hayward R, et al: Treatment of obstructive sleep apnoea using nasal CPAP in children with craniofacial dysostoses. *Childs Nerv Syst* 12:713–719, 1996.)

acclimatization period of anywhere from 1 day to 2 months, the patients were admitted for a trial of CPAP. The pressure level was started at 4 cm H_2O, then increased to reach satisfactory clinical and polygraphic improvement. Follow-up sleep studies were performed at intervals of up to 1 year.

Results.—Five of the 8 patients were successfully treated with n-CPAP, that is, they had marked clinical and polygraphic improvement immediately after starting the treatment. There was resolution of snoring and good maintenance of arterial oxygen saturation. One patient had a prolonged acclimatization period and was not admitted for an n-CPAP trial. Another child with a tracheostomy was withdrawn from the study. There was 1 true failure in a patient with enlarged adenoids completely blocking the upper airways; she was successfully managed with adenotonsillectomy and a nasopharyngeal airway (Table 1).

Conclusion.—Many patients with craniofacial dysostoses and obstructive sleep apnea can be safely and successfully managed with n-CPAP. This palliative therapy can be tolerated even by young patients, providing sufficient upper airway support until the child is old enough for surgical correction of the midface. Although it may take some time for the children to get used to n-CPAP, it seems to improve not only their breathing pattern during sleep but also their daytime performance.

▶ Numerous treatments for obstructive sleep apnea have been described for children with craniofacial dysostoses. Nasal continuous positive airway pressure is an important addition to the armamentarium. As correctly pointed out by these authors, the technique is generally well tolerated and can be used to bide time until more definitive procedures can be undertaken. Any craniofacial team dealing with these syndromes should have this treatment available to their patients.

S.P. Bartlett, M.D.

Maxillofacial

Total External and Internal Construction in Arhinia
Meyer R (Centre de Chirurgie Plastique, Lausanne, France)
Plast Reconstr Surg 99:534–542, 1997   1–14

Introduction.—Arhinia is a rare malformation of the middle third of the face, and there have been only 20 cases reported. When the olfactory system is absent as well, the condition is called total arhinia. The case of a child with arhinia, and his total external and internal nasal reconstruction, are reported.

> *Case Report.*—A male infant was born in Saudi Arabia without a nose. He required orotracheal intubation and mechanical ventilation because of difficulty breathing. Imaging studies showed complete absence of the nasal soft tissue, nasal cavity, and nasal septum. The child was eventually weaned off endotracheal intubation

and was able to breath through his mouth with an oral airway. A nasal passage was surgically created when he was 1 month old but became stenotic after 2 years.

The patient was seen in France for staged reconstructive surgery. Examination revealed complete choanal atresia and no sense of smell. The child was fully integrated with normal psychosocial development. In the first stage, an anterior septum and external nose was formed using a forehead flap and a triangular rib graft. Several weeks later, the internal nose was constructed by drilling out the 2 nasal cavities through solid bone. The new airway was lined at the floor with buccal mucosal flaps, and intermediate skin grafts were used to line the vaults of the anterior cavities and the ceiling of the posterior monocavity, including the neochoanae. After this stage, the child could breathe immediately and quickly learned to swallow properly. The next year, a third procedure was performed to enlarge the cavities and vestibules. The child did well after these procedures, although he did require silicone tubes for a prolonged period.

Conclusions.—A rare case of arhinia is reported. This child was managed by a 3-stage approach of total external and internal construction, consisting of construction of an external nose, drilling out and lining of the nasal cavities, and amplification of the cavities. The author recommends performing surgical construction before the child reaches school age, if possible. The patient in this report will require future attention to maintain the patency of the airway.

▶ Total arhinia is a rare condition indeed. Although conventional techniques of fabrication of an external nose are well known, this author puts forth a staged reconstruction that addresses not only the external appearance but also the nasal passages. Anyone dealing with nasal stenosis is aware that getting a nostril to remain patent over the long term is problematic. It will be interesting for the author to report on this patient some years hence, to see whether that goal has been achieved.

S.P. Bartlett, M.D.

Microsurgical Correction of Facial Contour in Congenital Craniofacial Malformations: The Marriage of Hard and Soft Tissue
Longaker MT, Siebert JW (New York Univ)
Plast Reconstr Surg 98:942–950, 1996   1–15

Objective.—It can be very difficult to correct facial asymmetry in patients with complex craniofacial malformations. Optimal reconstructive results depend on correction of both the skeletal deficiencies and the overlying soft tissue. The results of microsurgical correction of facial asymmetry in patients with congenital craniofacial malformations were reported.

Methods.—The 5-year experience included 19 patients who underwent microsurgical soft-tissue correction of facial contour, most after standard facial skeletal reconstruction. Fifteen patients had hemifacial microsomias, 2 had orbitofacial clefts, 1 had congenital temporomandibular joint ankylosis with micrognathia, and 1 had a lower midline mandibular cleft. The patients' ages at surgery ranged from 6 to 27 years. A total of 21 microvascular flaps were used for soft-tissue correction, including 19 de-epithelialized parascapular flaps, 1 superficial inferior epigastric flap, and 1 fibula with soleus muscle and large skin paddle for the patient with a facial cleft. For the 15 patients with hemifacial microsomias, treatment consisted of parascapular fasciocutaneous flaps in 10 patients, parascapular flaps with bone in 3, a parascapular flap with teres major muscle in 1, and a superficial inferior epigastric flap in 1.

Results.—At a minimum follow-up of 1 year, all patients had stable results (Fig 4). The only complications were limited hematomas and a partial skin paddle slough of the fibular flap. Most patients had ancillary procedures in an attempt to optimize the aesthetic results, such as nasoseptoplasty to straighten the deviated nose. Six patients had flap revisions performed no more than 3 months after operation.

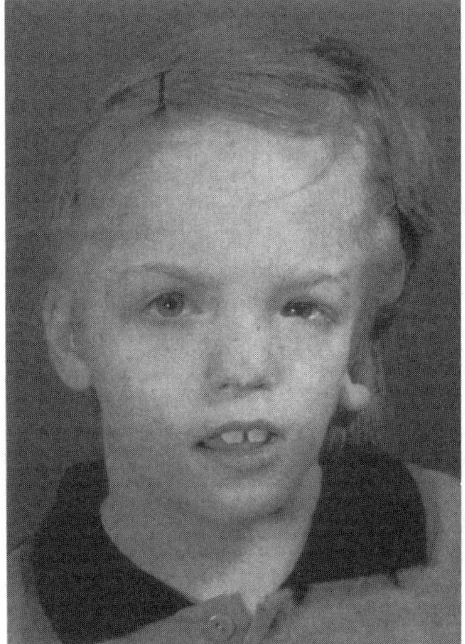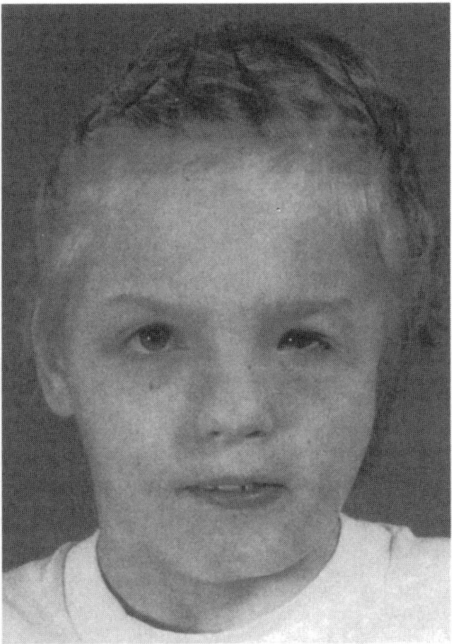

FIGURE 4.—A 7-year-old boy with left-sided Goldenhaar's syndrome (case 10). **Left,** preoperative frontal view. The patient has undergone previous surgery, including bone expansion of the left mandible. **Right,** postoperative frontal view 2 years after customized parascapular flap with vascularized bone flap to left mandible. (Courtesy of Longaker MT, Siebert JW: Microsurgical correction of facial contour in congenital craniofacial malformations: The marriage of hard and soft tissue. *Plast Reconstr Surg* 98:942–950, 1996.)

Conclusions.—Microsurgical techniques can correct facial asymmetry in patients with complex craniofacial malformations. Free flaps can be used to cover the remaining skeletal deformity while restoring symmetric facial contour. A combination of skeletal and microsurgical soft-tissue reconstruction is needed to optimize the aesthetic results and craniofacial contour in these difficult-to-manage patients.

▶ These authors correctly point out that there are several severe craniofacial malformations, primarily affecting the middle and lower face, that cannot be corrected by bony skeletal surgery alone. These congenital anomalies involve both the soft tissue and the bone, and accordingly, soft-tissue reconstruction is to be advocated. The question remains as to the optimal timing of such reconstruction. Traditionally, the bony skeletal framework has been treated initially, followed by any soft-tissue augmentation procedures. The authors correctly point out that individualization is important to improve not only function, but also appearance. Age does not appear to be a consideration because these procedures can be performed even in young children.

S.P. Bartlett, M.D.

Longitudinal Analysis of Mandibular Asymmetry in Hemifacial Microsomia

Polley JW, Figueroa AA, Liou EJ-W, et al (Univ of Illinois, Chicago; Cook County Hosp, Chicago)

Plast Reconstr Surg 99:328–339, 1997   1–16

Introduction.—The central skeletal deformity in patients with hemifacial microsomia is focused around the temporomandibular region. Little is known about the natural growth process of the mandible in this deformity. This information is crucial to development of an appropriate treatment protocol. Mandibular skeletal growth was analyzed longitudinally from childhood to adolescence in 26 patients with unoperated hemifacial microsomia.

Methods.—Medical records and posteroanterior cephalometric radiographs were reviewed retrospectively. Horizontal and vertical mandibular asymmetry were measured on radiographs, (Fig 1) and patients were classified by grade of mandibular deformity.

Results.—In 26 patients with skeletal mandibular asymmetry: 5 were grade I, 14 were grade II, and 7 were grade III. The average age for initial cephalometric records was 3.1 years and the average age for final cephalometric records was 16.7 years. Horizontal mandibular asymmetry as measured by protuberance menti (PM) and intercuspid point (IC) angles from initial to final measurement were minimal and not statistically different. Similarly, vertical mandibular asymmetry as measured by intergonial line (I-GO) angle showed a modest increment in the grade III deformities ($P < 0.05$) but in grades I and II increased minimally and was not

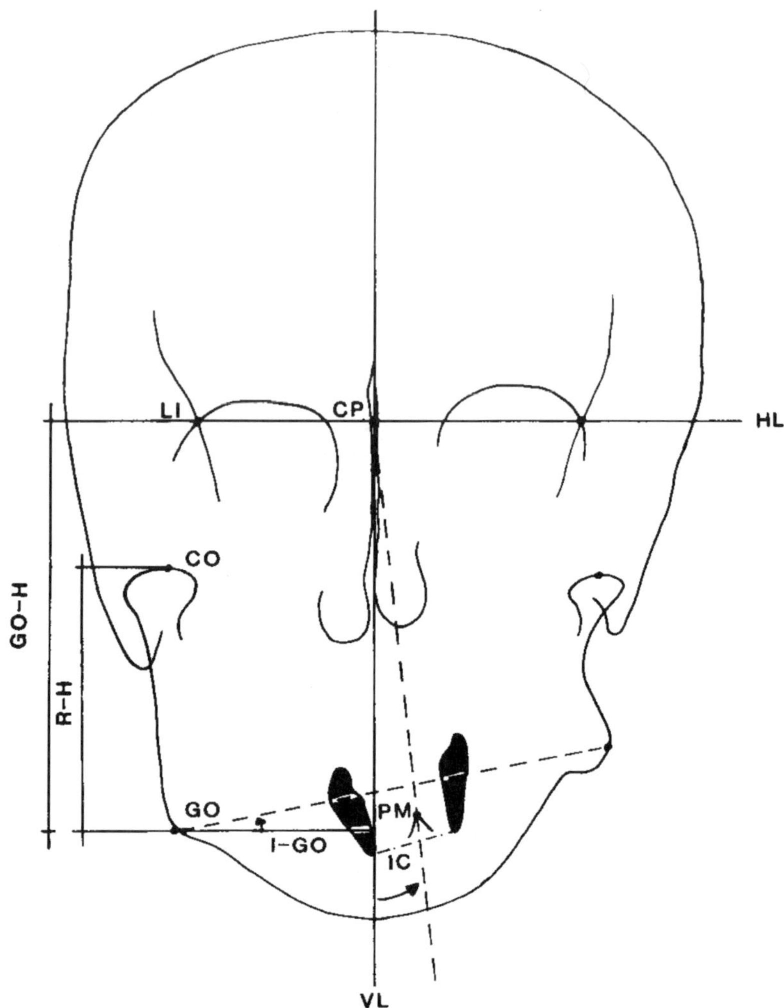

FIGURE 1.—Anatomic landmarks and reference lines. Landmarks: *LI*, linea innominata; *CP*, crista galli point; *CO*, condylion; *GO*, gonion; *PM*, protuberamce menti; *IC*, intercuspid point (half the distance between the mandibular cuspid root apices). Reference line and distances: *HL*, horizontal line; *VL*, vertical line; *GO-H*, gonial height; *R-H*, ramus height; *I-GO*, intergonial line, used to measure the angle between the intergonial line and the horizontal line. (Courtesy of Polley JW, Figueroa AA, Liou EJ-W: Longitudinal analysis of mandibular asymmetry in hemifacial microsomia. *Plast Reconstr Surg* 99:328–339, 1997.)

statistically significant (Fig 5). The skeletal mandibular asymmetry was not progressive in nature and growth of the affected side paralleled that of the nonaffected side (Fig 9).

Conclusion.—The question of facial growth potential is crucial in developing treatment strategies for patients with hemifacial microsomia. Most patients are treated by a combined surgical and orthodontic strategy in the teen years. Early extensive mandibular reconstruction in these

Ratio Changes

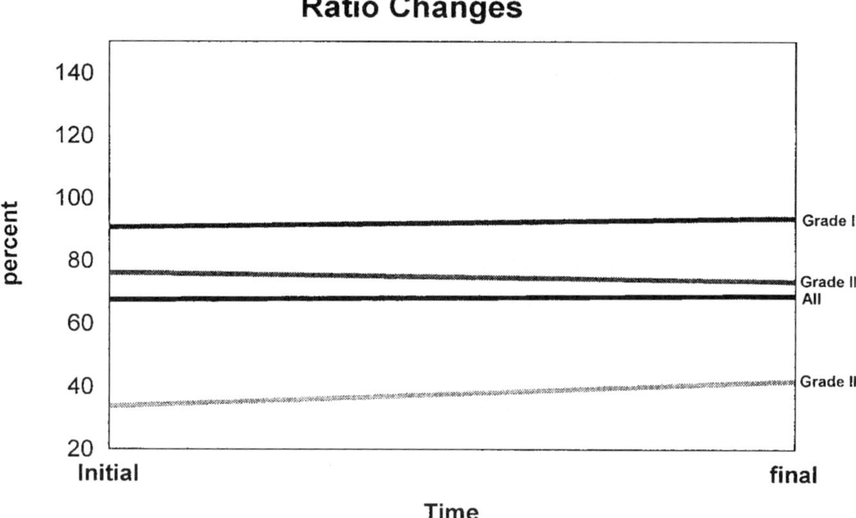

FIGURE 5.—The ratio changes from initial to final records between affected and nonaffected ramus heights. (Courtesy of Polley JW, Figueroa AA, Liou EJ-W: Longitudinal analysis of mandibular asymmetry in hemifacial microsomia. *Plast Reconstr Surg* 99:328–339, 1997.)

patients is not justified, as findings suggest that mandibular deformity does not progress over time.

▶ The timing and type of intervention for patients affected with hemifacial microsomia has been debated in the literature for years. Advocates of early intervention cite the need to release trapped skeletal parts to optimize overall growth and development, whereas those advocating late intervention believe that growth may be impeded if earlier intervention is undertaken.

This study corroborates earlier reports by Rune et al.[1] that the skeletal asymmetry in hemifacial microsomia is not progressive: skeletal proportions observed at birth continue into adolescence. As these authors correctly point out, despite early surgery, secondary procedures are generally required. This important bit of information should be used when informing patients of their choices. Indeed, the type and timing of intervention in this disorder are more often dictated by appearance-related needs than by functional needs.

The advent of the technique of distraction osteogenesis of the mandible presents new opportunities. However, the time and extent of distraction in these patients remains to be defined. Future studies are essential to determine whether early bony distraction has any salutary benefit on the development of adjacent craniofacial structures (muscles, soft tissue, etc.) or, alternatively, whether such intervention is counterproductive. The one reported in longitudinal studies of growth in the distracted patient such as those presented in this manuscript will be of paramount importance.

S.P. Bartlett, M.D.

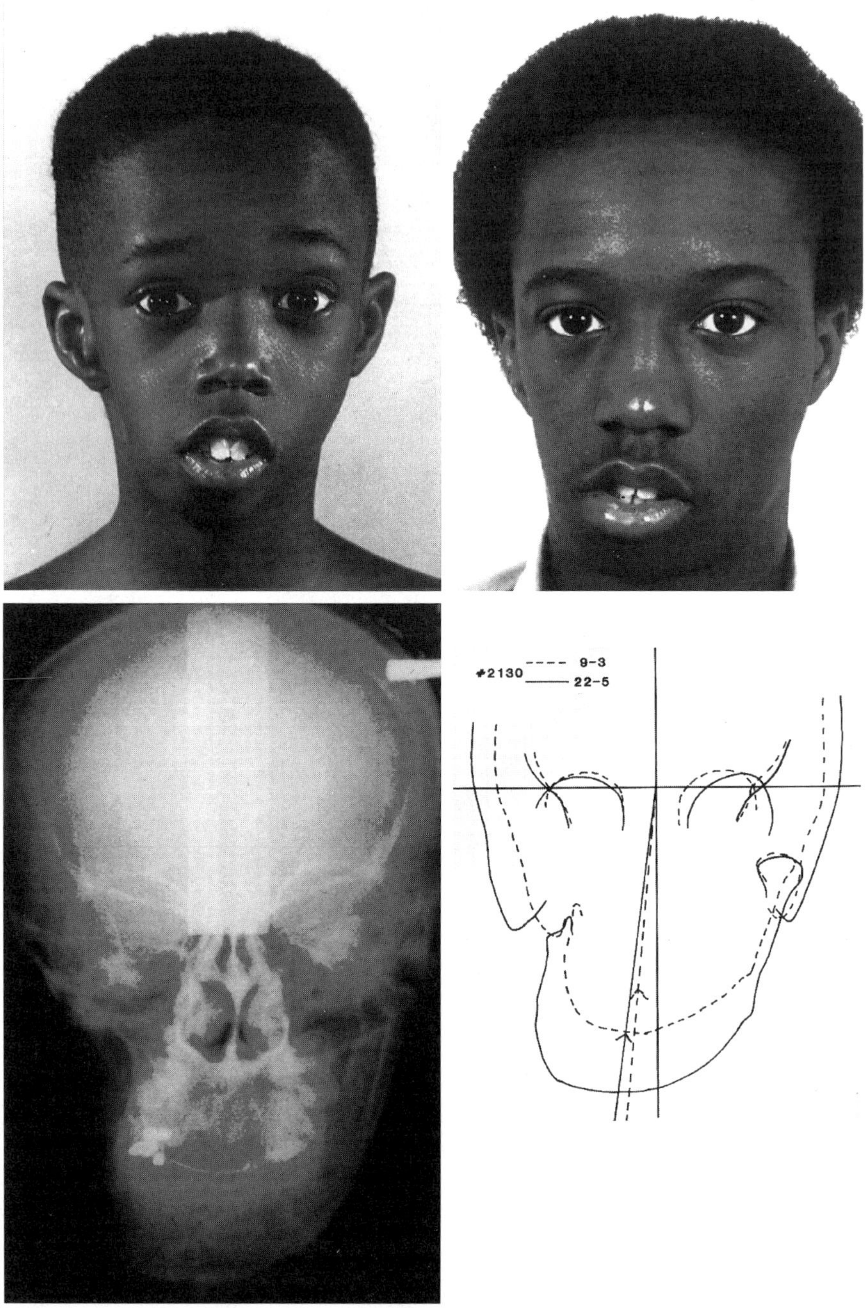

FIGURE 9.—*Case 4* (CFC 2130). Facial photographs (*above*) and corresponding PA cephalomctric radiographs (*below, left*) and tracings (*below, right*) at ages 9 years and 3 months and 22 years and 5 months. Note the stable right facial asymmetry with a 2-degree increase in the PM angle. (Courtesy of Polley JW, Figueroa AA, Liou EJ-W: Longitudinal analysis of mandibular asymmetry in hemifacial microsomia. *Plast Reconstr Surg* 99:329–339, 1997.)

Reference

1. Rune B, Selvik G, Sarnas KV, et al: Growth in hemifacial microsomia studied with the aid of roentgen stereophotogrammetry and metallic implants. *Cleft Palate J* 18:128, 1981.

Histopathologic and Biochemical Changes in the Muscles Affected by Distraction Osteogenesis of the Mandible

Fisher E, Staffenberg DA, McCarthy JG, et al (Univ of New Mexico, Albuquerque; Emory Univ, Atlanta, Ga; New York Univ)
Plast Reconstr Surg 99:366–371, 1997   1–17

Objective.—Distraction osteogenesis permits creation of new bone through gradual distraction after corticotomy or osteotomy. The histologic changes in distracted mandibular bone have been studied, but those in the mandibular soft tissues have not. A study was performed in dogs to study the effects of mandibular distraction osteogenesis on the muscles of mastication.

Methods.—An intraoral distraction device was used to lengthen the mandible of 10 dogs (Fig 1). At intervals of 3 days of lengthening to 20 days of lengthening and 48 days of fixation, biopsy specimens of the masseter and digastric muscles were obtained to evaluate distraction-related changes in those muscles over time. Control values were based on muscle biopsy specimens from the contralateral side obtained in 6 dogs. In addition to histologic examination, each specimen was spectrophotometrically analyzed for RNA, DNA, and protein content.

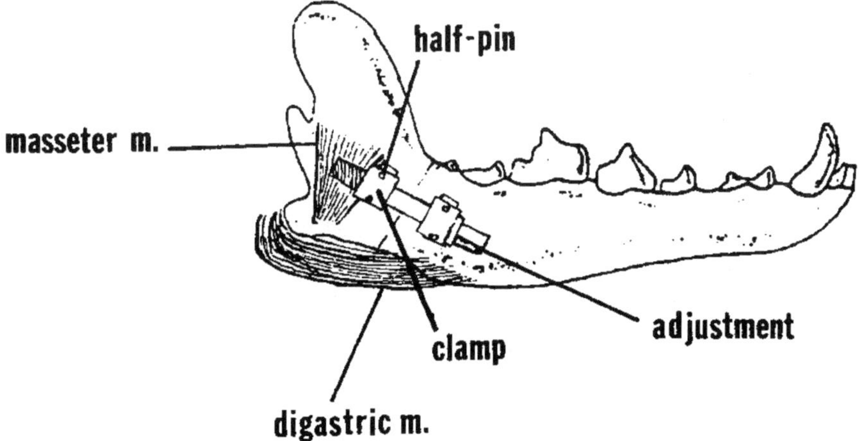

FIGURE 1.—The lengthening device after placement on the osteotomized mandible. Distraction of 1 mm/day is performed by turning the nut labeled "adjustment." The device does not impinge on the masseter muscle. (Courtesy of Fisher E, Staffenberg DA, McCarthy JG, et al: *Plast Reconstr Surg* 99:366–371, 1997.)

TABLE 2.—RNA/DNA

	3–11 Days of Distraction ($n = 4$)	20 to 48 Days of Fixation ($n = 6$)
Masseter	−5% (N.S.)	−9% ($p < 0.02$)
Digastric	+2% (N.S.)	+2% (N.S.)

Abbreviations: NS, not significant; +, increase from control group values; −, decrease from control group values.
(Courtesy of Fisher E, Staffenberg DA, McCarthy JG, et al: *Plast Reconstr Surg* 99:366–371, 1997.)

Results.—Temporary atrophy of the digastric muscle was noted at the start of distraction. However, by 48 days of fixation, this muscle regenerated completely. The masseter muscle began to atrophy with as little as 20 mm of distraction and showed continued atrophy during fixation. Masseter muscle atrophy was associated with significantly reduced protein synthesis, but digastric muscle atrophy was not (Table 2). The difference may have been related to the fact that the fibers on the digastric muscle ran parallel to the vector of distraction.

Conclusion.—In distraction osteogenesis, the associated muscles will show compensatory regeneration and hypertrophy if they line in the same plane or vector as the distraction. In contrast, persistent atrophy and reduced protein synthesis are noted for muscles that lie in a different plane. Regeneration and hypertrophy are likely to occur when a hypoplastic human mandible is distracted. This phenomenon could reduce the rate of relapse after single-stage orthognathic mandibular advancement.

▶ The very important finding that skeletal distraction in the same plane or vector of a muscle will lead to compensatory regeneration and hypertrophy deserves re-emphasis. However, I would question whether the finding that muscles lying in different planes show atrophy is truly correct. Could not this finding have been secondary to the irritative effects of surgery and distractor placement? As emphasized in the conclusion, the clinical importance of this is that the rate of relapse of distraction over conventional osteotomies is likely to be reduced.

Although no long-term positional stability studies have yet been undertaken, it is the clinical impression in those centers doing a large volume of distraction that this is, indeed, correct. Due to its current lack of precision, distraction will not replace conventional osteotomies but should be viewed as an additive and sometimes intermediate precursor technique.

S.P. Bartlett, M.D.

Clefts

The Effect of Cleft Lip Repair on Maxillary Morphology in Patients With Unilateral Complete Cleft Lip and Palate

Kapucu MR, Gürsu KG, Enacar A, et al (Hacettepe Univ, Ankara, Turkey)
Plast Reconstr Surg 97:1371–1375, 1996   1–18

Introduction.—Maxillary retrusion often is observed in patients treated for unilateral clefts of the lip and palate. These observations regarding the effects of surgery are made in patients who have undergone both repairs, but not in patients who have had cleft lip repair alone. The isolated effects of cleft lip repair on maxillary morphology were investigated in 40 adult patients with complete unilateral cleft lip and palate.

Methods.—All the patients were aged 16 years or older. Ten patients had undergone only cleft lip repair in childhood, followed by cleft palate repair in adulthood (group 1), and 30 patients had undergone both cleft lip and cleft palate repair in childhood (group 2). Twenty-four adults with normal lips and palates acted as control subjects. All the patients and normal control subjects underwent lateral cephalograms. Cephalometric values were compared for all 3 groups.

Results.—Patients in groups 1 and 2 had retrusion of the maxillary alveolus and basal bone. There were no significant differences between groups 1 and 2 in any measurements.

Conclusions.—Cleft lip repair can cause severe maxillary retrusion in patients with complete unilateral cleft lip and palate. There was no significant correlation between the magnitude of the retrusion and the presence of cleft palate repair in this patient series.

Timing of Hard Palatal Closure: A Critical Long-term Analysis

Rohrich RJ, Rowsell AR, Johns DF, et al (Univ of Texas, Dallas; Radcliff Infirmary, Oxford, England)
Plast Reconstr Surg 98:236–246, 1996   1–19

Introduction.—Controversy regarding the timing of cleft palate surgery focuses on the need for early palatoplasty for better speech versus delayed hard palate repair for undisturbed facial growth. There is no consensus on the preferred age or surgical technique. The Oxford Cleft Palate Study was performed to evaluate the long-term follow-up of patients with early versus late hard palate closure.

Methods.—A preliminary questionnaire was mailed to 91 patients who underwent early or late hard palate closure. Of 78 respondents, 44 were randomly selected to undergo interview and examination by a multidisciplinary team. The average patient age at follow-up was 17.5 years and the average length of follow-up was 12.8 years. Thirty-one and 13 patients, respectively, had unilateral and bilateral cleft types. There were 21 patients in the early closure group and 23 patients in the late closure group. The

TABLE 5.—Intelligibility Assessment

Speech Parameter	Rating Scale	Early Closure	Late Closure
Intelligibility	0 = normal	95%* ($n = 20$)*	65%* ($n = 15$)*
	1 = slightly impaired	5% ($n = 1$)	17% ($n = 4$)
	2 = moderately impaired	0	13% ($n = 3$)
	3 = grossly impaired	0	4% ($n = 1$)

*Statistically significant ($P < 0.02$).
(Courtesy of Rohrich RJ, Rowsell AR, Johns DF: Timing of hard palatal closure: A critical long-term analysis. *Plast Reconstr Surg* 98:236–246, 1996.)

average ages at follow-up for the early and late closure groups were 17 and 18.2 years, respectively. The overall average age at the time of cleft palate repair was 3.4 months. The ages at soft palate repair for early and late closure were 10.8 and 11.4 months, respectively. The hard palate was closed in the early and late closure groups at average ages of 10.8 and 48.6 months, respectively.

Results.—Patients with delayed hard palate closure had significantly greater speech deficiencies in articulation, nasal resonance, intelligibility (Table 5), and substitution pattern assessment, compared to patients with early closure. The persistent palatal fistula rates (Table 9) for early and late closure were 5% and 35%, respectively. There were no significant between-group differences in hearing or maxillofacial growth impairment.

Conclusion.—Patients with late hard palate repair had significantly greater speech deficiencies than patients with early closure. There is no benefit in delaying hard palate closure in patients with cleft palate.

▶ These 2 manuscripts (Abstracts 1–18 and 1–19) address the issue of the timing of intervention in the repair of clefts of the palate. Rohrich and co-workers demonstrated that delayed hard palate closure leads to greater speech deficiencies, a higher palatal fistula rate, and, importantly, no differences in ultimate maxillofacial growth. Kapucu and associates showed that the group with no palatal repair in childhood had no better anteroposterior maxillary growth than the group with palatal repair. As the reader is aware, other reports have argued against very early intervention in childhood, lest one disrupt the functional matrix and cause deficient maxillary growth. It appears that this point remains debatable, but these two manuscripts argue persuasively that "early" repair is to be preferred.

S.P. Bartlett, M.D.

TABLE 9.—Persistent Fistula Rate

Group	Persistent Fistula Rate	n
Early closure	5%	1*
Late closure	35%	8*

*Statistically significant ($P < 0.05$).
(Courtesy of Rohrich RJ, Rowsell AR, Johns DF: Timing of hard palatal closure: A critical long-term analysis. *Plast Reconstr Surg* 98:236–246, 1996.)

Comparison of the Hearing Histories of Children With and Without Cleft Palate

Broen PA, Moller KT, Carlstrom J, et al (Univ of Minnesota, Minneapolis)
Cleft Palate Craniofac J 33:127–133, 1996   1–20

Introduction.—Otitis media with effusion often is accompanied by mild to moderate conductive hearing loss. Middle ear effusion is secondary to eustachian tube dysfunction in all children, including those with cleft palate. Children with cleft palate almost always experience eustachian tube dysfunction before primary palatal repair. Otologic treatment and management was compared in 28 children with cleft palate and 29 children with no cleft palate.

Methods.—Children were evaluated at 3-month intervals from the age of 9 to 30 months. At each examination, middle ear function was assessed and hearing was screened. The timing of ventilation tube placement was recorded for both groups.

Results.—Children with cleft palate had ventilation tubes placed earlier and more often than children without cleft palate. Children with cleft palate were more likely to fail hearing testing. There was an association between age at first ventilation tube placement and number of failed hearing screening tests. Early ventilation tube placement was correlated with better hearing in children with cleft palate. Lack of ventilation tubes and non-functioning tubes were associated with middle ear effusion and poorer hearing.

Conclusions.—Without ventilation tubes, young children with cleft palate are not likely to have normal ear function. Hearing is depressed in the absence of normal middle ear function. Children with early placement of ventilation tubes had better hearing thresholds than children with later placement of tubes. Children with late tube placement failed tympanometry. Children who failed tympanometry failed hearing screening and had diminished hearing thresholds.

Secondary Alveolar Bone Grafting: Five-Year Periodontal and Radiographic Evaluation in 100 Consecutive Cases

Tan AES, Brogan WF, McComb HK, et al (Princess Margaret Hosp for Children, Perth, Western Australia; Univ of Western Australia, Perth)
Cleft Palate Craniofac J 33:513–518, 1996   1–21

Introduction.—All patients in Western Australia with cleft lip, cleft palate, or both are treated in Perth at the Princess Margaret Hospital for Children. A prospective trial was started in Perth in 1982 based on the Norwegian protocol for secondary bone grafting of the alveolar cleft. Treatment objectives include allowing teeth to erupt into or to be located in the cleft area; stabilizing and augmenting the bony support of the retained fissural teeth; stabilizing the maxillary segments, particularly in bilateral cases; augmenting and supporting the bone structure in bilateral cases; augmenting and supporting the bone structure at the alar base; providing closure of the palatal fistula if present; and simplifying or eliminating future dental prostheses. The 5-year results of periodontal and radiographic status of erupted teeth into grafted bone were evaluated in 100 consecutive children who had undergone secondary alveolar bone grafting.

Methods.—The mean patient age was 11.7 years. Clinical parameters included measurement of plaque and gingival indices, probing depth and gingival width, and septal bone heights. Fifteen of the 100 patients did not complete the 5 years of periodic documentation.

Results.—Ninety-eight percent of the patients who completed alveolar bone grafting had eventual eruption of the cleft-side cuspid/lateral incisor with acceptable parameters of tooth support.

Conclusion.—Secondary bone grafting in unilateral and bilateral cleft deformities is a highly predictable procedure when a strict clinical protocol involving a cleft lip and palate team is followed.

Prospective Evaluation of Morbidity Associated With Iliac Crest Harvest for Alveolar Cleft Grafting
Rudman RA (Univ of Florida, Gainesville)
J Oral Maxillofac Surg 55:219–223, 1997   1–22

Background.—Although the anterior iliac crest is considered the gold standard of donor sites for alveolar cleft grafting, the postoperative morbidity associated with this site has led surgeons to use cranial bone, mandibular symphysis, allogenic bone, and alloplastic materials. The morbidity associated with iliac crest bone harvesting for alveolar cleft grafting was assessed prospectively.

Methods.—Twenty-two consecutive patients were included in the study. The patients were 14 boys and 8 girls, aged 5–17 years. Sixteen patients had a unilateral cleft defect, and 6 had a bilateral alveolar cleft. All underwent alveolar cleft grafting with iliac crest bone harvest.

Findings.—All the patients tolerated the iliac harvest with no major complications. The volume of bone was sufficient in all but 1 patient. Ambulation occurred at an average of 3 hours and 18 minutes after surgery. Twenty-one children were discharged the day after the procedure, and 1 underwent surgery as an outpatient.

Conclusion.—These data are not consistent with previous reports of the morbidity occurring with iliac crest bone harvest. In this series, harvesting cancellous bone from the iliac crest did not result in delayed ambulation or extended hospitalization.

▶ This manuscript is a welcomed addition to the literature. Those of us who have been using bone from a variety of sources for a number of years would, I believe, agree with these findings. Morbidity associated with iliac crest harvesting in children and young adults has been overestimated, and in the majority of cases, this procedure can be performed simply without excessive pain or discomfort and can yield consistent quantities of bone for alveolar grafting.

The question remains unanswered as to whether this bone is superior to that from other sources. In our unit, we have found that iliac bone is superior to cranial bone in severe cleft deformities. Our experience, combined with the data presented here, makes an argument that iliac crest bone remains the material of choice in the majority of cleft reconstructions.

S.P. Bartlett, M.D.

Septoplasty for Obstructive Sleep Apnea in Infants After Cleft Lip Repair
Josephson GD, Levine J, Cutting CB (New York Eye and Ear Infirmary; New York Univ)
Cleft Palate Craniofac J 33:473–476, 1996   1–23

Introduction.—Children with unilateral cleft lip and palate commonly have a deviated nasal septum that does not cause difficulty. When the cleft lip is repaired, nasal resistance increases, and the child may have nasal airway obstruction that can be so severe that obstruction leads to apnea. Septoplasty is controversial in children because of concern for its effects on future craniofacial growth. The outcome in 2 children with cleft lip and palate who had obstructive sleep apnea after cleft lip repair and who underwent conservative septoplasty for relief of symptoms was reported.

Case Report 1.—Female infant, 3 months, was born with a complete unilateral cleft lip, alveolus, and palate. Parents reported symptoms of nasal obstruction with sleep pauses after cleft lip repair. The patient had a right inferior septal deviation, a septal spur, a build-up of scar tissue on the nasal floor, and chronic nasal drainage on that side. Sleep studies revealed obstructive sleep apnea. A conservative anterior septoplasty was performed and sleep apnea abated. At 17 months after surgery, the patient's developmental milestones were being met normally and she was asymptomatic of obstructive symptoms.

Case Report 2.—Male infant, 3 months, with unilateral cleft lip, alveolus, and palate, underwent cleft lip repair. The palatal cleft was closed 11 months later. The patient experienced obstructive symptoms during sleep. A significant septal deviation with scar tissue formation on the nasal floor was discovered. The symptoms became worse over time and a conservative septoplasty was performed. The nasal obstruction and sleep apnea resolved and the infant was asymptomatic at 1 year follow-up.

Conclusion.—This is the first known report on the rare occurrence of sleep apnea from a deviated septum after cleft lip repair. The 2 children treated with conservative septoplasty were relieved of obstructive symptoms and apnea and were doing well at short-term follow-up.

▶ Obstructive sleep apnea may have a variety of causes. In the patient with cleft lip and palate, these may include not only deformities consequent to the cleft of the lip and palate itself, but also associated anomalies. In this paper, attention is directed to 2 patients in whom obstructive sleep apnea developed after repair and who responded to conservative surgical correction of the septal deviation. To this reader's knowledge, this is the first documentation of such an occurrence and henceforth should be added to the list of etiologies of obstructive sleep apnea in this selected population of obligate nasal breathers.

S.P. Bartlett, M.D.

The Correction of Secondary Cleft Lip Deformities Using Dermofat Grafts

Richards AM, Withey SJ, Waterhouse N (Chelsea and Westminster Hosp, London)
Eur J Plast Surg 20:40–44, 1997   1–24

Introduction.—The lack of volume of repaired lips in patients who have undergone cleft lip repair often detracts from an otherwise pleasing result. The use of dermofat graft augmentation of the upper lip has not been previously described in patients with secondary cleft lip deformities. Results of this treatment approach are reported in 11 patients with secondary deformities.

Methods.—Patients underwent dermofat grafting with an approximate 30% overcorrection of the lip. Patients were asked to massage their upper lips regularly to help keep the graft soft. Evaluations were done at 1 and 6 months after surgery.

Results.—The mean age of 10 female patients and 1 male patient was 17 years (range, 13 to 37 years). Ten patients had a unilateral deformity and 1 patient had a bilateral cleft lip and palate. Patients had already undergone between 1 and 5 (average, 2.7) corrective procedures before dermofat graft augmentation. Five patients required either a Z-plasty or V-Y advancement to remedy local mucosal deficiencies. At follow-ups of 1 and 3½ years, there were no major complications. In 1 patient, a moderately hypertrophic submammary donor site scar developed that was successfully treated using intralesional steroid therapy.

Conclusions.—Dermofat graft augmentation may be used safely with good results in patients with mild to moderate upper lip tissue deformity after cleft lip deformity. This approach may be used in combination with local mucosal lengthening procedures.

▶ The technique of lip augmentation popularized in aesthetic surgery has been applied to residual deformities of cleft lip for a number of years. These authors provide long-term follow-up of the suitability of this technique. I would disagree with the authors that a submammary or groin incision is suitable; instead, all grafts should be taken from the dorsal integument because the dermis here is much thicker and provides substantially more volume. The buttock crease is the donor site of choice and can be used in nearly all patients. Additionally, it is essential that all scar in the central midline deformity be released and that the mucosa be rearranged by Z-plasties or other local rearrangement techniques. If these tenets are followed in addition to overgrafting by 30% to 50% of volume, satisfactory results can be expected for the long term.

S.P. Bartlett, M.D.

Surgical Management of Velopharyngeal Dysfunction: Outcome Analysis of Autogenous Posterior Pharyngeal Wall Augmentation
Witt PD, O'Daniel TG, Marsh JL, et al (St Louis Children's Hosp, Mo; Washington Univ, St Louis, Mo)
Plast Reconstr Surg 99:1287–1296, 1997   1–25

Introduction.—Patients with velopharyngeal dysfunction and a small coronal gap can benefit from posterior pharyngeal wall augmentation. There have been problems with nonautogenous augmentation, such as migration of alloplastic implants and resorption of injected materials. Despite a long history of use by Italian surgeons, there is little information on the results of autogenous posterior pharyngeal wall augmentation. An experience with this procedure for the treatment of velopharyngeal dysfunction was reported.

Methods.—The experience included 14 patients with velopharyngeal dysfunction that failed to respond to speech therapy. All patients had a coronal gap of less than 20%, seen on velopharyngeal nasendoscopy. Three patients had undergone prosthetic velopharyngeal management, including 2 patients with Robin sequence. All patients underwent autogenous posterior pharyngeal wall augmentation using a rolled, superiorly based pharyngeal myomucosal flap. Outcome evaluations included recorded perceptual, nasendoscopy, and fluoroscopic standard speech and airway evaluations. The tapes were evaluated in blinded fashion by independent raters. Parameters rated included resonance, auditory nasal emission, and visual characteristics of velopharyngeal closure.

Results.—Most patients were left with nasal turbulence after autogenous posterior pharyngeal wall augmentation, with intermittent to pervasive hypernasality. Resonance was improved in 17% of patients. The percent closure was slightly improved. However, analysis found that the patients' speech was not rated as any more normal postoperatively.

Conclusions.—In patients with velopharyngeal dysfunction and a small coronal gap, autogenous posterior pharyngeal wall augmentation does not produce impairment of the nasal airway. However, neither does it improve the patients' speech. The procedure has a low success rate in achieving normal velopharyngeal closure.

▶ The basic findings in this study are well outlined in the conclusions. Autogenous posterior pharyngeal wall augmentation does not result in speech improvement, but it does not impair the nasal airway. Clearly, what is required is the development of a method of augmenting the posterior wall in patients with a short but dynamic palate who can effect closure. This would lead to a decreased incidence of obstructive sleep apnea in patients currently treated with posterior pharyngeal flaps or related procedures.

S.P. Bartlett, M.D.

Vascular and Lymphatic

The Diagnostic Value of Magnetic Resonance Imaging in Combination With Angiography in Patients With Vascular Malformations: A Prospective Study
Hovius SER, Borg DH, Paans PR, et al (Univ Hosp Rotterdam, The Netherlands)
Ann Plast Surg 37:278–285, 1996   1–26

Background.—The Mulliken classification, based on cell kinetics, describes 2 major types of vascular birthmarks: hemangiomas and vascular malformations. The latter can be subdivided into capillary, venous, and arterial, with or without fistulas and lymphatic anomalies. Thirty-four patients with vascular malformations were prospectively studied with MRI and, when required, angiography as an additional test.

Methods.—The patients ranged in age from 2 to 48 years. Vascular malformations were located in the head and neck regions in 19 patients, the upper extremity in 7, the lower extremity in 7, and on the trunk in 1. Seventeen patients with evidence of high flow underwent angiography after MRI; 8 with low-flow lesions were studied with angiography as a control group. A single radiologist compared MRI and angiographic findings, together with histopathologic findings when available.

Results.—Magnetic resonance imaging clearly showed the anatomical location of all vascular malformations, which showed increased brightness on T2-weighted images. Lesions in the low-flow group appeared at MRI as a hyperintense meshwork of low-flow vessels (venous lakes). Angiography provided no useful information in these cases, and 4 studies indicated normal arterial findings. All 7 patients with high-flow lesions had hypertrophic high-flow vessels on MRI, with no venous lakes and little tissue matrix. The high-flow nature of the lesions was confirmed at angiography. These lesions were categorized as macrofistulous arteriovenous malformations. Ten patients were found to have combined-flow lesions, with MRI showing high flow next to a hyperintense, well-defined, low-flow mass. These lesions were classified as microfistulous arteriovenous malformations.

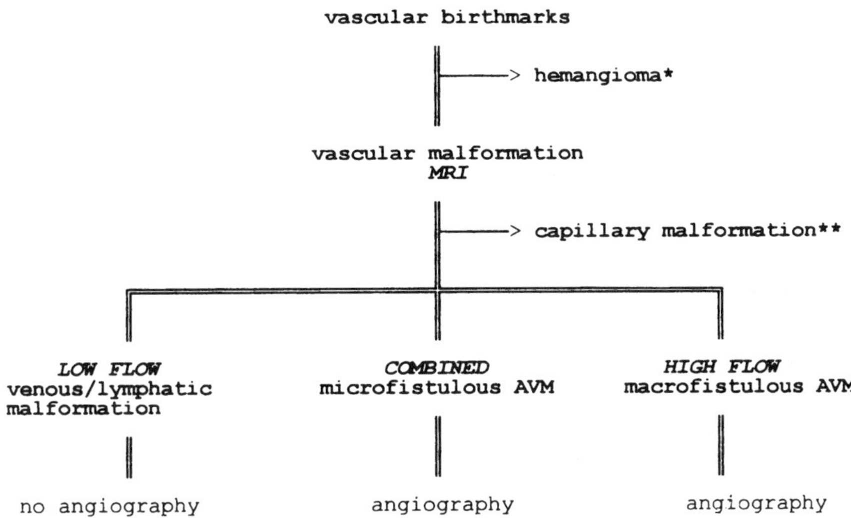

FIGURE 1.—Diagnostic flowchart for vascular birthmarks. After MRI, angiography exactly delineates the nidus and supplying vessels of combined-flow and high-flow lesions, which is essential for therapy planning (embolization, radical excision, or both). In low-flow lesions, on the other hand, no additional information is obtained with angiography. *Hemangiomas regress spontaneously in childhood. **Capillary malformations cannot be visualized on MRI: however, MRI is indicated for tracing possible coexisting lesions. *Abbreviation:* AVM, arteriovenous malformation. (Courtesy of Hovius SER, Borg DH, Paans PR, et al: The diagnostic value of magnetic resonance imaging in combination with angiography in patients with vascular malformations: A prospective study. Reprinted with permission from *Ann Plast Surg* 37:278–285, 1996.)

Discussion.—In all but 1 case, an extensive capillary malformation, MRI correctly established the flow character of these vascular malformations. Angiography added no relevant information in low-flow lesions, but delineated the nidus and supporting vessels in high-flow and combined-flow lesions. The location, extent, and flow characteristics of these lesions, as well as their relation to essential anatomical structures, are essential for the selection of appropriate therapy. No single imaging method provides as much information about the internal structure and flow characteristics of vascular malformations as MRI. A flowchart for the evaluation of vascular birthmarks starts with MRI (Fig 1).

▶ These authors provide us with valuable guidance in determining appropriate studies for visualization for vascular malformations. The algorithm they present will help the surgeon to get maximal information without unnecessary expenditure for tests that do not yield additional benefits. But, of course, the real challenge is not the *visualization*, but the *extirpation* of these difficult lesions.

R.L. Ruberg, M.D.

Port-Wine Stains: An Assessment of 5 Years of Treatment
Orten SS, Waner M, Flock S, et al (Univ of Arkansas, Little Rock)
Arch Otolaryngol Head Neck Surg 122:1174–1179, 1996   1–27

Background.—Many treatment methods have been used for port-wine stains (PWSs). Unfortunately, most have proved to be ineffective or are associated with adverse effects such as scarring. The outcomes of flashlamp-pumped dye laser treatment in patients with PWSs were reported.

Methods.—One hundred two patients with 118 PWSs were treated between 1989 and 1994. The patients ranged in age from 1 month to 66 years.

Findings.—Fifteen percent of the stains lightened by more than 90%, 65.3% by 50% to 90%, and 17.8% by 11% to 49%. Two stains (1.7%) were considered nonresponsive. Although clinical outcomes did not vary by age group, there were significant differences among lesions in different anatomical locations. Port-wine stains recurred in patients monitored for more than 1 year.

Conclusions.—In most patients with PWS, the flashlamp-pumped dye laser produces good to complete results. However, PWSs may gradually return over time. The tendency to recur approached a rate of 50% between 3 and 4 years after treatment was completed.

▶ The laser is preferred treatment for flat port-wine stains even if one needs to repeat this from time to time. Surgical excision and tattooing were helpful in their day but are rarely indicated anymore.

P.W. McKinney, M.D.

Other

An Operation for Stahl's Ear
Ono I, Gunji H, Tateshita T (Fukushima Med College, Japan)
Br J Plast Surg 49:564–567, 1996   1–28

Introduction.—The auricular malformation known as Stahl's ear is rare and difficult to treat when protrusion of the auricle is sharp. A new operation combines features of previously published techniques for correcting Stahl's ear. The status of 5 patients who underwent this operation has been followed from 6 to 18 months. In all cases, the ears had a satisfactory postoperative shape and no complications were noted.

Surgical Technique.—The procedure is done with the patient under general anesthesia. A wedge-shaped pattern, usually about 5–7 mm wide, is drawn around the third crus. The skin and cartilage of the abnormal prominence are then excised in the wedge shape and the cartilage on the flattened portion of the helix is excised beyond this excision. Incisions are made at the helix/scapha border to the cartilage as relaxation incisions. The posterior surface of the ear also should be incised to provide adequate advancement. Cartilage between the scapha and the anthelix is excised an additional 1 mm from the cut end of the skin, then sutured so that the auricle has a natural shape. Another cartilage graft harvested from the concha is fixed as a support on the posterior surface of the cartilage, allowing the scapha to maintain a normal concave shape. Suturing the helix edges under some tension gives the helix the same shape as that on the patient's normal side. To maintain shape postoperatively and prevent hematoma and excess edema, the ear is fixed with a bolster.

Discussion.—Nonsurgical treatment of Stahl's ear, using taping or an external prosthesis, can be effective if the deformity is mild and treatment is undertaken within the first year of life. Older patients or those with more severe deformity will require surgery. With the technique presented here, a normal auricular shape is created after wedge excision of the abnormal prominence of the third crus, including the skin and cartilage. This shape is maintained by means of an additional cartilage graft harvested from the concha and fixed as a support on the posterior surface of the cartilage.

▶ Characterized by a "third crus," Stahl's ear is indeed a rare deformity. Although anatomically it appears that this deformity would be quite simple to correct, the variety of procedures that have been described for correction argues otherwise. Two general approaches to the correction of the deformity have been advocated: cartilage excision (plus or minus skin) and cartilage manipulation. In general, both should be considered, depending on the degree of deformity. For severe folding of the third crus, anything short of excision is to be condemned. In these cases, the typically minimal scar of the anterior integument is an acceptable tradeoff for the correction of the cartilaginous deformity. Mild to moderate deformities may respond to a variety of postauricular approaches to cartilage manipulation and suturing. Each technique requires meticulous postoperative stenting and dressing care.

S.P. Bartlett, M.D.

Use of Lumbar Periosteal Turnover Flaps in Myelomeningocele Closure
Fiala TGS, Buchman SR, Muraszko KM (Univ of Michigan, Ann Arbor)
Neurosurgery 39:522–526, 1996   1–29

Background.—Myelomeningocele is the most common form of spina bifida cystica. A new technique for myelomeningocele closure was described.

Methods and Outcomes.—Bilateral lumbar periosteal flaps are used as an additional tissue layer in complex cases. The flaps reinforce the dural repair and protect the spinal cord. They also may help contain potential

CSF leakage from the primary repair of the cord, preventing pseudomeningocele formation. Bilateral thoracolumbar fascial flaps are developed in conjunction with periosteal flaps elevated from adjacent lumbar pedicles and transverse processes. This creates a composite tissue flap. The periosteally based flaps may be closed in a "pants-over-vest" manner to cover the spinal defect entirely and reinforce the repair (Fig 2). The outcomes in 2 representative patients were described. One underwent surgery in the early neonatal period for primary myelomeningocele repair, and the other

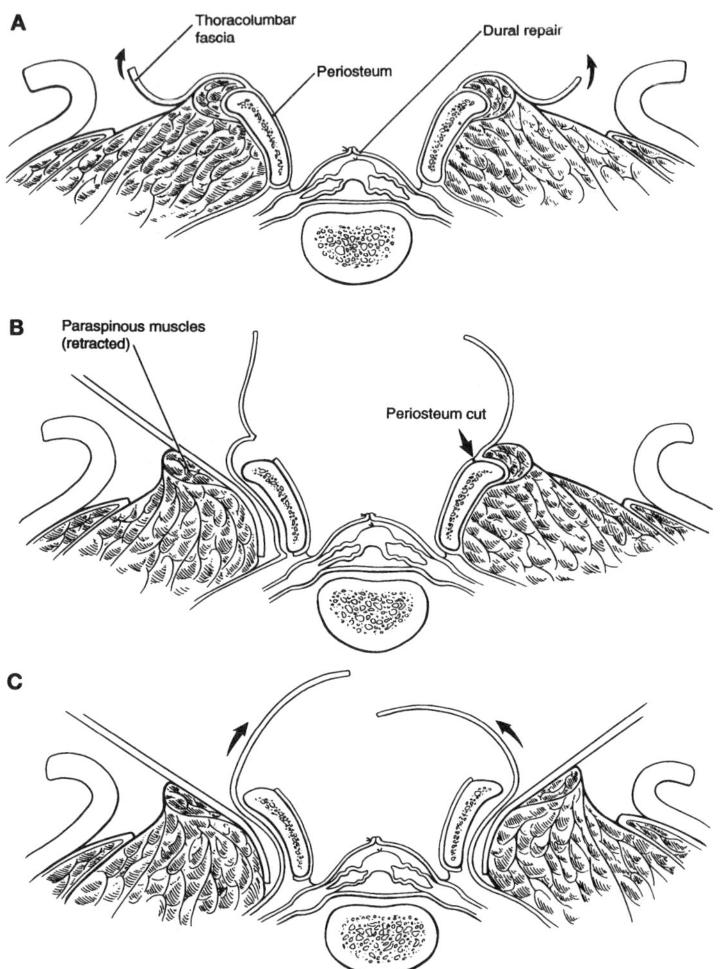

FIGURE 2.—A, after completion of the dural repair, the thoracolumbar fascia is incised laterally at its junction with the latissimus dorsi muscle and elevated from the underlying erector spinae muscles. B, periosteum on the bony pedicles is incised as medially as possible at the junction of the thoracolumbar fascia and periosteum. Subperiosteal dissection is performed on the lateral aspect of the bony pedicle, gaining additional flap length. C, bilateral lumbar periosteal flaps are developed and are ready for transposition (turnover) above the dural repair. (Courtesy of Fiala TGS, Buchman SR, Muraszko KM: Use of lumbar periosteal turnover flaps in myelomeningocele closure. *Neurosurgery* 39:522–526, 1996.)

at 5 years of age after a tethered cord release. In both patients, durable, stable soft-tissue coverage of the spinal cord was obtained. The patients were followed up for at least 12 months after surgery. The second patient had no recurrence of the pseudomeningocele found before surgery.

Conclusions.—In patients with myelomeningocele, the lumbar periosteal turnover flap may be used to reinforce tenuous spinal cord and dural repairs. The technique described provides a secure, watertight closure over the primary repair of the cord and an additional autologous tissue layer, and may help contain CSF leaks.

▶ This article provides a clever method of adding a potentially secure extra layer of closure in myelomeningocele repair. Unfortunately, several of the neurosurgeons who commented on the published article claimed that the additional layer was of limited value. My own concern about the technique was that subperiosteal dissection on the lateral aspect of the bony pedicle probably would not give much additional length to the flap and might compromise its vascular supply. At any rate, this seems like a useful concept that might be applicable in selected cases.

R.L. Ruberg, M.D.

The Repair of Myelomeningocele With Tissue Expanders

Celiköz B, Türegün M, Sengezer M (Gülhane Military Med Academy, Etlik, Ankara, Turkey)
Eur J Plast Surg 19:297–299, 1996   1–30

Background.—The use of local skin flaps, musculocutaneous flaps, or skin grafts for closing large myelomeningocele defects often is complicated by wound breakdown and varying amounts of skin necrosis. The use of tissue expansion, a relatively new approach in the treatment of this pathology, was described in patients with large myelomeningocele defects.

Methods and Outcomes.—Four children and 1 adult underwent tissue expansion to repair large myelomeningoceles. Ventriculoperitoneal shunting procedures were done first in the children because of hydrocephalus. After hydrocephalus regression, myelomeningocele closure was performed (Fig 1). Silicone tissue expanders were inserted on 1 or both sides of the lesion and inflated by saline injections once a week (Fig 2). The expanded skin and subcutaneous tissue permitted easy midline closure (Fig 3). No complications occurred after surgery. Outcomes were satisfactory in all patients.

Conclusions.—Tissue expansion in the repair of myelomeningocele defects delays the definitive reconstruction but reduces the risk of prolonged and troublesome problems associated with closure failure. The complications associated with tissue expansion usually are relatively minor and often do not interfere with successful completion of the expansion process.

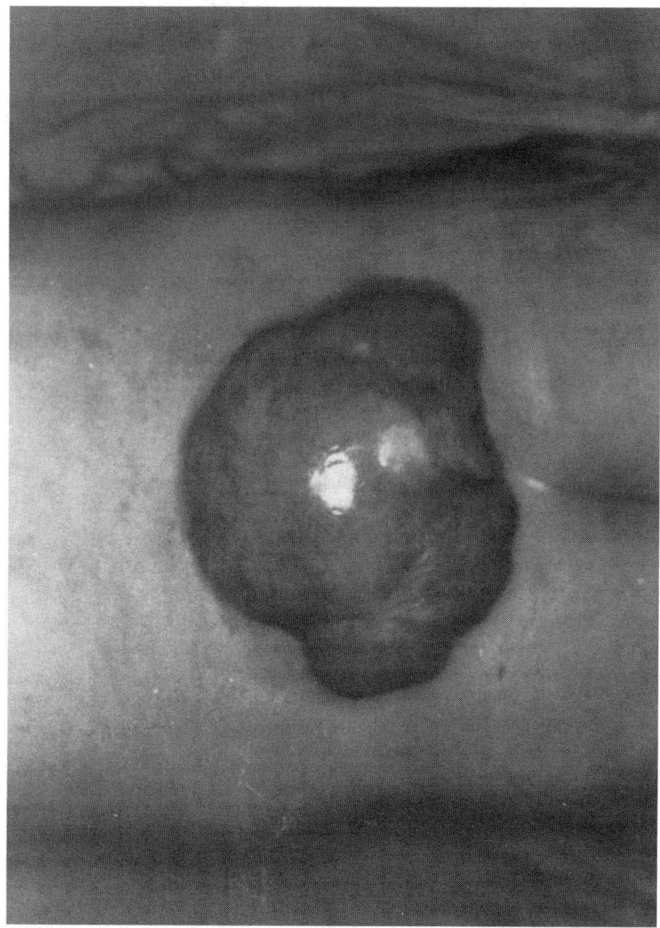

FIGURE 1.—Preoperative appearance of a large myelomeningocele in a child. (Courtesy of Celiköz B, Türegün M, Sengezer M: The repair of myelomeningocele with tissue expanders. *Eur J Plast Surg* 19:297–299, copyright 1996, Springer-Verlag.)

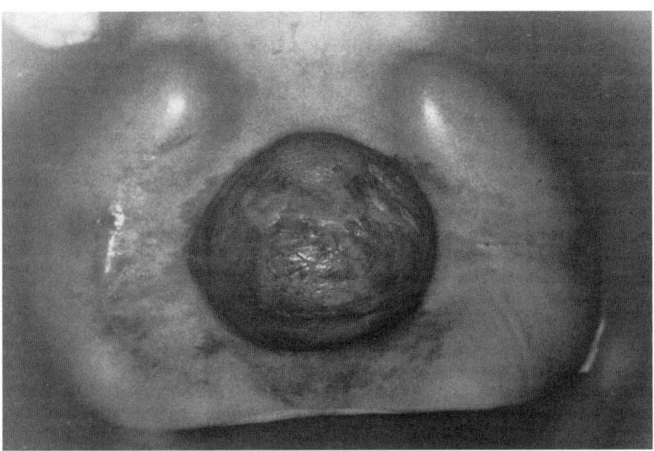

FIGURE 2.—Completion of tissue expansion in the same child. (Courtesy of Celiköz B, Türegün M, Sengezer M: The repair of myelomeningocele with tissue expanders. *Eur J Plast Surg* 19:297–299, copyright 1996, Springer-Verlag.)

▶ Although other techniques are available (and certainly require less time), the use of tissue expanders for really large myelomeningocele defects may have a place. My own use of tissue expanders in these patients generally is not for primary closure of the myelomeningocele defects, but much more commonly for closure after an orthopedic procedure such as kyphectomy. These patients may have "road map" scars of the back, as a result of multiple previous procedures, precluding the development of any logical local rotation or advancement flap. Tissue expansion before the projected orthopedic procedure provides a better opportunity for stable coverage.

R.L. Ruberg, M.D.

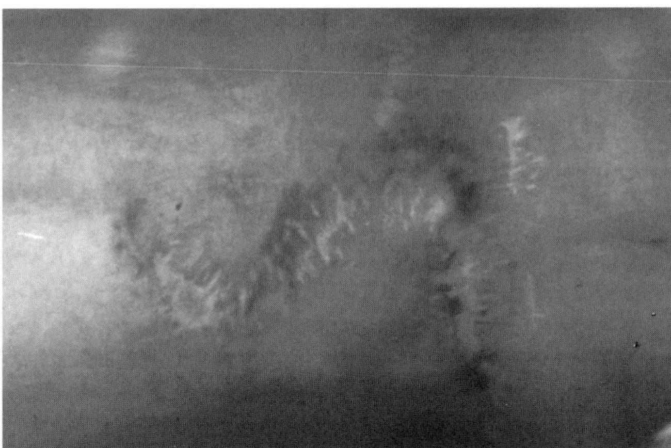

FIGURE 3.—Postoperative appearance of the back at 8 months, again in the same child. (Courtesy of Celiköz B, Türegün M, Sengezer M: The repair of myelomeningocele with tissue expanders. *Eur J Plast Surg* 19:297–299, copyright 1996, Springer-Verlag.)

Endoscopic Pediatric Plastic Surgery

Huang MHS, Cohen SR, Burstein FD, et al (Singapore Gen Hosp; Scottish Rite Children's Med Ctr, Atlanta, Ga)
Ann Plast Surg 38:1–8, 1997   1–31

Introduction.—Endoscopic technology is being used with increasing frequency in adult reconstructive and aesthetic surgery. Its use in the pediatric population has not been reported. This is surprising because its minimally invasive nature should be appealing for this age group. The initial experience with endoscopic pediatric surgery in 41 children was reported.

Methods.—The mean patient age was 5.6 years. Surgical procedures performed included insertion of tissue expanders (19 patients), excision of facial dermoids (7), torticollis release (5), excision of vascular lesions (4), and miscellaneous procedures (6).

Results.—The 19 children who were in the tissue expander group underwent 20 expander insertion procedures and received a total of 42 implants. The complication rate was 9.5% (4 of 42) and consisted of 2 infection, 1 rupture, and 1 extrusion. Seven children in the dermoid group had lesions situated in the lateral brow away from the upper eyelid (5 patients), nasal region (1), and midline of the forehead (1). Two patients with lateral periorbital lesions had infectious complications. One child in the vascular lesion group required reoperation of a large hemangioma, occupying the nasoglabellar and medial canthal regions, that may not have been completely removed by endoscopic-assisted excision. The lesion did not return after open excision. All 5 children who underwent surgical release of torticollis had satisfactory results at a mean follow-up of 2.8 years. Of 6 children who underwent miscellaneous procedures, all had favorable outcomes and no complications.

Conclusion.—Pediatric patients undergoing endoscopic procedures had favorable outcomes, with a complication rate no greater than that of conventional open surgery. The use of endoscopic-assisted surgery is likely to grow in popularity. Its use should always be tempered by critical review and its value by patient benefit.

Endoscopic Assisted Otoplasty: A Preliminary Report

Graham KE, Gault DT (Mount Vernon and Watford Hosps NHS Trust, Northwood, England)
Br J Plast Surg 50:47–57, 1997   1–32

Introduction.—Historically, the correction of prominent ears was performed through a postauricular incision. With endoscopy, the main skin incision can be transposed from the postauricular region to the scalp for patients with a known risk of abnormal scar formation. The outcome in 10 patients who underwent endoscopic-assisted surgery to correct prominent ears was reported.

Methods.—The age range of the 8 males and 2 females was 4–21 years. Eight patients had bilateral corrections and 2 patients had unilateral corrections. Ears were classified according to the degree of deformity of the antihelical fold and whether lobule prominence persisted after correction by finger pressure. Patients were excluded if the lobule prominence could not be corrected by finger pressure, as an additional procedure would be necessary for correction.

Surgical Technique.—No skin excisions were made. Instruments were inserted through scalp incisions. A custom-made abrader was used to weaken the posterior cartilage surface by abrasion, and a new antihelical fold was created. Nonabsorbable sutures were placed through 1 or 2 postauricular stab incisions to appose the scaphal cartilage and the mastoid fascia to retain the new fold.

Results.—The average operative time for bilateral procedures was 2 hours. The mastoid-helix distance was 16–31 mm before correction and 9–22 mm after correction. A single polypropylene suture extruded in an ear in 2 patients at about 6 weeks postoperatively. The sutures were removed without any loss of correction in either patient. Four corrections were not perfect but were acceptable.

Conclusion.—Prominent ears can be corrected using endoscopic-assisted techniques in selected patients. Transposing the main scar to the scalp reduces the signs of surgery and allows compression of hypertrophic or keloid scars if they develop.

Endoscope-Assisted Intraoral Approach for Masseteric Hypertrophy
Honda T, Sasaki K, Takeuchi M, et al (Tokyo Women's Med College)
Ann Plast Surg 38:9–14, 1997   1–33

Introduction.—Masseteric hypertrophy is typically treated by either an intraoral or extraoral approach. The intraoral approach involves a narrow visual field which makes resection of the mandibular angle difficult. The intraoral approach is superior to the extraoral approach in that it leaves no scars. Outcomes in 5 patients with bilateral masseteric hypertrophy who underwent surgery by the intraoral approach using an the endoscope were reported.

Surgical Technique.—Incision is made in the oral mucosa from the upper anterior border of the mandibular ramus toward the lateral side of the lower first molar. An incision is made on the dermal side to create a small canal opening into the oral cavity, and a Leibinger trocar is inserted through the canal for placement of the endoscope. With the surgeon viewing the monitor, an accurate oseotomy is possible with less risk of damage to soft tissue than with the conventional intraoral method. The muscle is divided into inner and outer layers and the inner layer is removed. An oblique-view endoscope allows secure resection by illuminating the muscle from the underside.

Results.—The endoscopic-assisted intraoral approach provided a clear view of the mandibular angle and facilitated accurate osteotomy on the mandibular angle, with low risk to surrounding soft tissue. Resection of the masseter was also enhanced by this approach. All 5 patients were treated successfully.

Conclusion.—All patients undergoing endoscopically assisted intraoral surgical correction of masseteric hypertrophy were treated successfully. The endoscope provided a safe and easy resection of the mandibular angle.

▶ In these 3 reports (Abstracts 1–32 to 1–34), the authors advocate the use of the endoscope in the treatment of conditions classically managed by open technique. The question remains as to whether the use of this instrument ultimately aids the patient or is just another expensive tool. Although Graham et al. (Abstract 1–33) show satisfactory results from the use of the endoscope for otoplasty and Honda et al. (Abstract 1–34) do likewise for the treatment of masseteric hypertrophy, neither group has shown the superiority of this technique over the more conventional open approach. Clearly, what is required is a blinded, prospective analysis comparing not only results of therapy, but complications, expense, and need for revision. It is hoped that this will be forthcoming.

Similar questions can be raised regarding the work of Huang et al. (Abstract 1–32). It is becoming well established that although the insertion of tissue expanders and the removal of large bulky subcutaneous lesions may be facilitated with the endoscope, excision of simple skin tumors via an open approach with well concealed incisions is likely to remain the procedure of choice. Anyone contemplating the use of the endoscope must first ask 2 basic questions: (1) Does it improve patient care (results, morbidity, and operative time)? and (2) Is it cost effective?

S.P. Bartlett, M.D.

2 Neoplastic, Inflammatory, and Degenerative Conditions

Premalignant and Malignant Skin Tumors

Long-term Efficacy and Safety of Jessner's Solution and 35% Trichloroacetic Acid vs 5% Fluorouracil in the Treatment of Widespread Facial Actinic Keratoses

Witheiler DD, Lawrence N, Cox SE, et al (Ohio State Univ, Columbus; Cooper Hosp Univ, Camden, NJ; Univ of North Carolina, Durham; et al)
Dermatol Surg 23:191–196, 1997   2–1

Background.—The long-term efficacy of fluorouracil (FU) or chemical peels for the treatment of actinic keratoses (AK) has not been well documented. The long-term outcomes of a medium-depth chemical peel and a standard regimen of topical FU in the treatment of widespread facial AK through 12 months were reported.

Methods.—Fifteen patients with severe facial actinic damage were included in the study. For 3 weeks, one side of the face was treated with one application of Jessner's solution and 35% trichloroacetic acid, and the other side was treated twice daily with 5% FU cream. The patients were examined at 1, 6, 12, and 32 months.

Findings.—Eight patients were available for the 32-month assessment. The number of AK was reduced on both sides of the face at 12 months, followed by an increased mean number of AK between 12 and 32 months. In biopsy specimens of clinically actinically damaged skin, improvements were seen in keratonicytic atypia, hyperkeratosis, parakeratosis, and inflammation at all treatment times on both sides of the face. Three squamous cell carcinomas developed, one on the peel side and 2 on the FU side. There appeared to be no association between sun exposure and clinical response.

Conclusions.—The 2 treatments studied are equally effective in the treatment of AK. However, AK reappear by 32 months after treatment. Despite this reappearance, the histologic improvements persist. Patients with widespread actinic keratoses should be reassessed every 1 or 1.5 years.

▶ We need to answer the question as to how much reduction of sun damage occurs with a resurfacing technique.

P.W. McKinney, M.D.

Recurrence of Thin Melanoma: How Effective Is Follow-up?
Moloney DM, Gordon DJ, Briggs JC, et al (Frenchay Hosp, Bristol, England)
Br J Plast Surg 49:409–413, 1996   2–2

Objective.—The incidence of malignant melanoma is increasing, largely because of increasing recognition of thin tumors and early-stage disease. The management and follow-up of these patients constitutes a significant workload for the surgical department. The benefits of 5-year follow-up for patients with thin malignant melanoma were analyzed.

Methods.—The retrospective study included 602 patients treated for thin malignant melanoma, all examined at least 5 years from the time of their primary surgery. The analysis sought to determine the tumor recurrence rate during follow-up and the effectiveness of surgical follow-up in detecting these recurrences.

Results.—The tumor recurrence rate was 4%, and the mean time to tumor recurrence was 53 months. Ten of the 24 recurrences developed after the 5-year follow-up. Just 5 surgically treatable recurrences developed within the 5-year period after surgery; 4 of those patients survived for longer than 5 years with appropriate further surgery. Thereafter, there were 4 surgically treatable recurrences, but their prognosis was poor (Table 3).

Conclusions.—Routine surgical follow-up for patients with thin melanoma provides little benefit in terms of detecting treatable recurrences. In this study, a 2-year follow-up detected all recurrences in which further surgery would have extended survival significantly. A better approach than

TABLE 3.—Surgically-treatable Recurrences Diagnosed After the Follow-up Period

Nature of recurrence	Time to recurrence (months)	Outcome after further surgery
Nodal recurrence	101	Death, melanoma, 24 months
Nodal recurrence	65	Death, melanoma, 6 months
Nodal recurrence	84	Death, melanoma, 24 months
Nodal recurrence	78	Death, other causes, 46 months

(Courtesy of Moloney DM, Gordon DJ, Briggs JC, et al: Recurrence of thin melanoma: How effective is follow-up? *Br J Plast Surg* 49:409–413, 1996.)

prolonged hospital follow-up may be patient education in self-examination and early self-referral when a recurrence is suspected.

▶ Most physicians still follow up patients with melanoma on a regular basis, with "routine" studies. This article supports my own belief that we don't make any significant difference in the final *medical* outcome for those patients with thin melanoma by doing all these studies. But is there a *psychological* benefit (both to the patient and maybe even the physician) from the performance of these follow-up studies? And if the answer to this question is "yes," can we still afford to keep doing this in the future?

R.L. Ruberg, M.D.

A Comparison Between Mohs Micrographic Surgery and Wide Surgical Excision for the Treatment of Dermatofibrosarcoma Protuberans
Gloster HM Jr, Harris KR, Roenigk RK (Mayo Clinic and Mayo Found, Rochester, Minn)
J Am Acad Dermatol 35:82–87, 1996   2–3

Background.—Increasing evidence suggests that Mohs micrographic surgery (MMS) is the treatment of choice for dermatofibrosarcoma protuberans (DFSP). Mohs micrographic surgery was compared with wide surgical excision in the treatment of this uncommon neoplasm.

Methods and Findings.—The medical records of 84 patients with DFSP treated at the Mayo Clinic by MMS or surgical excision were reviewed. Follow-up data were available on 15 patients undergoing MMS. The recurrence rate in this group was 6.6% at a mean of 40 months. The recurrence rate in the 39 patients undergoing wide excision was 10% at a mean follow-up of 36 months. In a review of the world literature, 11 studies were identified in which MMS was used to treat DFSP (Table 3). Neither local recurrences nor metastases were reported in these studies. Overall, including the Mayo series, the mean recurrence rate of DFSP after MMS was 0.6%. The total recurrence rate was 1.6%. Including the current series, 15 studies used wide excision to treat DFSP. Overall, the mean recurrence rate was 18%, and the total recurrence rate was 20%. In 8 published studies in which DFSP was surgically resected with undefined or conservative excisional margins, the mean recurrence rate was 43% and the total recurrence rate was 44%. Complete clearance of all tumors treated with MMS required a surgical margin of 2.5 cm to deep fascia. Twenty-two percent of the tumors removed had a margin of 0.5 cm; 50%, 1 cm; 67%, 1.5 cm; and 89%, 2 cm.

Conclusions.—The Mayo Clinic experience and previously published studies suggest that MMS, with its high cure rate and maximal conservation of tissue, is the best treatment for DFSP. With MMS, the surgeon can map the location of all tissue that has been removed and microscopically examine the entire deep and lateral margins of a horizontally sectioned excisional specimen, thus allowing precise margin control. Microscopic

TABLE 3.—Studies in Which Dermatofibrosarcoma Protuberans Was Treated With Mohs Micrographic Surgery

Author(s)	Year of Study	No. of Patients	Follow-up (mo)	No. of Patients with Local Recurrences	Recurrence Rate (%)
Mikhail and Lynn	1978	2	<60	0	0
Mohs	1978	7	<60	0	0
Peters et al.	1982	1	42	0	0
Hess et al.	1985	1	18	0	0
Robinson	1985	4	60	0	0
Hobbs et al.	1988	10	15–91	0	0
Hobbs and Ratz	1988	1	25	0	0
Weber et al.	1988	1	6	0	0
Rockley et al.	1989	1	18	0	0
Godberg and Maso	1990	1	12	0	0
Parker and Zitelli	1995	20	3–105	0	0
Current study	1995	15	5–96	1*	6.6
Total		64		1	1.6

*This patient was free of disease 65 months after the second Mohs procedure.
(Courtesy of Gloster HM Jr, Harris KR, Roenigk RK: A comparison between Mohs micrographic surgery and wide surgical excision for the treatment of dermatofibrosarcoma protuberans. *J Am Acad Dermatol* 35:82–87, 1996.)

extensions of tumor can be identified and removed with MMS while the maximal possible amount of normal tissue is conserved.

▶ The authors make a good case for the potential value of MMS for DFSP. They are careful, however, to say that this technique *may* be the treatment of choice (my emphasis). The article documents significant differences between the MMS group and the wide excision group, which make any statistical analysis impossible. (For example, there were significantly more patients in the wide excision group who had had previous, unsuccessful resections, perhaps indicating more aggressive tumors.) I think we can conclude that MMS works for DFPS; we need more convincing data before we conclude that it is *better* than the conventional approach of wide excision.

R.L. Ruberg, M.D.

▶ I believe the treatment of choice for dermatofibrosarcoma protuberans should be Mohs surgery. DFSPs have one of the highest recurrence rates for skin cancer even when resected with several centimeter margins of clinically normal skin. The subclinical spread of this cancer is not as an expanding mass but rather through asymmetric and numerous infiltrating "tentacles" spreading with ease among collagen bundles, fat, fascia, and muscle. Because the tumor spread is almost always asymmetric and importantly contiguous, its optimal treatment would logically be one that could, in a three-dimensional plane, examine all margins. This is the advantage that Mohs surgery provides and exactly what standard resection with routine pathologic analysis does not. Because of higher cure rates, dramatic tissue sparing (oftentimes a 5 mm margin is adequate around much of the tumor), and cost savings (no repeat surgeries, in-office surgery, no OR/hospital charges, potentially less involved reconstructive surgery, and no hospital pathology charge), Mohs surgery appears to offer a distinct advantage over conventional techniques for DFSP.

R.J. Siegle, M.D.

Dermatofibrosarcoma Protuberans (DFSP): Growth Characteristics Based on Tumor Modeling and a Review of Cases Treated With Mohs Micrographic Surgery
Haycox CL, Odland PB, Olbricht SM, et al (Univ of Washington, Seattle; Beth Israel Hosp, Boston)
Ann Plast Surg 38:246–251, 1997   2–4

Introduction.—Dermatofibrosarcoma protuberans (DFSP), a relatively rare cutaneous tumor, is highly invasive and aggressive locally but rarely metastasizes. Local recurrence is common and is not entirely prevented even by 3-cm wide local excision margins. Clinical features of DSFPs are discussed, together with histologic characteristics, treatment, and a review of cases treated with Mohs micrographic surgery.

Clinical Features and Histology.—Most DFSPs appear as plaque-like areas of cutaneous thickening. The tumors often have a reddish or blue color at the margins and may be initially symptomless. With increasing size, lesions are typically raised, firm, and multinodular and are fixed to the overlying skin but movable over deeper tissues. Untreated, DFSPs can attain massive dimensions. The classic anatomical locations are the trunk and proximal extremities. Infiltration of underlying adipose tissue, fascia, or musculature can occur at either the plaque or nodular stage. The tumor parenchyma is characterized by a distinct storiform pattern created by spindle-shaped cells arranged in an irregularly whorled pattern. Full-thickness incisional biopsies should be performed to establish the diagnosis.

Treatment.—The traditional treatment for DFSP has been wide and deep local surgical excision. Some surgeons have used margins of up to 5 cm of clinically normal tissue to prevent recurrence. Recently, however, Mohs micrographic surgical technique appears to be emerging as the treatment of choice. Of 169 cases reported to date at the University of Washington, the cumulative recurrence rate with the Mohs technique is 2.4%. The mean follow-up for 88% of these cases has been longer than 3 years. Mohs surgery achieves a low recurrence rate by precise margin control.

Discussion.—Tumor modeling based on microscopic observations shows that the standard wide local excision technique does not consider the complex growth characteristics of DFSP. Three-dimensional reconstructions of these tumors reveal shelflike nodular aggregates of tumor in the deep dermis and the deep subcutis, within or adjacent to the fascia. As previously reported, DFSPs have fingerlike projections into the subcutaneous fat and extend into underlying muscle. Mohs techniques offer the best functional and cosmetic results.

▶ Our experiences with DFSP at the Scripps Clinic are similar to those reported by the authors.

S.H. Miller, M.D.

Dermatofibrosarcoma Protuberans: Wide and Deep Block Excision Including Underlying Muscle

Kostakoğlu N, Özcan G, Gürsu KG (Hacettepe Univ, Ankara, Turkey)
Eur J Plast Surg 19:218–220, 1996   2–5

Objective.—Dermatofibrosarcoma protuberans (DESP) is a rare, slow-growing skin tumor that has a recurrence rate after excision ranging from 32% to 76%. Two cases of wide block resection of DESP tumors, including underlying muscles, were reviewed.

> *Case 1.*—Man, 32, with a recurrent left forearm mass 6 months after excision had the tumor resected with a 3-cm margin, including the extensor carpi radialis longus and brevis muscles. The area was covered with a pedicled flap. The man is tumor free after 4 years.
> *Case 2.*—Woman, 39, was seen with a right shoulder tumor after removal of an infected cyst 14 years previously and removal of a hypertrophic scar 10 years previously. The tumor was resected and covered with a rhomboid flap, and the patient is tumor free 3 years later.

Conclusion.—An aggressive approach to DESP tumor removal prevents recurrence.

▶ Wide excision, with inclusion of the deep fascia, has been the standard for surgical treatment of dermatofibrosarcoma protuberans. These authors have now extended the *deep* margin to include the underlying muscle. Does it work? With only 2 cases, and a short (3 to 4 year) follow-up, we really do not know. I would be inclined to try this approach, especially if sacrifice of the underlying muscle does not result in significant functional impairment.

R.L. Ruberg, M.D.

Head and Neck Reconstruction

Conchal Bowl Skin Grafting in Nasal Tip Reconstruction: Clinical and Histologic Evaluation

Rohrer TE, Dzubow LM (Boston Univ; Univ of Pennsylvania, Philadelphia)
J Am Acad Dermatol 33:476–481, 1995   2–6

Purpose.—Defects of the distal nose are commonly managed with full-thickness skin grafts taken from the periclavicular, pre-auricular, or post-auricular area. However, skin from these sites may not provide a good cosmetic match, largely because it lacks the highly sebaceous nature of the skin of the distal nose. The conchal bowl was evaluated as a site of donor skin to repair defects of the nasal tip.

> *Technique.*—The skin of the conchal bowl has a more "pebbled" appearance than the skin at other commonly used donor sites, and it also contains more sebaceous glands. It is readily available and often provides a better color match for the skin of the distal nose. Either full-thickness or composite grafts can be harvested and used. The full-thickness grafts provide excellent results in patients with superficial defects, such as those produced by Mohs micrographic surgery. The harvesting and suturing techniques are the same as those used for other full-thickness grafts. The graft is harvested just above the perichondrium, which is left behind to cover the cartilage; healing by secondary intention is allowed to occur. The donor site cartilage may be removed or perforated to permit healing. The cosmetic results are best when the graft used is slightly smaller than the defect to be covered.

Discussion.—Skin grafts from the conchal bowl provide excellent cover for defects of the skin of the distal nose (Figs 7 and 8). The conchal bowl is a reliable source of donor skin that provides a better cosmetic match than skin from the periclavicular, pre-auricular, and postauricular areas. The relative thinness and small size of conchal bowl skin grafts are limiting factors.

▶ This was initially described by Brent and Ott[1] as a means to add cartilage to nasal reconstruction. These authors promote the use of these grafts for defects of the tip of the nose because they provide color and texture match for replacement of the sebaceous skin of the nose. The limiting factors are the extent of the defect and its depth. Furthermore, leaving the donor site to close secondarily would likely be unacceptable to many patients.

S.H. Miller, M.D.

Reference

1. Brent B, Ott R: Perichondro-cutaneous graft. *Plast Reconstr Surg* 62:1–14, 1978.

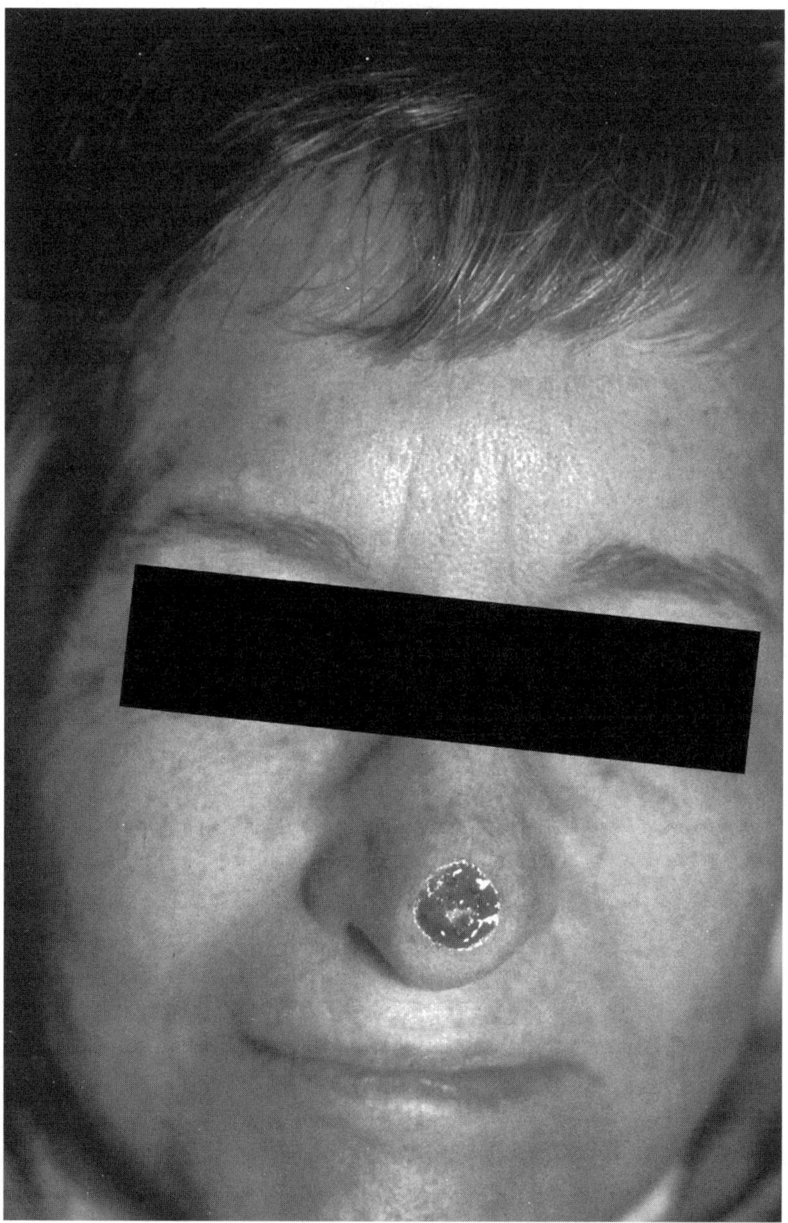

FIGURE 7.—Nasal defect after Mohs micrographic surgery. (Courtesy of Rohrer TE, Dzubow LM: Conchal bowl skin grafting in nasal tip reconstruction: Clinical and histologic evaluation. *J Am Acad Dermatol* 33:476–481, 1995.)

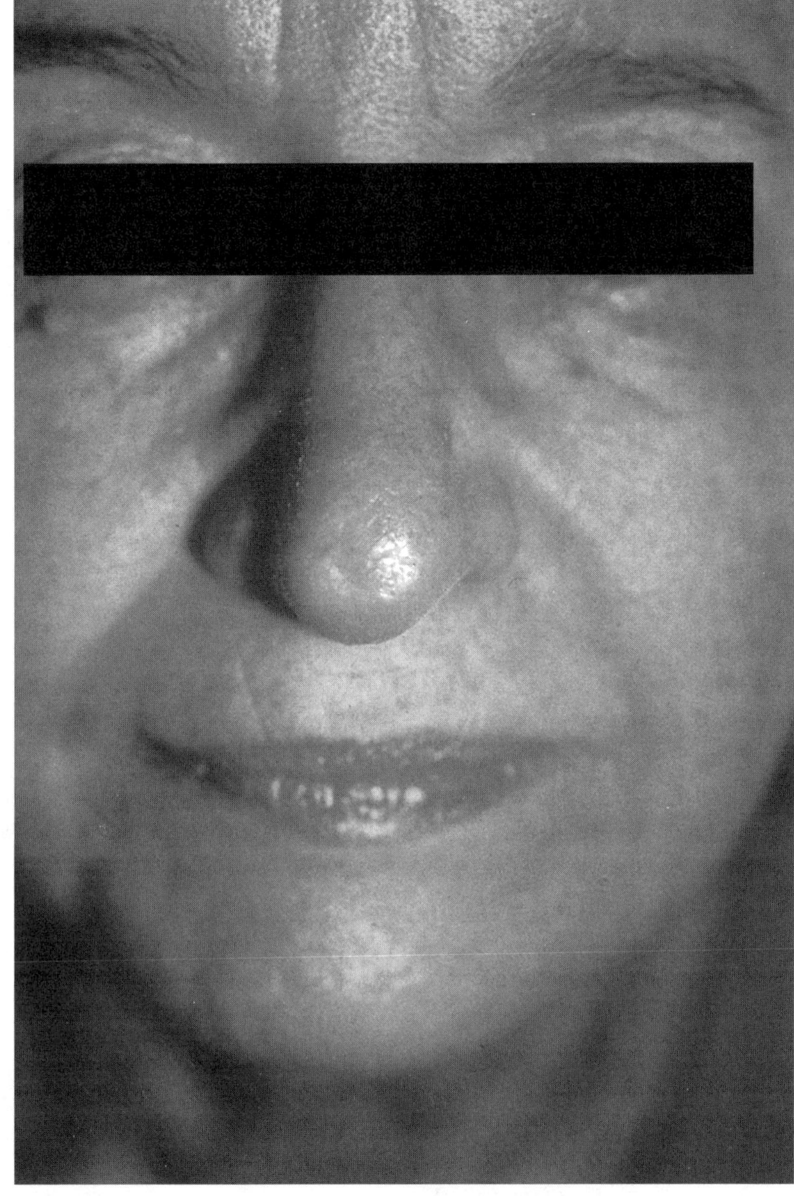

FIGURE 8.—Nasal tip 4 months after conchal bowl full-thickness skin graft. (Courtesy of Rohrer TE, Dzubow LM: Conchal bowl skin grafting in nasal tip reconstruction: Clinical and histologic evaluation. *J Am Acad Dermatol* 33:476–481, 1995.)

The Neurovascular Infrahyoid Muscle Flap: A New Method for Tongue Reconstruction

Remmert SM, Sommer KD, Majocco AM, et al (Med Univ of Luebeck, Germany)
Plast Reconstr Surg 99:613–618, 1997

Background.—Surgical treatment of tongue cancer results in extended functional failures in some patients. A neurovascular fasciomuscular flap derived from the infrahyoid musculature has been developed to reconstruct defects of the pharynx and tongue with a contractile muscle.

Methods and Outcomes.—Eleven patients with tongue cancer were treated. Five patients had stage T2 disease, 3 had T3, and 3 had T4. Four patients had total glossectomy, and 3 had hemiglossectomy. Half the tongue base was resected in 2 patients, and one fourth was resected in another 2 patients. In the patients undergoing total glossectomy, the tongue was reconstructed with the infrahyoid myofascial neurovascular flap from both sides of the neck. In all other patients, the new flap was only taken from 1 side of the neck. The glossectomy had to be combined with a laryngectomy in 1 patient. The tracheostoma could be closed 4 weeks after surgery in 10 patients. All were able to resume an oral diet. On electromyography, voluntary innervation of the reconstructed tongues was observed (Fig 4).

Conclusion.—Defects of the tongue base can be reconstructed successfully after partial resections or total glossectomies using the neurovascular

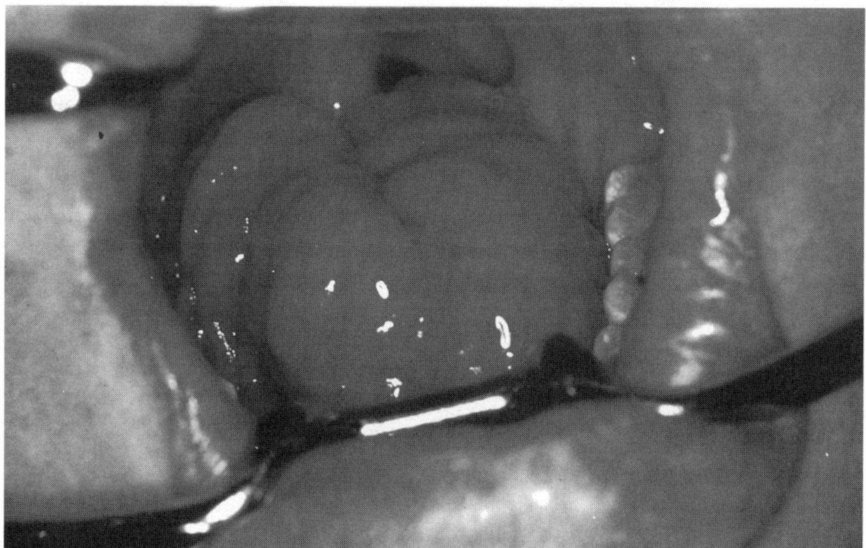

FIGURE 4.—Nine months after total glossectomy. The tongue has been reconstructed with infrahyoid flaps from both sides of the neck, which have been covered by a microvascular anastomosed jejunum patch. (Courtesy of Remmert SM, Sommer KD, Majocco AM, et al: The neurovascular infrahyoid muscle flap: A new method for tongue reconstruction. *Plast Reconstr Surg* 99:613–618, 1997.)

infrahyoid flap. The main advantages of this flap are the voluntary innervation by means of the ansa cervicalis and prevention of scarring and atrophy of the reconstructed tongue.

▶ This is a clever idea and fulfills a basic plastic surgical principle of replacing lost or excised tissues with like tissue.

S.H. Miller, M.D.

The Chondrocutaneous Ear Helical Free Flap for the Reconstruction of the Defects of the Nasal Tip, Columella and/or Ala
Bajec J, Gang RK (Ibn Sina Hosp, Kuwait)
Eur J Plast Surg 20:66–70, 1997
2–8

Background.—Reconstructing a full-thickness defect of the tip of the nose, columella, and ala is difficult. The use of local flaps often results in a bulky nose requiring additional surgery. The chondrocutaneous ear helical free flap in the reconstruction of such defects was described.

Methods.—Five patients with composite tissue defects of the tip, columella, and ala of the nose resulting from human bites underwent early reconstruction to avoid possible infection. The free flaps were designed and elevated from the upper part of the helix and concha of the opposite ear. The flap, which matched the traumatic defect on the nose, was based on the anterior auricular branches of the superficial temporal vessels. The free flap was sutured to the margins of the defect. In 4 patients, direct end-to-end anastomosis of both vessels was done, and in 1 patient, a venous graft was needed. Donor flap areas were closed directly. Follow-up ranged from 6 months to 5 years.

Outcomes.—In 4 patients, the contour, symmetry, and color match were considered satisfactory. Touch-up procedures were performed under local anesthesia to obtain the final aesthetic result. Deformity at the donor site was minimal. In the fifth patient, the free flap was lost because of venous thrombosis which could not be reversed.

Conclusion.—The chondrocutaneous free flap is a dependable vascularized composite tissue transfer that enables straightforward, 1–stage reconstruction of tissue defects of the tip, columella, and ala of the nose. Additional advantages include freedom in flap design and the structural similarity between the nose and ear, which makes the ear an ideal donor site for such defects.

▶ The results shown are good, but the donor deformity was real, the time required to perform the reconstruction was long, and most patients still required aesthetic touch-up procedures.

S.H. Miller, M.D.

Degenerative and Inflammatory Conditions

Microwave Heating in the Management of Postmastectomy Upper Limb Lymphedema

Gan J-L, Li S-I, et al (Ninth People's Hosp of Shanghai, China)
Ann Plast Surg 36:576–580, 1996

2–9

Background.—Lymphedema of the upper limb is one of the most distressing complications of breast cancer treatment. This condition is especially frustrating to treat. The outcomes of microwave heating of upper limb lymphedema after radical mastectomy were reported.

Patients and Outcomes.—Forty-five patients, aged 41 to 75 years, with postmastectomy lymphedema of the upper extremity, were treated. One was male. Treatment consisted of 60 minutes of heating each day for 20 days, with the course repeated after 2 weeks when necessary. The total treatment time for each patient was 40 hours. Follow-up ranged from 6 months to 2 years. The patients reported significant improvement in burning pain, swelling, heaviness, and mobility of the lymphedematous limb. The amount of edema was reduced significantly after microwave heating and compression bandaging. Inflammatory episodes also were significantly decreased by 2 courses of treatment. No complications were associated with the treatment.

Conclusions.—In this series of patients with postmastectomy upper limb lymphedema, treatment with microwave heating significantly decreased the amount of peripheral edema. The incidence and severity of secondary acute inflammation also were greatly decreased, and soft-tissue elasticity was restored.

▶ Lymphedema after treatment for breast cancer is far less common today. Nonetheless, it still does occur and may be recalcitrant to treatment. Although this therapeutic modality has been known in the United States, it has been infrequently used and never really studied. However, the authors report a significant reduction in edema and erysipelas, which does suggest that heating may be of benefit for treatment of postoperative and posttraumatic lymphedema. Confirmation of that benefit will require carefully controlled studies.

S.H. Miller, M.D.

Time Course of Bell Palsy

Qi WW, Yin SS, Stucker FJ, et al (Louisiana State Univ, Shreveport)
Arch Otolaryngol Head Neck Surg 122:967–972, 1996

2–10

Background.—The disease course and recovery from facial nerve palsy often are monitored by the results of electroneurography and facial grading. However, the association of electroneurography and the grading of facial function has not been determined quantitatively. In the current study, the time course of Bell's palsy and the relation between electroneurography and facial function grading were further characterized.

Methods.—Thirty-two patients with Bell's palsy were included in the study. Bilateral electroneurographic recordings in different stages in the disease course were repeated and compared with categorized videotaped facial movements using the House-Brackmann facial nerve grading system.

Findings.—A time gap was found between the percentage of electroneurographic response and the category of facial nerve grading during the same period of the disease process. A theoretical model of the time course and specific patterns of recovery was established. Three stages—preclinical, clinical, and postclinical—were defined. According to the findings of electroneurography and facial grading, the best period for prediction of recovery was 10 to 14 days.

Conclusions.—The specific pattern of the time course of Bell's palsy can be used to more reliably predict prognosis. Additional research involving larger numbers of patients is needed to characterize the theoretical model of the time course in complete facial paralysis and other facial nerve disorders.

▶ This is an interesting preliminary study of the course of patients with Bell's palsy. It is primarily of interest if the authors and others can find a useful model that will allow early and reliable prognostication of facial nerve recovery.

S.H. Miller, M.D.

Patterns of Coordinated Lower Facial Muscle Function and Their Importance in Facial Reanimation
Cacou C, Greenfield BE, Hunt NP, et al (Univ College London; Eastman Dental Hosp, London)
Br J Plast Surg 49:274–280, 1996   2–11

Background.—The individual action of facial muscles and their coordinated function in facial movement are not well understood. The electric activity of the lip and other lower facial muscles during movement was studied.

Methods.—Eleven healthy volunteers were assessed. Coordinated patterns of lower facial muscle activity were observed using 8-channel electromyography. Integrated electric activity was measured, and different muscle groups were compared during active, active-against-resistance, and passive movements.

Findings.—A contraction reflex was noted in 8 volunteers. Lower facial movements involved simultaneous bilateral activity in all muscle groups assessed bilaterally. These movements required a balance between dilator and constrictor forces.

Conclusions.—These findings have important implications for facial reanimation surgery. Reconstructing balanced constrictor and dilator forces is desirable, the latter having vector pulls upward, downward, and laterally, to reconstruct the normal mechanism of lower facial movement.

▶ Mimetic facial movements, especially those in the perioral region, result from finely balanced activity of several muscles, producing vector forces that pull the lips laterally as well as superiorly and inferiorly. In great part, failure of our facial reanimation procedures relates to our inability to replicate this balance.

S.H. Miller, M.D.

Postural Vasoregulation and Mediators of Reperfusion Injury in Venous Ulceration

He C, Cherry GW, Phil D, et al (Wound Healing Inst, Headington, Oxford)
J Vasc Surg 25:647–653, 1997   2–12

Introduction.—How persistence of venous ulcers is initiated and caused is unknown. The genesis of venous ulcers or their failure to heal may be related to ischemia-reperfusion injury. In this hypothesis, the dermal microcirculation of the lower legs of patients with venous hypertension has repeated and severe episodes of ischemia and reperfusion. At this site, biologically significant amounts of free radicals are generated. The effects of postural change on the microcirculation of ulcers and on levels of known mediators of reperfusion injury in their venous effluent were studied to test the hypothesis that ischemia and reperfusion injury may contribute to the cause or nonhealing of venous ulcers.

Methods.—In 10 patients with venous ulcers, a standard protocol of 20 minutes of stabilization, 1 hour of limb dependency, and 2 hours of re-evaluation was used. With a new laser-Doppler scanning technique, superficial blood flow in and around ulcers was repeatedly examined. Before dependency and at 1, 10, 30, 60, and 120 minutes after re-evaluation, blood samples from the saphenous vein or a tributary adjacent to the ulcer were taken and analyzed for tumor necrosis factor-α, interleukin-1RA, interleukin-1β, interleukin-6, platelet-activating factor, thromboxane B2, leukotriene B4, and P-selectin.

Results.—In 7 of 10 patients, there was a pattern of high ulcer blood flow which decreased on dependency and return to baseline levels on re-elevation and eventually exceeded initial values. In resting ulcer venous effluent, levels of platelet-activating factor, interleukin-1RA, and interleukin-6 were significantly higher than in systemic venous samples according to mediator assays. For P-selectin, the reverse was true. As a function of posture, ulcer size, or healing, there was no statistically significant change in effluent concentration of a mediator.

Conclusion.—In venous leg ulcers, postural vasoregulation causes relative ischemia and reperfusion. Changes in release of mediators known to be related to reperfusion injury in internal organs are not associated with this newly discovered development. Further studies should be conducted to determine the relationship between platelet-activating factor and healing. Angiogenesis and macrophage activation has been related to platelet-activating factor as well as a gain in tensile strength in experimental incisional skin wounds.

▶ I acknowledge the possible correlation between a possible vasoregulation with ischemia reperfusion and venous leg ulcers. Mark Ferguson in Manchester, England, has talked extensively about this, although his data have yet to be published. This article provides the first caution that I have seen on some of the discussions. The theory is intriguing, but as pointed out by Drs. He, Cherry, and Arnold, the final link has yet to be determined.

D.J. Smith, Jr., M.D.

3 Trauma

Head and Neck

Ear Replantation Without Microsurgery
Pribaz JJ, Crespo LD, Orgill DP, et al (Harvard Med School, Boston)
Plast Reconstr Surg 99:1868–1872, 1997   3–1

Objective.—There are few reports of successful reattachment of an amputated ear, particularly without the use of microsurgery. Use of the postauricular pocket principle has been advocated by Mladick et al. to enhance the success of replantation. The experience with 6 patients is described.

> *Case 1.*—Man, 21, had complete avulsion of the left ear. No suitable vessels for microsurgical reattachment were found. The epidermis, outer dermis, and skin margin at the stump were removed by dermabrasion and excision while the cartilage was left well covered. The ear was reattached in layers using Vicryl sutures and buried under a scalp flap for 2 and one half weeks. The ear was removed from the pocket and, within 10 days, had re-epithelialized. The ear has retained its shape for 5 years (Fig 1).

Discussion.—When microsurgical reattachment of an amputated ear is not possible, performing dermabrasion, but leaving the cartilage well covered to prevent distortion, followed by reattachment and burial under a scalp flap allows the ear to revascularize quickly before scarring can cause distortion. Five of 6 amputated ears were salvaged in this manner. The sixth became necrotic after infection developed.

▶ The value of this article is not the reporting of the "pocket principle technique"—that technique has been described for more than 20 years. The value is the evidence that the principle works in a high percentage of cases. There are many articles describing different techniques for ear reattachment, almost all of which are accompanied by single case reports of success. In this article, we find that the appearance and the function of 5 of 6 reattached ear parts were normal using the pocket principle, which is a pretty good success rate!

R.L. Ruberg, M.D.

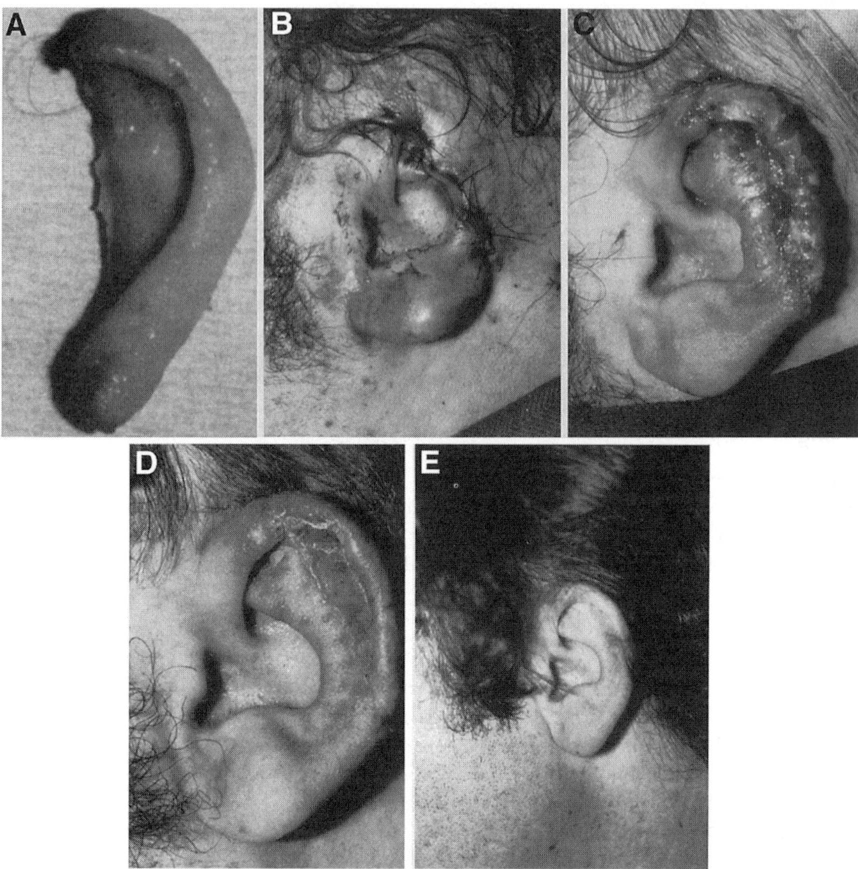

FIGURE 1.—(*Above, left*) Amputated ear segment after débridement and dermabrasion. (*Above, center*) The de-epithelialized ear is sutured back into its anatomical location and has been buried beneath a postauricular flap. (*Above, right*) Two and one half weeks later the ear has been extracted from the pocket. Active bleeding is seen in all areas of the dermis of the reattached segment. (*Below, left*) At 1 month, complete spontaneous re-epithelialization is evident. (*Below, right*) At 12 months, the reattached ear had a satisfactory appearance and had good contour and projection. (Courtesy of Pribaz JJ, Crespo LD, Orgill DP, et al: Ear replantation without microsurgery. *Plast Reconstr Surg* 99:1868–1872, 1997.)

Reconstruction of the Microtic External Ear in Adults Using Porous Polyethylene Implant

Sengezer M, Türegün M, Işik S, et al (Gülhane Military Med Academy, Ankara, Turkey)

Eur J Plast Surg 19:314–317, 1996

3–2

Introduction.—The ideal ear framework must be preformed, sterilized, nontoxic, and capable of becoming vascularized. Porous polyethylene has recently proved clinically acceptable in the maxillofacial region and for ear reconstruction because it allows vascularization and appears to be resis-

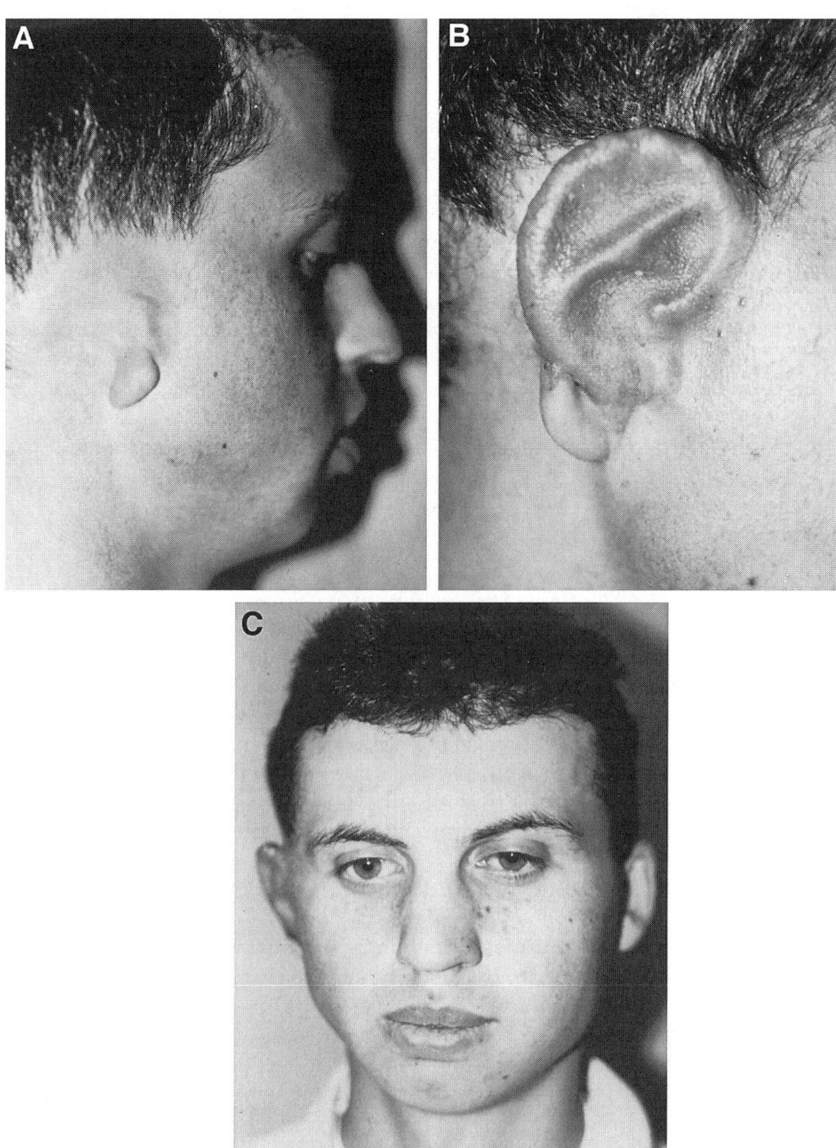

FIGURE 3.—A, preoperative view of a patient with microtia; **B** and **C,** postoperative views after 2 stages at 9 months. (Courtesy of Sengezer M, Türegün M, Işik S: Reconstruction of the microtic external ear in adults using porous polyethylene implant. *Eur J Plast Surg* 19:314–317, 1996. © Springer-Verlag 1996.)

tant to infection and extrusion. Porous polyethylene ear implants were performed in 10 21-year-old men with microtia who had no previous ear surgery.

Surgical Technique.—A vertical incision was made on the ear remnant using local anesthesia. The cartilage remnants were removed and a subcutaneous pocket was created just above the temporoparietal fascia and mastoid fascia. The implant was soaked in an antibiotic solution before it was inserted. It was placed into the pocket but not sutured to the tissues. The skin was closed and a small-diameter suction drain was placed. No dressing was used. The drain was removed in 5 days. Two months later the framework was elevated and the posterior aspect of the ear and mastoid region skin grafted. The skin flap was sutured to the helical rim of the framework to avoid contraction of the flap. The earlobe was transposed to its correct position. Average operative times for the first and second stages of surgery were 40 and 45 minutes, respectively. Average patient follow-up was 13 months.

Results.—Most patients were satisfied with their reconstructions (Fig 3). There were 2 exposures because of contraction of the ventral skin flap of the helical rim of the frame. The exposures were corrected by removal of enough framework to permit direct closure without tension. An infected implant was salvaged using antibiotic solution irrigation in the first postoperative week. One of 4 biopsies obtained showed bleeding from the implant with vascularization and soft tissue ingrowth.

Conclusion.—Porous polyethylene implants have a very high rate of satisfaction in patients with microtia. The implant provided an ideal shape for ears and surgery was performed using local anesthesia. Surgical time was short and patients did not require hospitalization.

▶ This technique offers promise because of the difficulty in finding noncalcified cartilage to use for autologous ear reconstruction in adults. If this is shown to be a material that can be prepared before surgery without the morbidity associated with harvesting rib cartilage yet provide equivalent results, it is certainly worthy of consideration for all ear reconstructions.

S.H. Miller, M.D.

High-Energy Ballistic and Avulsive Facial Injuries: Classification, Patterns, and an Algorithm for Primary Reconstruction
Clark N, Birely B, Manson PN, et al (Univ of Maryland, Baltimore)
Plast Reconstr Surg 98:583–601, 1996   3–3

Introduction.—During World Wars I and II, many advances were made in the treatment of high-energy ballistic and avulsive facial injuries. Some of the management principles developed during wars are now applied when results of civilian weapons are seen in city emergency departments. Instead of delayed reconstruction, however, a more aggressive policy toward primary reconstruction now seems appropriate. A 17-year experience (1977 to 1993) with "ballistic wound" surgical management of gunshot, shotgun, and high-energy avulsive facial injuries was described.

Methods.—The essential difference between most blunt facial injuries and ballistic or avulsive facial injuries is missing or severely damaged soft tissue. In high-energy ballistic or avulsive injuries, soft-tissue loss results in devascularization of bone. Management in such cases involves immediate stabilization in anatomical position of existing bone, primary closure of existing soft tissue, periodic "second look" serial débridement procedures, and definitive early reconstruction of soft-tissue and bony defects. Patients reviewed in this series had 250 gunshot wounds, 53 close-range shotgun wounds, and 15 high-energy avulsive facial injuries.

Results.—Most gunshot victims were young men; the most common age was 25 years, with another peak at 55 years. About one third were suicide attempts and the rest were assaults. Four general patterns of involvement were noted for both gunshot and shotgun wounds and 3 for avulsive facial injuries. Treatment, prognosis, and complications vary according to these patterns. In gunshot wounds, patterns include the frontal cranium, the orbit, the lower midface, and the mandible. Patterns of shotgun wounds are the lateral mandible, the central face, the lateral midface and orbit, and the lateral cranium and orbit. In avulsive high-energy wounds, the mandible is the area of tissue loss in 27%; the mandible and the maxilla in 27%; and the mandible, maxilla, and orbit in 47%.

The treatment algorithm begins with identification of zones of injury and loss for both soft and hard tissue. Whereas gunshot wounds are best classified by location of the exit wound, shotgun and avulsive facial wounds are classified by the zone of soft-tissue and bone loss. The most common major defect in initial treatment planning was underestimation of the need for replacement of vascularized lining. In avulsive facial injuries, the major management problem was not appreciating that these wounds are subject to tissue loss and necrosis.

Conclusions.—High-energy ballistic and avulsive facial injuries present a challenge to the reconstructive surgeon. With an aggressive treatment program that emphasizes initial primary repair of existing tissue, serial conservative débridement, and early definitive reconstruction, many patients can have a reasonable functional outcome.

▶ This is a valuable contribution and extends the authors' philosophy for management of blunt facial injuries. The ability to provide vascularized tissue after staged débridement is critical to the success of early reconstruction of these devastating injuries.

S.H. Miller, M.D.

Combined Paresis and Restriction of the Extraocular Muscles After Orbital Fracture: A Study of 16 Patients

Mauriello JA Jr, Antonacci R, Mostafavi R, et al (Univ of Medicine and Dentistry–New Jersey Medical School, Newark, NJ)
Ophthal Plast Reconstr Surg 12:206–210, 1996   3–4

Objective.—A small subset of patients with orbital fracture have diplopia resulting from combined paresis and restriction of the entrapped muscle, despite timely and appropriate repair of the fracture. Findings were reported for a group of 16 such patients.

Methods.—Patients eligible for the study had satisfied 3 criteria: (1) before orbital fracture repair, positive forced ductions were present such that the eye could not be pulled away from the field of action of the entrapped muscle; (2) CT of the orbit revealed a muscle adjacent to or within the fracture site; and (3) shortly after orbital floor fracture repair, there was significant weakness in the field of action of the paretic muscle and improved function in the field of action of the antagonist of the entrapped muscle. The 16 patients who met study criteria ranged in age from 4 to 80 years.

Results.—Causes of orbital fracture were blunt trauma during a fistfight in 7 patients, motor vehicle accidents in 5, and a fall in 2; 1 patient was injured by a soft ball and another by the impact of a coiled garage door opener. Before surgery, all patients had significant motility disturbance. The time from injury to orbital repair ranged from 1 week to 8 months. Single extraocular muscles were involved in 13 patients and 2 extraocular muscles in 3 patients. A deviation in primary position was present in 3 patients before orbital surgery. In all 16 cases, the restricted extraocular muscle was released from the incarcerated fracture site; time required for the actual release was 10 minutes or less. A silicone implant material was used in 10 patients and a layered Vicryl mesh in 6. Seven patients had good recovery of function of the paretic muscle and 3 additional patients required no further treatment. Six patients, including all 3 with 2-muscle involvement, had significant deviations in primary position; 3 underwent strabismus surgery and 3 had prism therapy.

Conclusions.—All 16 patients with combined paresis and restriction of the extraocular muscle(s) after blunt orbital trauma experienced severe motility restriction. All underwent orbital exploration and release of the incarcerated tissues, confirmed by the intraoperative forced duction test. It was not possible to determine whether surgically induced trauma contributed to the transient paresis of the involved muscle.

▶ Here is an important issue to consider preoperatively in patients with periorbital trauma. Perhaps all patients with muscle, visualized on CT scan, adjacent to or within an orbital fracture site should be evaluated by an ophthalmologist preoperatively.

S.H. Miller, M.D.

Upper Extremity

Electrodiagnostic Testing in Hand Surgery

Campion D (Univ of California, Los Angeles)
J Hand Surg [Am] 21A:947–956, 1996

3–5

Background.—The electrodiagnostic examination (EDX) can provide useful, objective information on the progression of nerve entrapment syndromes over time and recovery after surgery. Whereas the hand surgeon is the best person to decide which tests are needed for appropriate diagnosis, it is more often the EDX physician who selects the type of EDX to be performed. Techniques in EDX were reviewed from the perspective of the hand surgeon.

Electrodiagnostic Examination Techniques.—To test the motor nerves, the nerve is stimulated and the electrical response recorded using a small surface electrode placed on the muscle and a reference electrode placed off the muscle. The compound muscle action potential (CMAP) is recorded as the trigger for muscle contraction as it moves out along the muscle fiber from the neuromuscular junction. When the response is maximal—even with additional current—it is known as the supramaximal CMAP. Successful EDX of motor nerves requires accurate electrode placement and the ability to determine a maximum stimulus. Sensory nerve EDX is done by recording the nerve action potential from pickup electrodes placed over the sensory nerve. The sensory distal latency is shorter than the motor distal latency because the action potential is not conducted along muscle.

Carpal Tunnel Syndrome.—In the diagnostic evaluation of carpal tunnel syndrome (CTS), EDX can only show the presence or absence of slowed conduction at the carpal ligament. The order of abnormalities—from median palmar latency to denervation of the thenar muscles—is very important in deciding on the need for further testing. The differential diagnosis includes radiculopathy, a more proximal median nerve entrapment, diabetic neuropathy, and median nerve damage in the palm.

Ulnar Nerve Neuropathy.—In ulnar nerve neuropathy, the ulnar nerve is stimulated at the wrist and above and below the elbow, and the conduction velocity is calculated from wrist to elbow and across the elbow. In contrast to CTS, in which sensory conduction is affected before motor conduction, slowing of either suggests ulnar nerve neuropathy (UNN) at the elbow. The site of the lesion can be localized in most patients, especially with sensory and mixed nerve conduction testing. Testing the ulnar nerve at intervals of 1–4 cm can identify the compressed site more precisely.

Radial Nerve Entrapment.—Radial nerve entrapment is best assessed by needle examination of radial innervated muscles of the forearm. The extent of denervation in these muscles indicates the severity of axonal damage. Repeated EDX studies over time can provide information on the onset of reinnervation and determine the percentage of surviving motor units.

Brachial Plexopathies.—Brachial plexopathy can be assessed by EDX of the upper extremity. Testing should be delayed for a few weeks after symptom onset to allow time for denervation of the muscles supplied by the degenerating axons. Decreased amplitude of the sensory nerve responses shows sensory axonal loss.

Thoracic Outlet Syndrome.—The diagnosis of thoracic outlet syndrome is suspected in patients who have no apparent focal lesions and are considered unlikely to have radiculopathy. Sensory evoked responses are the most valuable form of EDX for making this diagnosis, which is recognized mainly in Southern California and Colorado. However, the diagnosis is difficult to make and remains primarily a clinical one.

Radiculopathy.—The major EDX finding in radiculopathy is denervation related to motor axon damage (the diagnosis cannot be made if only sensory axons are affected). The reinnervation that follows radiculopathy is reflected on EDX by the finding of long, large motor units. This condition is sometimes confused with CTS or UNN.

Peripheral Neuropathy.—Entrapment neuropathies are more likely to be found in patients with underlying polyneuropathy, and EDX can provide a great deal of information on the form of polyneuropathy. The diagnosis of CTS in a patient with mild diabetic neuropathy must be made with caution. Nerve conduction studies of the lower extremity will tell whether there is any widespread neuropathy.

The EDX Report.—The final EDX report should state whether there are any abnormalities of latency or conduction on needle examination and describe the probable pathophysiologic processes. Too often these reports only describe a pattern of slight abnormalities without reference to the patient's clinical condition. Electrodiagnostic physicians and hand surgeons should share concepts and ideas to improve the value of EDX for hand surgery.

▶ It is easy to fall in the trap of simply sending a patient for "nerve studies." This article reminded me of the importance of understanding exactly what one is searching for, both in presentation of the physiology and pathophysiology and in what can be expected in certain syndromes. I was particularly impressed with the discussion of thoracic outlet, radiculopathy, and peripheral neuropathy and with the overall EDX report.

D.J. Smith, Jr., M.D.

Bilateral Fast Magnetic Resonance Imaging of the Operated Carpal Tunnel

Pierre-Jerome C, Bekkelund SI, Mellgren SI, et al (Tromso Univ, Norway)
Scand J Plast Reconstr Hand Surg 31:171–177, 1997   3–6

Introduction.—After operation for carpal tunnel syndrome, intracarpal soft tissue changes and modification of the size of the canal are among the factors associated with painful wrists. Although the presence of edema and ischemia of the median nerve has been identified with magnetic resonance imaging, the modifications of the size of the carpal tunnel have not been identified. A bilateral volumetric study of the carpal tunnel from inlet to outlet before and after release was conducted to determine the modifications of the size of the carpal tunnel.

Methods.—There were 28 patients with a mean age of 54.7 years who had 31 operations for carpal tunnel syndrome. Abnormal conduction studies were evident in all patients. Using 2 fast imaging sequences, turbo spin echo and fast field echo, magnetic resonance imaging of both wrists was conducted before and after operation. The values of the relative signal intensity of the median nerve before and after operation were quantified, and the postoperative intracarpal changes were assessed objectively.

Results.—In 31 wrists with carpal tunnel syndrome, the mean volume of the tunnel was 11,511.7 (2,857) mm$_3$ before and 13,803.4 (3,934.8) mm$_3$ after surgery. Preoperatively, the mean relative signal intensity of the median nerve was 1.7 (1.8) and postoperatively, it was 1.3 (1.1). Persistent nerve enlargement (21 wrists), misalignment of the tendons (20 wrists), fat tissue deposits (21 wrists), fibrous tissue deposits (20 wrists), and muscle edema (6 wrists) were other postoperative changes.

Conclusion.—The use of an endoscopic procedure in the treatment of carpal tunnel syndrome is recommended due to the modifications of the carpal canal as a consequence of open surgical release (including increased volume and displacement of the flexor tendons). Functional outcomes were more quickly achieved with the endoscopic approach in previous studies that compared open surgery with endoscopic carpal tunnel release.

Median Nerve Compression Can Be Detected by Magnetic Resonance Imaging of the Carpal Tunnel

Horch RE, Allmann KH, Laubenberger J, et al (Albert Ludwigs Universität, Freiburg, Germany)
Neurosurgery 41:76–83, 1997

3–7

Introduction.—Interest in the anatomical correlation of median nerve compression has surged since the introduction of minimally invasive techniques in the surgical decompression of carpal tunnel syndrome. A new diagnostic tool was studied to determine therapeutic options in patients without measurably impaired nerve conduction values. Little is known about dynamic morphological changes in patients with carpal tunnel syndrome, and there has never been a direct comparison to healthy volunteers. Static and dynamic changes in the carpal canal in patients with carpal tunnel syndrome were analyzed and compared with those in asymptomatic volunteers.

Methods.—Twenty patients with carpal tunnel syndrome and pathologic nerve conduction values had MR imaging performed, and the results were matched to those in 20 healthy volunteers. In patients, preoperative and postoperative T2-weighted signal intensity of the median nerve was measured.

Results.—Healthy volunteers tend to have larger cross-sectional areas of the carpal tunnel than patients with carpal tunnel syndrome. At the pisiform and hamate level, the cross-sectional area of the carpal tunnel decreases. At the level of the pisiform, the cross-sectional area decreases during wrist extension. It increases at the level of the hamate during extension. In 94% of the patients, the distal flattening of the median nerve recovered postoperatively. The motor latency recovered in only 39% of patients, despite the signal intensity of the median nerve on T2-weighted images decreasing by 67%.

Conclusion.—The space available for the median nerve narrows during flexion and extension, which may lead to potential median nerve compression. For diagnosis and postoperative follow-up of carpal tunnel syndrome, MR imaging is accurate and reliable and may help in making a decision for surgical decompression.

► These 2 articles (Abstracts 3–6 and 3–7) take different tacks for the analysis of carpal tunnel syndrome. One studies the median nerve compression at the wrist utilizing analysis with MRI. The study by Horch et al. shows comparisons between patients and healthy normal volunteers and shows how an MRI may be useful in determining whether surgery would be of benefit. All of us would welcome this information should this correlation prove to be valid. On the other hand, it appears that Pierre-Jerome et al. have taken the analysis too far too quickly. They relate their results with MRI analysis and use these as a mechanism to support endoscopy as opposed to open release. The jury is still out.

D.J. Smith, Jr., M.D.

Single-portal Endoscopic Carpal Tunnel Release: Agee Carpal Tunnel Release System
Elmaraghy MW, Hurst LN (Univ of Western Ontario, Canada)
Ann Plast Surg 36:286–291, 1996   3–8

Background.—Few studies have assessed the efficacy and safety of the redesigned Agee carpal tunnel release system (CTRS). Outcomes of the single-portal endoscopic carpal tunnel release (ECTR) using the redesigned Agee CTRS were reported.

Methods.—Eighty-six procedures were performed in a cohort of 69 patients. Objective motor/sensory assessments and clinical questionnaires were completed at 10 days, 6 weeks, and 10 weeks after surgery.

Findings.—By the tenth postoperative day, the subjective symptoms of carpal tunnel syndrome—including paresthesia, numbness, and pain— were improved substantially. Less than 2% of the patients were symptomatic at 10 weeks. By 6 weeks after surgery, the percentage of patients with normal, static, 2-point discrimination in median nerve distribution was significantly improved. Preoperative grip and 3-point pinch strength were recovered by 6 weeks. Lateral pinch was markedly improved at this time. Patients with workers' compensation returned to work at a mean of 40.8 days, and those without workers' compensation returned in 22.2 days. Time to return to activities of daily living were comparable between these 2 groups, at a mean of 13.5 days. No major neurovascular injuries occurred. The most important complications were mild reflex sympathetic dystrophy, occurring in 1 patient, transient digital neuropraxias in 3, and superficial wound infection in 1.

Conclusion.—Single-portal ECTR using the redesigned Agee CTRS is effective and safe when performed by appropriately trained surgeons. Such training may include attending the 3M surgical skills workshop. Further research is encouraged.

▶ The single-portal ECTR continues to enjoy wide recognition. The single-portal technique with the new Agee system appears to have some advantages, and the authors discuss these. The avoidance of the palmar incision clearly avoids possible complications and tenderness. The numbers in this study are too small to provide clear differences. The lack of complications and morbidity is impressive.

D.J. Smith, Jr., M.D.

Vein-graft Wrapping for the Treatment of Recurrent Compression of the Median Nerve

Sotereanos DG, Giannakopoulos PN, Mitsionis GI, et al (Univ of Pittsburgh, Pa)
Microsurgery 16:752–756, 1995   3–9

Background.—Managing recurrent compressive neuropathy of the median nerve from cicatrix is very difficult. Preliminary experience with the autogenous vein graft wrapping method has been promising in patients with chronic compressive neuropathy after other treatments have failed. Experiences with 3 patients were described.

Patients and Outcomes.—In 1993 and 1994, 3 patients with chronic median nerve entrapment in the distal forearm and wrist were seen at 1 center. Two patients had had more than 3 failed procedures for decompressing the median nerve at the carpal tunnel. The third patient had been injured traumatically in the forearm and wrist. The patients were treated with vein-graft wrapping and studied for a mean of 2 years. After surgery, significant improvement was noted on the electromyograms of all patients. Both subjective and objective assessments indicated an excellent outcome in 1 patient and a good outcome in 1.

Conclusion.—Autogenous vein-graft wrapping performed as a supplementary technique in patients with chronic nerve compression is a simple technique that causes no complications in the donor area. This technique can also be applied to the treatment of chronic nerve compression other than carpal tunnel syndrome. The preliminary outcomes of this procedure have been encouraging.

The Histologic Effect of Barrier Vein Wrapping of Peripheral Nerves
Ruch DS, Spinner RM, Koman LA, et al (Wake Forest Univ, Winston Salem, NC; Duke Univ, Durham, NC)
J Reconstr Microsurg 12:291–295, 1996   3–10

Background.—To date, no one has documented the effect of glutaraldehyde vein wrapping on peripheral nerves. In the current study, the effect of glutaraldehyde-preserved allograft vein wrapping of normal peripheral nerves was assessed and compared with the effect of fresh autogenous vein wraps.

Methods.—The sciatic nerve was exposed in 24 Sprague-Dawley rats, followed by sham isolation, irrigation, and wound closure (group 1); barrier vein wrapping of the nerve using glutaraldehyde-preserved allograft inferior vena cava (group 2); or barrier vein wrapping of the nerve with femoral vein autograft from the contralateral extremity (group 3). The rats were killed 4 months later for histologic study.

Findings.—Epineural scar formation in group 2 was 10 times that in group 3. No significant differences among groups were found in epineural thickness and the number of degenerating axons. Inflammatory cells in group 2 increased 100 times compared with those in group 3. All allografts but none of the autografts showed continuity with the underlying epineural layer grossly and microscopically.

Conclusions.—Glutaraldehyde-preserved allograft vein wraps apparently incite a substantial inflammatory response, with epineural scarring and adherence to the underlying nerve. Autograft vein wraps do not provoke this response.

▶ The first article (Abstract 3–9) presents three clinical cases where a simple vein graft wrapping gave excellent results. I have not adopted this method but rather have used hypothenar, pedicle flaps, or free fat grafts to protect the nerve. This looks like an easy method that should be adopted. It is interesting to note that these authors talk about no idea of the histological evaluation and the subsequent article deals with this. The subsequent article (Abstract 3–10) is interesting in that the amount of glutaraldehyde reaction appears unusual, particularly with previous work on heart valves, flexor tendons, and interpositional upper extremity materials. What is more intriguing is the non-adherence of the autograft veins to the nerves. This is an interesting observation and may go a long way to explain the clinical results of the first article.

D.J. Smith, Jr., M.D.

Tubular Versus Conventional Repair of Median and Ulnar Nerves in the Human Forearm: Early Results From a Prospective, Randomized, Clinical Study
Lundborg G, Rosén B, Dahlin L, et al (Univ of Lund, Malmö, Sweden)
J Hand Surg [Am] 22A:99–106, 1997   3–11

Introduction.—The regeneration of an injured peripheral nerve involves local synthesis and release of key neurotrophic factors. These include nerve growth factor, brain-derived neurotrophic growth factor, and ciliary neurotrophic factor. The authors have been using a principle of tubulization—encasing the 2 cut ends of the nerve to allow neurotrophic factors to accumulate. Early results of a randomized trial of this approach for the repair of transected nerves in the human forearm are reported.

Methods.—Eighteen patients with transected median or ulnar nerves of the distal forearm were studied. All of the transections were located at the wrist or within 10 cm of the wrist. They were randomized to tubulization or conventional microsurgical repair. In the tubulization group, the 2 cut ends were attached to the inside wall of a silicone tube, with a 3 to 4-mm gap left between the ends. The patients were followed up closely for 1 year, including tests of motor and sensory function.

Results.—At follow-up, the 2 groups were similar in most measures of recovery, including the Tinel sign, the results of tactilometry, and tactile gnosis. The exception was touch perception as measured with the Semmes-Weinstein monofilaments, which was better at 3 months in the tubulization group. One patient underwent surgical re-exploration to remove the tube at 11 months. In this case, the gap between the proximal and distal nerve ends had been replaced by regenerated nerve tissue. The replacement was so complete that it was impossible to pinpoint the location of the previous injury.

Conclusions.—Good early results are reported with a tubulization approach to the repair of transected peripheral nerves. This technique emphasizes the intrinsic healing capacity of the cut nerve, providing an optimal environment for nerve healing while minimizing surgical trauma. The results are comparable with those achieved with conventional microsurgical repair. The authors plan further studies to refine their approach, including the development of bioresorbable materials that will not interfere with the axonal regeneration process.

▶ The idea of tubular repair in peripheral nerves is not new. It has certainly been investigated aggressively in the literature. Personally, I have a problem with not repairing an anatomic structure when tension and local factors prohibit. This article begins to dispel some of my biases by randomizing peripheral nerve injuries in humans to one of two groups and following them closely for one year. Certainly this review begins to force me to re-think my approach to peripheral nerve injuries. At the present time, I will not change but will certainly be much more mindful of the literature available to see if further reports verify this information.

D.J. Smith, Jr., M.D.

Long-term Follow-up Evaluation of Cold Sensitivity Following Nerve Injury

Collins ED, Novak CB, Mackinnon SE, et al (Washington Univ, St Louis)
J Hand Surg [Am] 21A:1078–1085, 1996   3–12

Background.—Patients often report cold sensitivity after nerve injury. Although some authors have suggested that this sequela declines with time and with the return of sensibility, few have reported the long-term outcomes of patients with cold sensitivity associated with nerve injury. The long-term follow-up of 50 patients with upper-extremity peripheral nerve injuries was documented.

Patients and Findings.—The 36 men and 14 women (aged 24–82 years) were followed up for 5–42 years after injury (mean, 10 years). Cold sensitivity was the most common persistent symptom, reported by 38 patients. Thirty-three of these patients described moderate or severe symptom intensity. Typically, cold sensitivity developed within months of the initial injury. It resolved in only 2 patients. The incidence of this symptom did not differ significantly between patients with subjectively normal sensation and those with abnormal hand sensibility. Cold sensitivity severity scores were associated with patients' subjective ratings of cold sensitivity intensity and change in job status or occupation because of injury. The incidence of cold sensitivity was unrelated to age, mechanism of injury, smoking, and level of nerve injury. Cold sensitivity was significantly associated with digital amputation injuries.

Conclusions.—Cold sensitivity is a common sequela of nerve injury that usually does not diminish with time. Patients should be cautioned about this symptom and advised to reduce their exposure to cold temperatures.

▶ This article has significantly altered the way I approach patients with nerve injuries. Whereas I previously, rather cavalierly, told them that their cold sensitivity would improve, I now caution them that there is a distinct possibility that the cold sensitivity will be a long-term and permanent sequela of the nerve injury. When the patient lives in a relatively cold climate, this has obvious work implications.

D.J. Smith, Jr., M.D.

Cold Intolerance Following Peripheral Nerve Injury: Natural History and Factors Predicting Severity of Symptoms

Irwin MS, Gilbert SEA, Terenghi G, et al (Queen Victoria Hosp, East Grinstead, UK; Northwick Park Hosp, Harrow, UK)
J Hand Surg [Br] 22B:308–316, 1997   3–13

Background.—Hand injury can lead to severe, debilitating cold intolerance. Little is known about the natural history and the factors predicting symptom severity of cold intolerance. Cold intolerance was studied in a large group of patients who had had surgical repair of a peripheral nerve in the upper limb.

Methods and Findings.—Questionnaires were sent to all 814 patients with upper limb peripheral nerve injuries occurring in a 12-year period. Patient records were also reviewed. Three hundred ninety-one patients completed the first questionnaire, for a response rate of 57%. Eighty-three percent reported cold intolerance. Of this subgroup, 23% reported that their symptoms were mild; 41%, moderate; 15%, severe; and 4%, extreme. Symptom onset was within 1 month of the initial injury in 48%. Fifty-nine percent of the original group responded to the second questionnaire. At a mean follow-up of 51 months, 21% reported improved symptoms and 18% reported deterioration. Cold intolerance was more likely to develop in smokers and less likely to develop in patients sustaining a sharp injury. Symptom severity was significantly increased with complete nerve division, median and ulnar nerve division, and an associated vessel injury. Improvement in symptoms was significantly more likely to occur in nonsmokers. Deterioration was most likely in patients with a high severity score.

Conclusions.—This study provides insight into the natural history of cold intolerance after peripheral nerve injury. Several factors were associated with the development and severity of symptoms, such as smoking.

▶ The authors of this article substantiate the findings by Mackinnon et al. (Abstract 3–12) regarding the continued problem with cold intolerance after injury. They further evaluated their group to note that symptom improvement was significantly more likely in nonsmokers and deterioration with a higher severity score. Obviously, increasing information verifying the maintenance of cold intolerance after nerve injury is accumulating. In addition, we are learning more about what predictors may influence outcome.

D.J. Smith, Jr., M.D.

Can Cast Immobilization Successfully Treat Scapholunate Dissociation Associated With Distal Radius Fractures?
Tang J-B, Shi D, Gu YQ, et al (Nantong Med College, Jiangsu, China)
J Hand Surg [Am] 21A:583–590, 1996   3–14

Introduction.—Carpal instability can be produced by varying malalignments of the carpal bones after the distribution of ligamentous restraints. There have been reports of fractures of the distal radius with concomitant scapholunate dissociation. Although closed reduction and cast immobilization have been accepted treatment for fractures of the distal radius, it is not well known whether the same treatment is effective for a concomitant scapholunate dissociation. By examination of a cohort of 20 patients with fractures with persistent clinical signs of scapholunate dissociation over a 1-year period, the clinical consequences of scapholunate dissociation associated with fractures of the distal radius and their impact on wrist function were investigated.

Methods.—Twenty patients with fractures of the distal radius who also had evidence of scapholunate dissociation were examined. Over a 1-year period, the sequential changes of radiographic abnormalities of the scapholunate joint were observed. One year after injury, wrist functions were evaluated.

Results.—At the time of injury, the scapholunate gaps were 3.5±0.5 mm; immediately after closed reduction, they were 3.2±0.4 mm; after removal of fixation, they were 3.4±0.5 mm; and 1 year later, they were 3.0±0.4 mm. One year after injury, 4 patients had poor wrist function, 14 had fair; 2 had good, and none had excellent wrist function. Compared to a selected group of 228 wrists with no signs of intercarpal ligament disruptions, the wrists with scapholunate dissociation had significantly worse function. One year later, there were clinical signs in the scapholunate joint and positive radiographic findings of dissociation in all 20 patients with signs of scapholunate dissociation on radiographic examination at the time of injury. For relief of symptoms, 8 of 20 patients had surgery after 1 year. There was disruption in the scapholunate interosseous ligament according to arthrography results in patients with persistent symptoms.

Conclusion.—Cast immobilization of the fracture is not adequate treatment for scapholunate dissociation with concomitant fractures of the distal radius. For the concomitant scapholunate dissociation, early operative treatment should be instituted.

▶ The authors' conclusions are shared by others who have followed the explosion of knowledge in the diagnosis and treatment of severe wrist injuries. Early surgical intervention provides a much better opportunity for good results than late salvage procedures.

R.E. Salisbury, M.D.

Gliding Resistance of Extrasynovial and Intrasynovial Tendons Through the A2 Pulley

Uchiyama S, Amadio PC, Coert JH, et al (Mayo Clinic and Mayo Found, Rochester, Minn)
J Bone Joint Surg Am 79A:219–224, 1997   3–15

Background.—The use of a free tendon graft may be indicated when primary repair of the flexor tendon in the finger is not possible. Recent research has shown that extrasynovial tendon grafts are associated with more adhesions to the surrounding tissue than are intrasynovial tendon grafts. The gliding ability of an extrasynovial tendon may be inferior to that of an intrasynovial tendon. A system to directly measure gliding resistance between the tendon and the pulley was developed.

Methods and Findings.—Fourteen digits and the ipsilateral palmaris longus tendons from 14 cadavers were included in the study. The gliding resistance between the A2 pulley and the flexor digitorum profundus tendon, an intrasynovial tendon, was compared with that between the A2 pulley and the palmaris longus tendon, an extrasynovial tendon. The mean gliding resistance at the interface between the palmaris longus tendon and the A2 pulley was significantly higher than that between the flexor digitorum profundus tendon and the A2 pulley when loading conditions were similar.

Conclusion.—The gliding ability of the palmaris longus tendon appears to be inferior to that of the flexor digitorum profundus tendon in vitro. The poor gliding ability of the palmaris longus tendon may explain the adhesions associated with the use of extrasynovial tendon grafts.

▶ I often wondered why choices for flexor tendon grafts have previously primarily been based on availability and size match. This analysis should make us all think about inherent characteristics of the tendon that may contribute to the success of the graft.

D.J. Smith, Jr., M.D.

Burns

Reduced Resuscitation Fluid Volume for Second-degree Burns With Delayed Initiation of Ascorbic Acid Therapy

Tanaka H, Matsuda H, Shimazaki S, et al (Kyorin Univ, Tokyo; Cook County Hosp, Chicago; Univ of Illinois, Chicago)
Arch Surg 132:158–161, 1997   3–16

Background.—Treatment with high-dose antioxidant ascorbic acid has been found to decrease edema in burned and unburned tissue, lipid peroxidation, and the subsequent requirement for resuscitation fluid volume in experimental burn models. The hemodynamic effects of delayed initiation of antioxidant treatment for second-degree burns were investigated.

Methods.—Twelve guinea pigs were subjected to subxiphoid immersion in 100°C-water for 3 seconds to produce burns over 70% of their body surface area. Ringer's lactated solution was administered using the Parkland formula beginning from 0.5 to 2 hours after injury to resuscitate the animals. Thereafter, the resuscitation fluid volume was decreased to 25% of the Parkland formula. The animals were given Ringer's lactated solution with or without ascorbic acid.

Findings.—The 2 groups did not differ significantly in heart rates or blood pressure during 24 hours of observation. None of the guinea pigs died. The group given ascorbic acid had significantly lower hematocrit levels and significantly higher cardiac output values 7 hours after burn injury and at intervals thereafter.

Conclusion.—Delayed initiation of high-dose ascorbic acid treatment resulted in a 24-hour fluid resuscitation volume reduced to 32.5% of the Parkland formula. Adequate cardiac output values were maintained.

▶ This work is extremely interesting. Further investigations will be needed to determine the mechanism of action and whether the effect is all the result of the antioxidant efficacy of vitamin C or because of its action as an antihistamine.

R.E. Salisbury, M.D.

Burn Resuscitation: Crystalloid Versus Colloid Versus Hypertonic Saline Hyperoncotic Colloid in Sheep
Guha SC, Kinsky MP, Button B, et al (Univ of Texas, Galveston)
Crit Care Med 24:1849–1857, 1996   3–17

Background.—The value of early colloid use in burn victims has not been definitively established. It was hypothesized that initial and early use of a colloid or hyperosmotic colloid decreases fluid requirements and edema.

Methods.—Eighteen female sheep were studied in the blinded, controlled study. The sheep were scalded and treated by 1 of 3 regimens. Lactate Ringer's solution, hetastarch, or hypertonic saline dextran, 10 mL/kg in each case, were infused 30 minutes after injury at a rate to restore and maintain the baseline oxygen delivery value.

Findings.—Scalding caused an initial 30% decline in cardiac output, a 20% decrease in mean arterial pressure, and a 10% to 15% increase in hematocrit. All the solutions restored and maintained baseline oxygen delivery within 1 hour, but hetastarch and hypertonic saline dextran decreased the net fluid volume by 48% and 74%, respectively, over 8 hours, compared with lactated Ringer's solution. Treatment did not affect burn wound edema. Hypertonic saline dextran decreased edema in nonburned skin, compared with lactated Ringer's solution and hypertonic saline dextran. The hetastarch and hypertonic saline dextran groups had significantly higher plasma colloid osmotic pressures. The lactated Ringer's solution and hetastarch groups had a continuous decline in plasma sodium concentrations from baseline values over 8 hours. Plasma sodium levels were increased at 4 hours in the hypertonic saline dextran group but normalized within 8 hours.

Conclusion.—Initial resuscitation of large body surface area burn injury with a colloid can markedly decrease net volume loading. Further reductions can be achieved by using hypertonic saline colloid. Hyponatremia occurred in the isotonic crystalloid-treated and colloid-treated sheep but not in sheep given hypertonic saline colloid.

▶ This excellent study begs for a sequel that will track resuscitation longer during the first 24 hours. Specifically, the capillary leak extends for more than 8 hours, and it would be instructive to know how these groups responded over a longer interval than the first 8 hours. The authors rightly point out that finding a resuscitation that would lead to less edema and volume load is extremely important in the patient with a very large burn and/or an inhalation injury or antecedent cardiorespiratory compromise. Different resuscitation regimens that are presently in use will all achieve the desired result: keeping the patient out of shock.

Complications occur most commonly when beginners attempt to mix the regimens or experiment with a resuscitation regimen with which they are not familiar. Each has its own vagaries and problems. Interestingly, no study has been devoted to fluid management beyond the first 36 hours, when the patient is attempting to unload large volumes of excess salt-containing solutions.

R.E. Salisbury, M.D.

Prognostic Indicators in the Elderly Patient With Burns
Covington DS, Wainwright DJ, Parks DH (Univ of Texas, Houston)
J Burn Care Rehabil 17:222–230, 1996   3–18

Introduction.—The treatment of burn injury is particularly challenging in the elderly, who are more adversely affected by burns. Although survival has increased among these patients, the cost to them and to society is considerable. To identify prognostic indicators in the elderly burn-injured patient, a large group of such patients was evaluated for the impact of preinjury health conditions, mechanisms of injury, and postinjury complications.

Methods.—The retrospective study reviewed the records of patients 55 and older who were admitted to a burn unit from November 1979 through April 1991. Data collected included demographic information, pre-existing medical conditions, cause and size of burn, acute clinical and operative management, complications, survival, and disposition. The treatment protocol consisted of fluid resuscitation in all cases, commonly followed by wound débridement, excision of deep second- and third-degree burns, and immediate coverage with split-thickness autografts. Patient care also included aggressive enteral parenteral nutritional support and physical and occupational therapy. In some cases, when immediate survival and a meaningful life after injury were highly unlikely, the attending physician and patient's family decided not to proceed with aggressive resuscitation and care.

Results.—The study group included 252 patients: 120 aged 55–65 years (group I); 62 aged 66–75 years (group II); 49 aged 76–85 years (group III); and 21 aged 86–96 years (group IV). Mortality was higher in groups III and IV (60.1%) than in groups I and II (33.9%), despite a similarity in overall burn size among groups. Most injuries were caused by accidents at home. The most common cause of injury was flame (69.0%), and this cause was associated with the largest surface area involved (average 34.4%) and the highest mortality rate (46.5%). Patients in groups III and IV accounted for 70.0% of scald injuries. More than two thirds of patients had some type of preinjury medical condition, and the incidence of complications was significantly higher among those with 2 or more preinjury conditions. Cardiovascular conditions, present in 64.2% of patients, were associated with the highest complication (60.7%) and mortality (53.3%) rates. Patients in older age groups were more likely to have infections (76.2% in group IV) and a fatal outcome when systemic sepsis occurred (100% in group IV).

Conclusion.—Advanced age is an important determinant of survival after burn injury. Even with smaller burns, elderly patients are more likely than younger patients to have infections, sepsis, and complications. Preinjury medical conditions also influence outcome and are more common with advancing age. A knowledge of these predictors of poor outcome is helpful in treating the elderly burn-injured patient and in counseling the family.

▶ This type of article is extremely valuable in stimulating a thoughtful discussion among burn team members to deal with sensitive subjects that affect the patients and their families. The obvious danger of this paper is that it is open to misinterpretation and misuse by individuals whose only agenda is to cut patient care costs.

R.E. Salisbury, M.D.

Energy and Protein Provisions for Thermally Injured Children Revisited: An Outcome-based Approach for Determining Requirements
Prelack K, Cunningham JJ, Sheridan RL, et al (Shriners Burns Inst, Boston; Massachusetts Gen Hosp, Boston; Harvard Med School, Boston)
J Burn Care Rehabil 18:177–181, 1997   3–19

Introduction.—Because of advances in the management of burn injury, previous estimates of the energy needs of moderately to severely burned patients may need to be revised downward. The energy and protein requirements adequate for wound healing and weight maintenance were determined retrospectively in a group of severely burned children.

Methods.—The 27 children had all been admitted with a greater than 40% total body surface area burn. Mean age of the group was 8 years. Energy requirements were calculated using predicted basal metabolic rate (PBMR) and the table by Altman and Dittmer, with an added injury factor of 1.75 to account for energy requirements above basal needs. Target protein goals were 3 g/kg for children from birth to 6 years and 2.5 g/kg for those older than 6 years. Nutrients were delivered by a combination of parenteral and intragastric enteral tube feedings. Calorie and protein intakes were monitored during a 4-week period while wounds were progressively closed. The children were divided into 3 groups on the basis of mean energy intake (Em) during these 4 weeks (Em less than or equal to PBMR $\times$ 1.2; Em greater than PBMR $\times$ 1.2 but less than PBMR $\times$ 1.7; and Em greater than or equal to PBMR $\times$ 1.7).

Results.—Mean energy intake during the study period averaged 140% of the PBMR; mean protein intake was 2.8 g/kg daily. During week 1, actual energy intakes closely matched the PBMR for many patients. An increase occurred during weeks 2 through 4, when energy intakes approximated PBMR $\times$ 1.5. Protein intakes averaged 80% of targets during week 1, then increased to a mean of 112% of target during week 2 and 101% of target during weeks 3 and 4. Twelve children needed some level of parenteral nutrition during the entire study period so that energy targets would be met, but all had satisfactory wound healing and recovered from their injuries. The mean weight at the end of the 4-week period was 91% of admission weight. Comparison of the 3 Em groups showed a significant effect of Em on 4-week weight status. Discharge weights were significantly higher among children whose energy intake was greater than PBMR $\times$ 1.7 for at least 1 of the 4 weeks.

Conclusions.—Patients with burns were once administered large quantities of nutrients, but modern approaches emphasize weight maintenance rather than weight gain for children during the acute phase of recovery. These children did well clinically with approximately 86% of the recommended daily allowance for energy. Wound closure can occur at intakes of PBMR $\times$ 1.2 when provided with a high nitrogen diet, but targets approximating PBMR $\times$ 1.7 can enhance weight status.

▶ This paper should be read carefully because it emphasizes a very practical approach that underscores a change in philosophy in the past 25 years. Specifically, the authors emphasize that if skin grafts take, donor sites heal, and weight is maintained, then caloric intake is satisfactory. What is particularly interesting is that even when intake fell below PBMR $\times$ 1.2, good graft take and healing were achieved.

R.E. Salisbury, M.D.

Ornithine α-Ketoglutarate Metabolism After Enteral Administration in Burn Patients: Bolus Compared With Continuous Infusion

Le Bricon T, Coudray-Lucas C, Lioret N, et al (Hôpital St-Antoine, Paris)
Am J Clin Nutr 65:512–518, 1997   3–20

Introduction.—A durable hypermetabolic state with increased protein turnover is associated with burn injury. The dramatic body wasting observed in patients with severe burns is caused by increased muscle protein breakdown and energy expenditure. In the treatment of burn patients, nutritional support plays a key role. The use of specific nutritional therapies, such as arginine, branched-chain amino acid, and ornithine α-ketoglutarate supplementation, has benefited burn patients. In a large group of severely burned patients, a prospective kinetic study was performed to determine the appropriate mode of administration and dose of ornithine α-ketoglutarate and to study its metabolism and metabolite production.

Methods.—In 42 consecutive burn patients, the pharmacokinetic parameters of ornithine and the appearance of metabolites were studied 7 days post burn. Patients were randomly assigned to receive ornithine as a continuous gastric infusion of 10, 20, or 30 g/day 21 hours or to receive ornithine as a single bolus of 10 g.

Results.—In these patients, ornithine, having an absorption constant of 0.028 $^{-1}$ and an elimination half-life of 89 minutes, was extensively metabolized. It was associated with the production of glutamine, arginine, and proline, with proline being the main metabolite. Proline production was dose dependent and quantitatively similar in the 2 groups. In the bolus group, glutamine and arginine production were higher than in the infusion group, and they were not dose dependent.

Conclusion.—Ornithine was well absorbed and metabolized after enteral administration in burn patients, and it led to the production of proline, glutamine, and arginine. A higher metabolite production, however, was seen in the bolus mode when compared with continuous infusion, particularly for arginine and glutamine. Further investigation is necessary to determine the clinincal efficacy and dose dependency of different modes of enteral administration of ornithine.

▶ This study is fascinating in its results but is also quite perplexing. The production of glutamine and arginine was influenced by the mode of ornithine delivery. The authors do not know why and speculate on various reasons. Studies are ongoing and, hopefully, the answer will be forthcoming. That enterally administered ornithine is efficiently metabolized in burn patients is highly significant.

R.E. Salisbury, M.D.

Skin Expansion in Burn Patients: Problems, Rules and Indications
Echinard C (Marseille, France)
Eur J Plast Surg 19:178–184, 1996   3–21

Introduction.—Functional and cosmetic problems are often the result of deep second and third degree burns. Tissue expansion can be used for patients who do not respond to early excision with immediate grafting, rapid rehabilitation, or pressure therapy. Tissue expansion has resulted in as many as 60% of patients having complications. Skin expansion problems are more frequent in burn patients than in other patients.

Problems.—In the first stage, complications caused by silastic implant include skin sensation, wrinkling of the silastic envelope, hematomas inside the pocket, infection, and traumatization of fragile skin. Problems related to the inflating system include access to the port becoming difficult, folding of the inflation tube, and leakage from the inflating system. In the second stage, in which the expander has been removed, problems include insufficient skin gain, hematomas or infection under the flap, necrosis of the advancement flap, and enlargement of the scars.

Indications.—It helps to wait until the scar is mature, to use radial incision, to undermine in the good plane, to maintain sterility, to use external ports, to control the smoothness of the balloon, to use large expanders, to perform long and slow expansion, to use safe flaps, and to drain during the first and second stages. Tissue expansion in indicated for hypertrophic scars, for contractures, and for tissue destruction.

Conclusion.—For scar revision, skin resurfacing, or remodeling, skin expansion is a current technique; however, it has more complications with burn patients because of the modest quality of the skin, the greater susceptibility to infection, the residual bad general conditions, and the greater tendency to hemostasis disorders. Complications have decreased dramatically with experience and by paying attention to certain rules.

▶ This article presents no new information, but it is an excellent review. The incidence of complications jumps geometrically in the hands of surgeons who do not appreciate the differences between burn patients and those with different indications for the use of tissue expanders.

R.E. Salisbury, M.D.

A Randomized Prospective Trial of Hyperbaric Oxygen in a Referral Burn Center Population
Brannen AL, Still J, Haynes M, et al (Med College of Georgia, Augusta)
Am Surg 63:205–208, 1997   3–22

Background.—The effect of hyperbaric oxygen (HBO) has been studied in a wide variety of diseases. Animal and clinical studies of its value in the treatment of burns have yielded conflicting findings. Few controlled studies have been done in humans.

Methods and Findings.—The effect of HBO was further investigated in a randomized study of 125 burn victims assigned to HBO or no HBO. All patients had been hospitalized within 24 hours of injury. The treatment and control groups were matched by age, burn size, and presence of inhalation injury. The treatment group received their first HBO treatment within 24 hours of injury and were treated with 2 atmospheres of pressure for 90 minutes twice daily for at least 10 treatments and a maximum of 1 treatment per total body surface percent burn. The control group received similar treatment but without HBO. Analysis of outcomes demonstrated no significant between-group differences in mortality, number of operations, or length of stay among survivors.

Conclusion.—The use of HBO in this series of burn victims appeared to have no significant benefit. The mortality rate was 11% in both the treatment and control groups. The need for surgery and length of hospitalization were also comparable in the HBO-treated and untreated groups.

▶ These authors are to be congratulated for making a good attempt at a controlled clinical study of the use of HBO in burn patients. Previous clinical studies have been impressionistic, anecdotal, and far from convincing. In fact, they have not added luster to the star of HBO, which is beneficial in certain defined conditions. Although experimental data seem to suggest the efficacy of HBO treatment of burns, most definitive answers will, hopefully, be forthcoming in future studies involving patients with large total-body-surface burns and increased fluid needs.

R.E. Salisbury, M.D.

The Index of Deep Burn Injury: An Analysis of 66 Extremity Sites in 15 Children
Zhu X, Donelan M, Sheridan R (Jiamusi Med College, China; Harvard Med School, Boston)
Burns 23:11–14, 1997   3–23

Introduction.—A better classification system than "fourth degree burn" is needed to define deep burn injury. Objective criteria need to be generated from a detailed analysis of the structures involved. The Index of Deep Burn Injury (IDBI) was created from an anatomical analysis of 17 cadavers with deep burn injuries of the extremities. The IDBI assigns structural and functional values to quantify the severity of damage to individual vessels, nerves, tendons, bones, joint capsules, muscles, and ligaments. Deep burn injuries of 66 extremity sites in 15 children were evaluated retrospectively to determine the usefulness of the IDBI as a comparative and prognostic tool.

Methods.—Medical records of 1,903 children with severe burn injury were evaluated. Of these, 15 children had an index of deep burn injury that was greater than 2 and medical records with complete photographic documentation. The 66 deep burn injuries were evaluated in these patients using the IDBI.

Results.—The average patient age was 13 years. The mechanisms of injury were high-voltage (9 patients), fire (3), explosions (2), and hot liquid (1). The IDBI increased progressively in each wound during the 7 days after injury (mean increase, 3.2; range, 0–15). Twenty-six extremities were lost (12 digital; 14 more proximal sites). Of 40 sites requiring repair, 13 were repaired with 12 flaps (7 abdominal pedicle flaps, 2 local flaps, 1 cross-leg flap, and 2 free flaps). One free flap did not survive. The remaining 27 sites underwent closed debridement and autografting. There was an inverse relationship between grade of IDBI and outcome.

Conclusion.—The IDBI is useful in describing deep burn injury. It is a tool that provides a meaningful grading system for injury severity.

▶ If the authors' goal is to develop an index that would allow all of us to be describing the same types of injuries by the same nomenclature, then they have probably succeeded. I question the assertion that the management of these deep injuries is controversial. Most surgeons now agree that early excision and wound closure is the goal. Although techniques of closure may differ, most patients and their families will opt for every effort to be made to salvage the extremity. It is doubtful that using this index will change the clinical efforts of limb salvage.

R.E. Salisbury, M.D.

Emotional and Psychosocial Factors in Burn Patients During Hospitalization

Franulic A, González X, Trucco M, et al (Hosp del Trabajador, Santiago, Chile)
Burns 22:618–622, 1996   3–24

Introduction.—The emotional response shown by patients with burn injury during the period of inpatient treatment includes restlessness, fear, anxiety, and even psychotic behavior. Later they can become depressive and their emotional reactions make care managements stressful for the medical team. The relationship between severity of the injury, personality factors, and previous adjustment, along with the presence of emotional symptoms during the hospital stay, was investigated.

Methods.—In 25 consecutive patients with burn injury, psychological symptoms, previous psychosocial adjustment, and severity of injury were recorded. The patients were evaluated by a psychiatric consultation-liaison team and their burns were all work-related. They took the Hamilton Scales of Anxiety and Depression, Cloninger's Tridimensional Personality Questionnaire, Goldberg's General Health Questionnaire, and a modified version of Schooler's Adjustment Scale.

Results.—There was no significant correlation between anxious or depressive symptoms and the extent and severity of burns. There were no severe and extensive injuries, and all burns varied from mild to moderate.

In the Tridimensional Personality Questionnaire, there was a significant correlation found between anxiety and the harm avoidance dimension. Great anxiety symptoms were found with patients with poor psychosocial adjustment. The income level and degree of anxiety symptoms had a significant negative correlation.

Conclusion.—Probable factors of psychological symptoms after burn injury are the relevance of previous psychosocial adjustment and personality. The absence of depression may be a result of its measurement early in the illness, because usually depression becomes a factor later in the illness.

▶ This population is uniform (all had workers' compensation injuries), is prospective, and properly identifies the importance of pain control.

R.E. Salisbury, M.D.

Critical Pathways to Enhance the Rehabilitation of Patients With Burns
Staley M, Richard R (Shriners Burns Inst, Cincinnati, Ohio; Miami Valley Hosp, Dayton, Ohio)
J Burn Care Rehabil 17:S12–S14, 1996   3–25

Background.—The optimal result from care for an individual who has sustained a burn injury is total rehabilitation, defined as a return to preinjury level of function in all domains—physical, social, emotional, mental, and spiritual. Critical pathways, which are guidelines designed for treatment of an "average" patient, extend over a long period of time in burn injuries. Few approaches currently used in burn units have been validated by research.

Methods.—The figure in this article consists of a flow chart based upon the American Burn Association's Musculoskeletal Desired Burn Care Outcome A: "The patient will maintain/attain optimal level of function." Six clinical indicators are presented: range of motion; muscle strength; functional ambulation; demonstration of prescribed exercise program by patient/caregiver; demonstration of correct application, care, and use of splints by patient/caregiver; and the patient's performance of activities of daily living appropriate for type of burn injury. After treatment for desired outcomes, the patient's progress is assessed and treatment continued or modified. Subsequent assessments of progress and outcome may indicate areas in need of investigation, either as a performance improvement project or research study.

Discussion.—During rehabilitation of a patient with burns, critical pathways can help to identify and quantify differences between expected and actual outcomes. For a given clinical indicator, a burn facility may modify or expand the description for an individual patient's needs. Thus the "optimal outcome" may be that the patient is functional in ambulation in his or her own home and community. A table is provided to show how a patient may transition through the third clinical indicator with a clinical pathway format. Adoption of critical pathways by burn care facilities can help to rehabilitate patients in a judicious and cost-effective manner.

▶ This article warrants reading because it discusses issues that all burn centers will be addressing in the next few years. Economic necessities will drive the provider to prove the efficacy of a given treatment.

R.E. Salisbury, M.D.

Competence and Physical Impairment of Pediatric Survivors of Burns of More Than 80% Total Body Surface Area
Moore P, Moore M, Blakeney P, et al (Univ of Texas, Galveston)
J Burn Care Rehabil 17:547–551, 1996   3–26

Introduction.—Children are surviving severe burn injuries that would have been fatal a decade ago. Survivors are challenged to adapt to as normal a life as possible with extreme disfiguring and debilitating injuries. There are no reports examining the association between physical impairment and psychosocial adjustment of children with extensive burns. The relationship between psychosocial adjustment and physical impairment was evaluated in 19 children with severe burn injuries.

Methods.—Children aged 4–19 years who survived a burn injury of more than 80% total body surface were given physical impairment scores based on range-of-motion measurements of upper and lower extremities according to American Medical Association guidelines. Competence was calculated by parental report using the Child's Behavior Checklist and the child's self-report on the Youth Self-Report.

Results.—The mean physical impairment score was 52%, ranging from 2 patients with no physical impairment to other patients with more than 90% impairment. The mean scores for the left upper, right upper, left lower, and right lower extremities were 25%, 24%, 10%, and 9%, respectively. Competence scores assessed by parents were within normal limits. Parents reported no significant problem behaviors or syndromes and normal competence in academic performance, social situations, and activities. There was a significant negative correlation between total physical impairment and parental report of activity competence, suggesting that children with the most impairment were less involved with organized activities and athletics. Competence scores reported by 11 of 19 children were within normal limits. Children reported themselves to be as competent as their peers in social situations and activities. There was a negative correlation between self-report of activity competence and lower extremity impairment.

Conclusion.—Children who survived severe burn injuries and their parents reported competence in school and interpersonal relationships. The children with the greatest physical impairment were the least physically active. Severe physical impairment in children with burn injuries does not necessarily lead to poor psychosocial adjustment.

▶ This series is unique in the world literature and the papers that are generated from this group should be studied carefully. This particular subject may help us know more about what survivors are able to do, instead of focusing on their deficits.

R.E. Salisbury, M.D.

Applying What Burn Survivors Have to Say to Future Therapeutic Interventions
Robert R, Berton M, Moore P, et al (Shriners Burns Inst, Galveston, Tex)
Burns 23:50–54, 1997   3–27

Introduction.—Burn survivors are the experts on postburn issues. If universal concerns of burn survivors can be determined, then caregivers can be prepared to address patient concerns. A psychological assessment tool was used to determine whether universal concerns of the postburn survivor can be assessed using a sentence completion task.

Methods.—Sixty survivors of pediatric burn injuries were randomly selected. Age range of participants was 6–19 years. The mean number of years after burn was 3.2 years. The incomplete sentences for children (ISC) is a nonstandardized incomplete sentences form consisting of 30 sentence stems. A subject or subject and verb are provided for each sentence stem and participants are expected to complete the sentence as desired.

Results.—Five major themes of postburn life emerged from the ISC: (1) preoccupation with health, (2) struggle for internal acceptance, (3) reconstruction of one's life map, (4) changing relationships, and (5) redefining the world.

Conclusion.—Response to the ISC by children with severe burn injuries has provided a valuable tool for caregivers. Listening, mirroring, normalizing, educating, and articulating internal conflicts are interventions that can help incorporate the information provided by survivors of severe burn injury. Successful listening and use of the patient's own words to guide responses can enhance the patient's adaptation and caregiver's expertise.

▶ Considering the sporadic and often mediocre studies nationwide, this type of paper represents an encouraging effort. It would be interesting if this same population were followed up and the study repeated in 3 years.

R.E. Salisbury, M.D.

Topical 2% Lidocaine Gel Versus Placebo in Burn Wound Debridement Pain

Maxwell D, O'Brien J, Sparkes G, et al (Dalhousie Univ, Halifax, NS)
Can J Plast Surg 4:109–110, 1996

3–28

Introduction.—In awake patients, burn wound débridement hurts, and the usual solution is offering parenteral analgesics or general anesthesia. An efficacious and cost-effective alternative may be local anesthetics. Topical 2% lidocaine gel has been found anecdotally to be useful in decreasing the pain of skin abrasion. Whether topical 2% lidocaine gel was superior to placebo in decreasing the pain of burn wound débridement was determined in a double-blind study, in which patients were their own controls.

Methods.—There were 19 patients with burn wounds who were admitted to a burn unit. They had no history of allergy to local anesthetics, were not pregnant, and did not have severe liver disease. The burn wounds were débrided 4 times, twice with placebo and twice with lidocaine, so that the patients could act as their own controls.

Results.—In decreasing the pain of burn wound débridement, topical 2% lidocaine gel was found to be superior to placebo. With lidocaine, the mean pain score was 2.42 and with placebo it was 4.14 on a scale of 1–10. With lidocaine, the total pain score was 100 and with placebo, it was 165.

Conclusion.—The 2% lidocaine was applied to the burn wound 1 hour before débridement, because the literature shows this to be the most effective timing of application. However, in a busy burn unit, application times of less than 1 hour would be more practical, and should be tested clinically.

▶ This study warrants further investigation and is encouraging. Obviously, if no anesthesia is given, meals will not be missed, therapy sessions will not be cancelled, and rehabilitation can be optimized.

R.E. Salisbury, M.D.

Procedural Burn Pain Intensity Under Conditions of Varying Physical Control by the Patient

Sutherland S (California State Univ, Sacramento)
J Burn Care Rehabil 17:457–463, 1996

3–29

Background.—Despite the use of medication and cognitive strategies, burn victims continue to experience pain during dressing changes. The effect on perceived pain-intensity scores of allowing the patient to have control over the dressing change has not been investigated. Such scores associated with patient washing vs. nurse washing during burn dressing changes were compared.

Methods and Findings.—Ten hospitalized adults with major burn injuries were enrolled in the study. Repeated-measures analysis of variance of verbal numeric pain scores obtained at regular intervals during the procedure showed that each patient had significantly less pain when washing themselves during dressing changes, compared with nurse-performed washing. The quality of washing did not differ significantly between the 2 conditions. The amount of opioid medication given was also comparable.

Conclusion.—Self-washing enables burn victims to avoid the frequent pain spikes of nurse washings and to feel in control of their pain experience. The nurse's role during patient washings is to observe, teach, and supervise the dressing change. Nurses can also finish the dressing changes for patients who cannot self-inflict pain in the amounts needed to accomplish débriding.

▶ Articles concerning pain and the burn patient should not just be relegated to the psychosocial literature. Considering the number of new alternatives for pain control, too few clinical studies on pain control reach our literature. The techniques suggested here, however, must be balanced against the patient's ability to participate and the available time a nurse has to coach the patient through the dressing change.

R.E. Salisbury, M.D.

Structural Changes and Cell Viability of Cultured Epithelium After Freezing Storage

Hibino Y, Hata K, Horie K, et al (Nagoya Univ, Japan)
J Craniomaxillofac Surg 24:346–351, 1996   3–30

Introduction.—Cultured epithelial grafting is a valuable technique in plastic and reconstructive surgery. Recent studies have shown that it is possible to graft cultured epithelium that has been frozen and thawed. However, it is uncertain whether the cultured epithelium retains its normal structure and viability after freezing. The morphology and cell viability of cultured mucosal epithelial sheets were studied after freezing.

Methods.—Cultured mucosal and epidermal sheets were prepared for testing. In addition to evaluating the effects of freezing per se, the study looked at the effects of storage temperature and cryoprotectants. All sheets were frozen at a fixed, slow cooling rate. Cell viability was tested by flow cytometry.

Results.—When dimethyl sulfoxide was used as a cryoprotectant, significant vacuolar degeneration and other structural changes were noted in cultured mucosal sheets that had been frozen. These changes were more pronounced after storage at −80°C than at −196°C. In contrast, sheets stored with glycerin as the cryoprotectant showed little morphological change. Viability studies suggested that more than 62% of the cells retained their viability after freezing in all groups.

Conclusions.—Under some conditions, some structural changes occur in cultured epithelial sheets after freezing. Cell viability is good under any freezing conditions. The results suggest that the best way to store cultured epithelium is by slow freezing with glycerin as a cryoprotectant and a temperature of −196°C.

▶ Cultured epithelial grafts have received increased attention as a treatment for both acute and chronic wounds. Some practitioners have used cryopreserved grafts for these treatments with clinical success. This paper addresses 2 issues: (1) the viability of cells within these grafts after cryopreservation and (2) the optimal storage temperature for cryopreservation. The results support the use of low-temperature (liquid nitrogen) storage, a fact that has been documented in numerous other studies of frozen cell viability. In general, either freezing technique resulted in viable cells. The results support the continued use of frozen cells as investigators determine the role of these products in wound treatment.

W. Garner, M.D.

Controlled Clinical Study of Skin Donor Sites and Deep Partial-thickness Burns Treated With Cultured Epidermal Allografts
Rivas-Torres MT, Amato D, Arámbula-Alvarez H, et al (Traumatology Hosp Magdalena de Las Salinas, Mexico City; Centro Médico Nacional, Mexico City; Centro de Investogación y Estudios Avanzados del IPN, Mexico City)
Plast Reconstr Surg 98:279–287, 1996   3–31

Background.—Several studies have been done in an attempt to increase the limited shelf life of cultured epidermal allografts and to make them easily available for burn treatment. Conditions for banking the cultured epidermal grafts have been previously reported. These conditions permitted high viability and colony-forming efficiency levels of the stored allografts similar to those of epidermal grafts that were not stored. The results of using banked cultured epidermal allografts for 2 clinical indications in burn victims were described.

Methods.—In the first part of the study, 10 patients with burn injury undergoing donor split-thickness skin harvesting were included in a controlled, blinded, randomized trial. Each patient received a cultured epidermal allograft and a control dry dressing in a side-by-side comparison. Ten patients with 18 deep partial-thickness burn wounds were treated in the second study.

Findings.—Banked cultured epidermal allografts resulted in faster wound re-epithelialization in the first study. Epithelialization occurred at a mean of 6.9 days, compared with 11.1 days for control wounds. The decrease in time to heal was 37.8%. Allografted sites were less erythematous than control sites and showed a greater tendency to normopigmentation. In the second study, complete re-epithelialization of wounds treated with cultured allografts occurred in 3–6 days.

Conclusion.—Banked cultured epidermal allografts permit significantly faster epithelialization of donor sites and deep partial-thickness wounds.

These data support the practice of routine cultured allograft use for improving burn therapy and shortening treatment time.

▶ This technique deserves further exploration in patients with life-threatening injuries and limited donor skin. The ability to frequently recrop limited donor skin in reduced time intervals would be extremely valuable. Likewise, rapid healing of deep second-degree burns in a patient with a large total-body burn is potentially lifesaving.

R.E. Salisbury, M.D.

Clinical Trials of a Biosynthetic Temporary Skin Replacement, Dermagraft-transitional Covering, Compared With Cryopreserved Human Cadaver Skin for Temporary Coverage of Excised Burn Wounds
Hansbrough JF, Mozingo DW, Kealey GP, et al (Univ of California, San Diego; U S Army Inst of Surgical Research, Fort Sam Houston, Tex; Univ of Iowa, Iowa City)
J Burn Care Rehabil 18:43–51, 1997   3–32

Background.—Human cadaver allograft skin (HCAS) is commonly used to cover excised burn wounds in patients with limited donor sites or under conditions that do not permit immediate grafting with autologous skin. However, the supply of HCAS is limited, the quality is variable, immune rejection can occur, and bacterial and viral disease transmission is a risk. Thus, a dependable substitute for HCAS is needed. Dermagraft-TC (DG-TC) is made of human neonatal fibroblasts cultured on a synthetic dressing consisting of nylon mesh fabric covered with a thin layer of silicone rubber membrane, which provides an epidermal barrier. The material, which is semitransparent, is stored frozen and thawed just before use. The efficacy of this biosynthetic analogue of human skin to temporarily close excised burn wounds was studied in humans.

Methods.—Ten patients with a mean age of 33.5 years were included in the study. Burn wounds covering a mean 39.9% of the total body surface area were surgically excised. Two variants of DG-TC skin analogues were used: 1 cryopreserved to maintain fibroblast viability and 1 frozen without effort to maintain fibroblast viability. One area on each patient was treated with cryopreserved HCAS to serve as a control site.

Findings.—Wound adherence and subsequent autograft take were excellent with both variants of DG-TC. The efficacy of this material was at least equal to that of HCAS. There was no evidence of immune rejection with DG-TC. By contrast, the HCAS control sites in 4 patients showed epidermal sloughing/rejection, limiting persistence of those grafts on the wound.

Conclusion.—Dermagraft-TC is safe and effective as a temporary covering for excised burn wounds prepared for eventual autografting. Because DG-TC is semitransparent, subgraft appearance can be inspected directly and fluid accumulation detected.

▶ This initial work is very encouraging. Several different skin replacements or temporary skin dressings are now available. Further work needs to be done to determine which product should be used in each situation. Cost will unquestionably help determine which techniques are adopted most quickly by burn centers.

R.E. Salisbury, M.D.

Free Flap Reconstruction in Massive Upper Extremity Burns
Muuronen E, Asko-Seljavaara S, Tukiainen E, et al (Helsinki Univ)
Eur J Plast Surg 20:7–10, 1997   3–33

Background.—Early excision and free flap reconstruction is limb saving in some patients with massive burns. One experience with a group of patients with deep, massive upper extremity burns undergoing free flaps was presented.

Methods and Outcomes.—Eleven patients were treated between 1979 and 1993. Eight reconstructions were acute or subacute, and 3 were late reconstructions. Rectus femoris microneurovascular musculocutaneous free flaps were used in 2 patients; latissimus dorsi free flaps in 4; rectus abdominis free flaps in 3; and the gluteal thigh flap, lateral arm flap, and serratus flap in 1 each. The gluteal thigh flap was lost and subsequently replaced by a rectus abdominis flap. Reanastomosis was performed in 3 patients. Nine patients underwent functional late reconstructions. The limb was saved with satisfactory functional recovery in all 11 patients.

Conclusion.—The use of a free musculocutaneous or muscle flap is recommended, proximal to the wrist, if tendons, bone joint, or major vessels are exposed after careful excision of nonviable tissue. The rectus femoris musculocutaneous flap is useful for restoring extensor musculature of the forearm after extensive injury.

▶ It is never clear in this article what constitutes massive burn injuries. The summary of the cases never presents the extent of total body burn or the amount of third degree or fourth degree burn injury. Thus, it is very hard to determine whether these patients could have been treated by other means. Exposed muscles, nerves, and tendons can often be covered by split thickness skin grafts without the necessity for flaps in the acute period. In an isolated, small, total body burn of the upper extremity that leaves an open joint and large exposed neurovascular bundles, this may be the only alternative.

R.E. Salisbury, M.D.

Recombinant Neutral Endopeptidase Decreases Oedema in the Skin of Burned Guinea-Pigs

Neely AN, Imwalle AR, Holder IA (Univ of Cincinnati, Ohio)
Burns 22:520–523, 1996   3–34

Background.—Increased vascular leakage after burn injury causes edema, which results in significant problems. The efficacy of local application of a recombinant neutral endopeptidase (rNEP) in reducing the increased vascular permeability resulting from burn injury was investigated.

Methods and Findings.—Guinea pigs were used in this study. Treatment with rNEP was found to reduce burn-induced extravasation in a dose-dependent manner. This effect also depended on the peptidase being enzymatically active. In addition, rNEP treatment reduced plasma leakage from direct injection of bradykinin into the guinea pigs. The effect of rNEP on bradykinin-induced leakage depended on both the dosage of rNEP used and on its being enzymatically active.

Conclusion.—The findings are consistent with the notion that rNEP reduces burn-induced plasma extravasation. Treatment with rNEP appears to effect this reduction by degrading bradykinin. Further exploration of the potential of rNEP for decreasing plasma extravasation in burned hosts is indicated.

▶ This is a fascinating study and warrants further investigation in larger mammals.

R.E. Salisbury, M.D.

Essential Microminerals and Their Response to Burn Injury

Gamliel Z, DeBiasse MA, Demling RH (Harvard Med School, Boston)
J Burn Care Rehabil 17:264–272, 1996   3–35

Introduction.—To maintain homeostasis, trace elements or microminerals are essential, and these include aluminum, chromium, copper, iron, manganese, nickel, selenium, and zinc. Little is known about the role they play in a burn injury, which necessitates nutritional requirements. Altered intestinal absorption, altered body losses, and altered distribution among body tissues are side effects of the mechanisms that can be altered by stress. The role that several trace elements have in critical illness was assessed.

Trace Elements.—Aluminium has been associated with Alzheimer's disease, impairment of renal function, hypochromic microcytic anemia, and encephalopathy. Intravenous albumin solutions contain high levels of aluminum, and patients with burn injuries at high risk of renal impairment are at risk of aluminum toxicity. Chromium deficiency affects glucose tolerance and results in insulin resistance. In neutrophils of patients with burn injuries, chromium uptake is increased. Copper reduction results in a decrease in collagen syntheses and synthesis of superoxide dismutase, neutropenia, leukopenia, and other immune disorders. Acute trauma causes a decrease in serum copper. Iron has a role in oxygen-carrying proteins and has a strong influence on intestinal absorption. Impaired immune function is associated with iron deficiency and overload. After burns, free iron not bound appears to be increased and can be harmful.

More Trace Elements.—Manganese is essential for glucose utilization, metalloenzymes involved in gluconeogenesis, and for glycosyltransferases. Stress influences manganese metabolism and its deficiency after burns is not understood. A rise in serum nickel, which can cause coronary vasoconstriction, has been seen in burn-injured patients. In rats, nickel depresses myocardial contractility. Selenium is needed for tissue oxygenation and protection against lipid peroxidation. It also plays a role in cell-mediated immunity. In burn injuries, there is a selenium deficiency. Zinc helps more than 200 metalloenzymes function, and is beneficial for wound healing as it may contribute to new growth. Immune function is also affected by zinc, and in burn victims, there is a decrease in zinc.

Conclusion.—In healthy populations, the requirement levels for most of the micronutrients have not been defined, although recommended dietary allowances of 11 vitamins and 7 minerals have been established. In critically ill patients, the effects of trace elements may be far-reaching.

▶ Hopefully, this article will stimulate further research into trace element needs in the critically ill. Conflicting results, unsupported claims by industry, and lack of good research have led to much confusion.

R.E. Salisbury, M.D.

4 Aesthetic

General

Patients' Health Related Quality of Life Before and After Aesthetic Surgery

Klassen A, Jenkinson C, Fitzpatrick R, et al (Univ of Oxford, England; Radcliffe Infirmary, Oxford, England)
Br J Plast Surg 49:433–438, 1996
4–1

Background.—According to the World Health Organization, health involves complete physical, psychological, and social well-being. Evidence of the effectiveness of various medical treatments is important to medical resource allocation. In the National Health Service, access to some aesthetic surgery is limited because it is believed to be trivial and less important than other medical treatments. Data were collected to provide evidence of the benefits of aesthetic surgery.

Methods.—Patients aged 16 years or older who had specific operations of the abdomen, breast, chest, ear, or nose were enrolled. Questionnaires were mailed before surgery and 6 months after surgery. The Short Form 36 Health Survey Questionnaire, the 28-item General Health Questionnaire, and the Rosenberg Self-Esteem Scale were used. The information was compared with information collected from a random sample of the general population.

Results.—Before surgery, questionnaires were mailed to 656 individuals and completed by 443 individuals. After surgery, questionnaires were sent to 259 and completed by 198 individuals. Overall, the greatest change was seen in self-esteem. Patients in all surgical groups reported significant improvement in self-esteem. Patients who had breast reduction surgery reported significant improvement in self-esteem on all 3 health status instruments.

Discussion.—These findings showed that individuals who had aesthetic surgery had improved social, psychological, and physical functioning. The majority of individuals were very pleased with the outcome of their surgery and the effect the change had on their lives. Health status instruments are reliable and valid for evaluating the effect of health care interventions.

▶ In the era of outcome studies, this is valuable documentation of our contribution as aesthetic surgeons to the quality of life—something we have always known, and our patients have felt, but others tell us to prove it.

P.W. McKinney, M.D.

Teaching Aesthetic Surgery at the Resident Level
Linder SA, Mele JA III, Capozzi A (San Francisco)
Aesthetic Plast Surg 20:351–354, 1996   4–2

Objective.—Because the field of plastic surgery continues to broaden its scope, it is difficult for residents to receive sufficient training in all areas in 2 years. A plastic surgery clinic is important for the "hands on" experience necessary for developing the aesthetic sense, surgical approach, and competency of the chief resident.

Methods.—A 2-page survey was sent to 40 plastic surgery residents recently graduated from western U.S. programs to determine the best ways to enhance aesthetic skills and competence. Thirty-one responses were received.

Results.—Only 51.6% of programs had a chief resident aesthetic clinic. Of those surveyed, 52% felt there were not enough aesthetic cases, 42% said there was insufficient "hands on" experience, 35.5% were uncomfortable performing a majority of aesthetic procedures, and 25% believed they did not have enough practice in aesthetic cases during residency. More than half were not comfortable performing rhinoplasty/septoplasty and laser/endoscopic surgery. More than one third were not confident performing peels, dermabrasions, and injections, and almost one third were uncomfortable performing blepharoplasty and/or browlift procedures.

Conclusion.—Approximately half of western U.S. plastic surgery programs do not have aesthetic clinics. More than half of residents surveyed felt that more "hands on" experience was needed. Approximately a third to a half of all residents felt uncomfortable performing 1 or more procedures.

▶ We have had a resident clinic at Northwestern since the inception of the program in 1969. It is an invaluable learning experience as the patient is seen first by the resident, and at the second visit is presented to the attending surgeon who is present for none or all of the surgery, depending on many factors. The resident then follows the patient postoperatively with the attending supervision. This is worth a thousand "ghost surgeries," but it has not been easy and it requires a tremendous dedication by the faculty. At several points the university claimed the clinic did not exist, citing the dual standard of care for patients. This comment stemmed from various reasons. Essentially our method at Northwestern has allowed the patient to achieve a higher level of care and the resident a high level of education. Times have changed, and we hope that any of you setting up this form of teaching will not run into the obstacles that we did in the mid-80s.

P.W. McKinney, M.D.

Mini-slit Graft Hair Transplantation Using the Ultrapulse Carbon Dioxide Laser Handpiece

Ho C, Nguyen Q, Lask G, et al (UCLA Med Ctr, Los Angeles; Skin Cancer Found of California, Santa Monica)
Dermatol Surg 21:1056–1059, 1995   4–3

Background.—Mini-, micro-, and slit hair grafting techniques have improved the esthetic results of hair transplantation. The Ultrapulse CO_2 laser with a slit handpiece can produce ultrashort high-energy pulses that minimize thermal damage to adjacent tissues and may be useful in doing mini-slit graft hair transplant.

Methods.—Twenty-five patients underwent laser hair transplantation using the newly developed slit handpiece with the Ultrapulse CO_2 laser. The donor strips were strip harvested from the occipital area with a triple-blade scalpel and divided into 1×2-mm minigrafts. The recipient sites were made with the Ultrapulse laser at settings of 300–450 mJ, 10–15 W, and 0.8–sec pulse durations. The sites consistently measured 2×0.2 mm. Biopsy specimens from some sites were obtained to assess thermal damage of adjacent tissues. The patients were followed up for 4 to 6 months.

Results.—The optimal laser setting was 350 mJ, 12 W, and 0.8-sec pulse durations. Approximately 2.5–3 hours of operative time was required for 200–400 minigrafts. Intraoperative bleeding and charring were minimal. The recipient slits accepted the grafts well with minimal compression. There was no excessive pain or swelling. Crusting lasted up to 2 weeks. More than 98% of the grafts took. There was good long-term hair regrowth from the transplant sites. The biopsy specimens revealed minimal thermal damage to the adjacent tissues.

Conclusions.—The Ultrapulse Co_2 laser with the slit handpiece is effective in performing mini-slit graft hair transplantation procedures. Its advantages over conventional scalpel techniques include minimal bleeding, reduced operative time, consistent recipient slit sizes, easier graft handling, less compression, and minimal adjacent tissue damage. Its disadvantages include its cost, the safety and fire hazard requirements, and the prolonged crusting.

▶ We have to weigh adjacent tissue necrosis vs. potential hematoma, either of which can interfere with graft take.

P.W. McKinney, M.D.

Skin

Are All 585 nm Pulsed Dye Lasers Equivalent?: A Prospective, Comparative, Photometric, and Histologic Study

Jackson BA, Arndt KA, Dover JS (Harvard Med School, Boston)
J Am Acad Dermatol 34:1000–1004, 1996   4–4

Background.—The 585-nm flashlamp-pumped pulsed dye laser is used to treat port-wine stains and other cutaneous vascular lesions. These lasers were initially sold by a single manufacturer, Candela Corp. of Wayland, Mass. Since 1992, a second manufacturer, Cynosure Inc., of Bedford, Mass., has been marketing flashlamp-pumped pulsed dye lasers. However, the lasers from these 2 manufacturers have given strikingly different results at equivalent fluences. The photometric and histologic effects of these apparently similar laser systems from different manufacturers were compared.

Methods.—Two Candela SPTL-1 lasers and 2 Cynosure Photogenica V lasers were studied. For the first part of the study, laser beam profiles were measured for both the Candela and the Cynosure lasers. For the second part of the study, 3-, 5-, and 7-mm spots with fluences of 3, 5, and 7 J/cm^2 were placed on normal buttock skin of 8 human volunteers, using a single pulse of 1 of the Cynosure lasers. Twenty-four punch biopsy specimens were obtained immediately thereafter and evaluated for histologic changes. The results were compared with those on record for the Candela laser.

Results.—Measurement of the laser beam profiles revealed that the diameter of the 5-mm spot made with the first Candela laser was actually 5.8 mm, or 35% larger than expected, and that made with the second Candela laser was actually 5.7 mm, or 30% larger than expected. The laser beam profiles of the Cynosure lasers were 8% and 4% smaller than expected. Neither beam profile was uniform. The Candela laser maintained its gaussian-like beam profile, whereas the Cynosure laser's beam profile resembled a top hat. Examination of the biopsy specimens showed that the vascular specificity was maintained and that there was no thermal tissue damage.

Conclusions.—To achieve consistent treatments when using 585-nm pulsed dye lasers from different manufacturers for the treatment of port-wine stains and other cutaneous vascular lesions, placement of a single spot of energy onto burn paper and measurement of its diameter is recommended.

▶ With the popularity of lasers, it is important to recognize the variabilities of any of the tools with which we work. I think these instruments vary even from the same company and with usage, because we have to replace the canister from time to time.

P.W. McKinney, M.D.

Laser Hair Transplantation
Fitzpatrick RE (Encinitas, Calif)
Dermatol Surg 21:1042–1046, 1995   4–5

Introduction.—The use of the pulsed CO_2 laser for small graft hair transplantation has been proposed as a solution to some of the potential problems, such as intraoperative bleeding, graft compression, elevation, depression, and difficult graft insertion. The results of small graft hair transplantation using various laser parameters were compared with the results using standard micrografting and minigrafting techniques. In addition, residual thermal damage occurring with the various laser parameters was evaluated histologically.

Methods.—Eight adult males with male pattern alopecia were treated with transplantation of 100 micrografts and minigrafts obtained from the occiput. For each patient, 20 grafts each were done as follows: micrografts into 18-gauge needle puncture recipient sites, minigrafts into 14-gauge needle puncture recipient sites, micrografts with laser-created recipient sites, minigrafts with laser-created recipient sites, and slit grafts with laser-created recipient sites. Dilators were used in all needle-created recipient sites. The following power settings were used for all laser sites in 2 patients each: 15, 20, 30, and 50 W. The patients were examined monthly for 6 months.

Scalp tissue obtained during scalp reduction surgery done with laser power settings at 5-W intervals between 5 and 50 W were examined histologically to determine the zone of thermal damage.

Results.—Crusting and healing resolved more slowly at the laser sites, compared with the conventional sites, with the crusting and healing time correlating with laser power. The hair yield was greater and the onset of growth was earlier at conventional sites than at laser sites. At laser sites, hair yield decreased with increasing power settings. The operative time was reduced by 50% for the laser recipient sites but was increased for the laser donor sites because of the need to avoid thermal damage to adjacent hairs.

Thermal necrosis increased with increasing laser power settings. Necrosis zones of less than 100 μm could only be achieved with laser powers of 5 and 10 W or repetition rates of less than 20 Hz. The necrosis zone was greater than 200 μm with a laser power setting of 50 W.

Conclusions.—Optimal results of laser hair transplantation can be achieved using a small beam size, continual beam movement, and a power setting of 15 W. These settings minimize lateral thermal necrosis and crusting and healing time and maximize hair growth.

Histologic Effects of the High-energy Pulsed CO_2 Laser on Photoaged Facial Skin

Stuzin JM, Baker TJ, Baker TM, et al (Univ of Miami, Fla; Univ of Pennsylvania, Philadelphia)
Plast Reconstr Surg 99:2036–2050, 1997

4–6

Objective.—There is a dearth of information about the histologic effects of pulsed laser resurfacing of photoaged skin. Results of a comprehensive histologic study of the structural changes induced by CO_2 laser resurfacing are presented.

Methods.—In Part 1, two 3-mm areas on the right side of the face of each of 5 patients were treated with the UltraPulse CO_2 (Coherent) laser at 300 mJ before they underwent a facelift for severe photodamage. One site received 2 passes, and the other side received 4 passes. A similar treatment using 500 mJ was performed on the left side of the face. These test sites were examined histologically for the depth of injury. In Part 2, 10 patients, aged 51–85 years, with photodamaged skin, underwent laser resurfacing of the right preauricular area using 2 passes at 500 mJ. Fifteen days to 6 months later, after rhytidectomy, a skin section containing laser-resurfaced and untreated skin was removed and examined histologically. In Part 3, the hypopigmentation effect was histologically examined after 3 months in 3 blacks aged 30, 60, and 62 years, after 2 passes at 500 mJ.

Results.—In Part 1, the depth of injury was found to be dose-dependent (Fig 3). In Part 2, the treated site was smoother, more uniform in texture and clarity, and firmer than the nonresurfaced site. Re-epithelialization occurred within 7–10 days, and normal color returned in 2–3 months. The epidermis regenerated, and large, uniform keratinocytes formed. The melanocytic density, quantity, and distribution returned to normal. The dermis had a more normal appearance. New collagen formed, and glycosaminoglycans diminished (Fig 9). In Part 3, re-epithelialization occurred within 7–10 days. Although treated skin was lighter than untreated skin initially, normal color returned at 4 months. These older black individuals had a high degree of skin damage.

Conclusion.—Laser resurfaced photoaged skin is histologically similar to photoaged skin treated with phenol chemical peeling in the short term. Long-term effects have to be assessed. The hypopigmentation effects of laser resurfacing of black skin gradually resolved by 4 months.

► Here is an important communication suggesting an improvement in elastic tissue via laser resurfacing; the authors found the same improvement previously using phenol peels. We have, however, studied phenol vs. dermabrasion in a mini pig model and, at 6 months, found that the elastic tissue completely returned in the dermabraded pigs but was severely impeded in phenol-treated skin. Unequivocally in the authors' previous study,[1] it was found that elastic tissue did return, as opposed to our experimental model. It is particularly germane here that the authors have shown the capability of the melanocytes to be defunctionalized with a laser, whereas the phenol

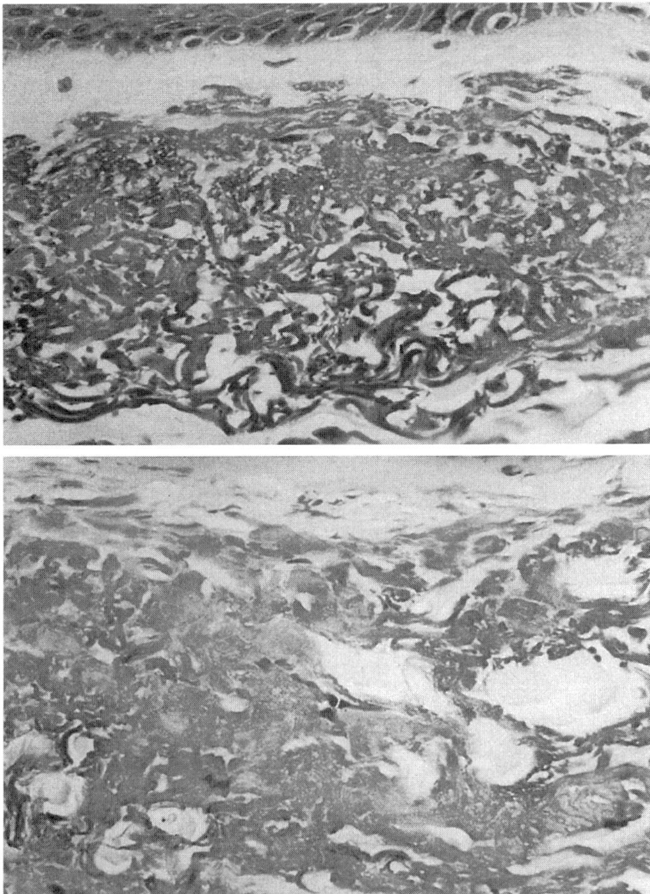

FIGURE 3.—Immediate effect of 2 passes with 300 mJ. (**Above**) Untreated area. This specimen is typical of photoaged skin. Note the atrophic dysplastic epidermis, beneath which lies a thin band of normal collagen (the Grenz zone). A mass of tangled, abnormal elastic tissue extends deeply into the dermis below the Grenz matrix. This is the appearance of marked elastosis, reflecting severe actinic damage to the dermal matrix. (**Below**) Treated test spot. The epidermis and the underlying Grenz zone have been destroyed completely. The elastotic tissue in the upper to middle dermis shows the coagulative effects of thermal injury. The elastotic fibers are no longer apparent, having been converted into an amorphous, coagulated mass. Note that the deeper portions of the elastotic tissue present in the middle dermis also appear to have been affected by the laser energy, even though this area is not completely necrotic. (Courtesy of Stuzin JM, Baker TJ, Baker TM, et al: Histologic effects of the high-energy pulsed CO_2 laser on photoaged facial skin. *Plast Reconstr Surg* 99:2036–2050, 1997.)

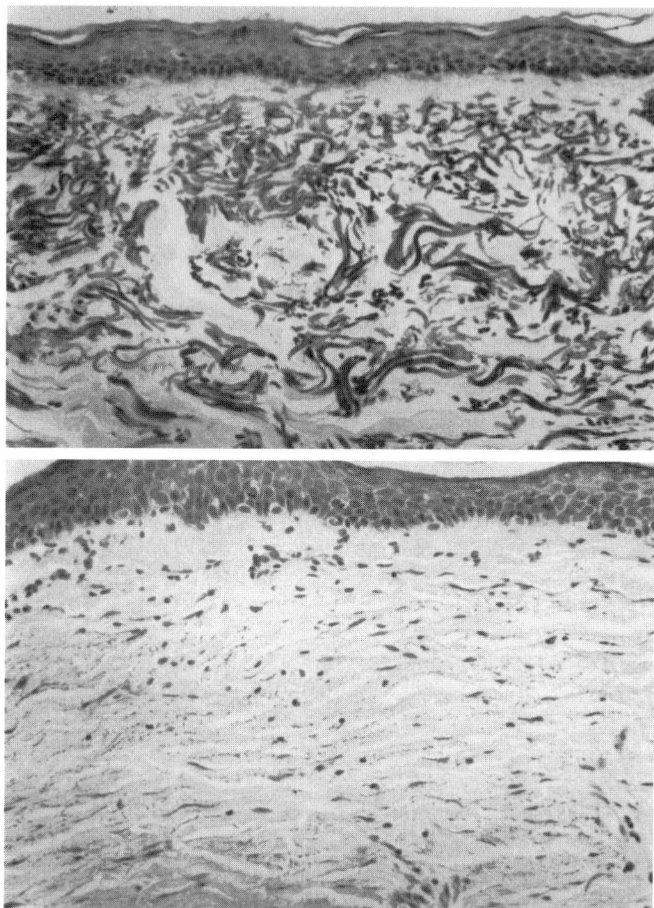

FIGURE 9.—(**Above**), untreated specimen. Typical appearance of photoaged skin. Marked elastosis is evident in the deeper dermis, whereas a thin Grenz zone of normal collagen appears beneath the atrophic epidermis. (**Below**), six months after laser resurfacing, the elastotic tissue has been completely replaced by new bundles of normal collagen. Fibroblasts are numerous. Under higher power (not visible here), there are new elastic fibers interspersed among the collagen bundles. This histologic picture represents essentially normal epidermis and dermis. (Courtesy of Stuzin JM, Baker TJ, Baker TM, et al: Histologic effects of the high-energy pulsed CO_2 laser on photoaged facial skin. *Plast Reconstr Surg* 99:2036–2050, 1997.)

allows melanocytes to regenerate but they do not function with pigment formation.

P. W. McKinney, M.D.

Reference

1. Kligman AM, Baker TJ, Gordon HL: Long-term histologic follow-up of phenol face peels. *Plast Reconstr Surg* 75:652–659, 1985.

Combined Use of Superpulsed Carbon Dioxide Laser and Cryotherapy for Treatment of Facial Rhytids

Nasri S, Newman JP, Goode RL (Stanford Univ, Calif)
Arch Otolaryngol Head Neck Surg 122:1169–1173, 1996   4–7

Purpose.—Although the carbon dioxide (CO_2) laser has been used widely for cosmetic resurfacing of the facial skin, control of thermal damage to the adjacent skin poses challenging problems. The superpulsed laser mode addresses this problem by vaporizing the tissue in a short enough time that heat is not transferred to the adjacent tissues. Cryotherapy is used for the treatment of many different types of cutaneous lesions. The superpulsed CO_2 laser alone was compared with cryotherapy plus the superpulsed CO_2 laser for the treatment of facial rhytids.

Methods.—The randomized, prospective trial included 20 patients with perioral rhytids. They were assigned to treatment with the superpulsed CO_2 laser alone or a combination of the laser and cryotherapy. In the laser group, the shoulders of the rhytids first were spot-treated with the superpulsed CO_2 laser. After the area was wiped and rehydrated, a second pass was made over the entire area. The shoulders then were treated with a third pass, if necessary. In the combined treatment group, initial treatment was with cryotherapy, with a single pass over the entire perioral region. The skin then was treated by the superpulsed CO_2 laser, as in the other group. The results were assessed using a skin wrinkle grading system, preoperative and postoperative photographs, and a patient satisfaction questionnaire.

Results.—The postoperative wrinkling scores were similar in the 2 groups. There were no significant differences in the anesthetic requirements or complication rate. Most patients in both groups were satisfied with their procedure.

Conclusions.—The superpulsed CO_2 laser is an effective mode of therapy for perioral rhytids. The results are no different with or without the addition of cryotherapy. There are no differences in results, complication rate, or patient satisfaction.

▶ Resurfacing for fine wrinkles, particularly non–muscle-induced wrinkles, is a successful technique, but we must understand that resurfacing by any method produces a second-degree burn and the wound will behave that way. It does not matter whether we do it with temperature, chemicals, or friction.

P.W. McKinney, M.D.

Treatment of Facial Rhytides With a High-energy Pulsed Carbon Dioxide Laser

Alster TS, Garg S (Georgetown Univ, Washington, DC)
Plast Reconstr Surg 98:791–794, 1996   4–8

Background.—The utility of traditional treatment modalities for facial rhytides has been limited by the complications of scarring or pigment changes. The results of treatment with a high-energy pulsed carbon dioxide laser were reported.

Methods.—Two hundred fifty-nine patients with facial rhytides were treated. Rhytides were perioral in 104, periorbital in 83, glabellar in 53,

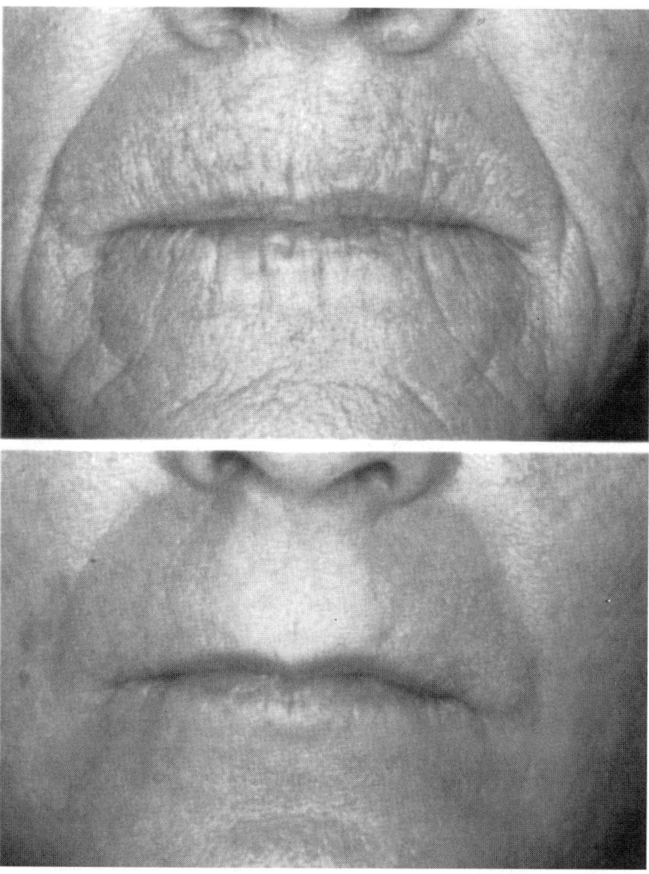

FIGURE 1.—A 72-year-old woman with perioral rhytides of moderate severity before (**above**) and 10 weeks following (**below**) 1 treatment with the high-energy pulsed carbon dioxide laser. (Courtesy of Alster TS, Garg S: Treatment of facial rhytides with a high-energy pulsed carbon dioxide laser. *Plast Reconstr Surg* 98:791–794, 1996.)

TABLE 3.—Side Effects After Laser Treatment

Location	Duration of Erythema	Hyperpigmentation	Hypopigmentation	Infection	Scarring
Perioral	2.36 mos.	31%	0	0	0
Periorbital	1.86 mos.	31%	0	0	0
Glabella	2.47 mos.	32%	0	0	0
Forehead	2.11 mos.	26%	0	0	0
Total	2.20 mos.	30.8%	0	0	0

(Courtesy of Alster TS, Garg S: Treatment of facial rhytides with a high-energy pulsed carbon dioxide laser. *Plast Reconstr Surg* 98:791–794, 1996.)

and on the forehead in 17. Outcomes were evaluated for up to 24 weeks after the treatment.

Findings.—Clinical response rates were uniformly excellent but varied by location. On average, all areas showed a 90% improvement. The best results were achieved in the periorbital regions, with a 93% improvement (Fig 1). The lowest response rates (87%) were associated with the most severe rhytides and those caused by excessive muscle movement. No scarring occurred, but erythema lasted for 1–3 months (Table 3). Transient postinflammatory hyperpigmentation, lasting an average of 3 months, occurred in 30% of patients. This was not limited to those with darker skin tones.

Conclusions.—High-energy pulsed carbon dioxide laser treatment for facial rhytides is effective and safe. The excellent results appear to be long-lasting. Treatment can be done on an outpatient basis with no need for general anesthesia.

▶ We welcome these studies on the laser that investigate competitive advantages and/or disadvantages with mechanical and/or chemical resurfacing techniques. The difference so far seems to be possibly prolonged erythema and a higher incidence of hyperpigmentation; however, the laser seems to have a lower incidence of hypopigmentation compared with chemical means. The laser is overall very competitive with mechanical means including dermabrasion using a wired-brush diamond face and/or sand paper, which may take a little longer but may avoid the hyperpigmentation and/or erythema problems seen so far with lasers.

P.W. McKinney, M.D.

Laser Skin Resurfacing

Lowe NJ, Lask G, Griffin ME (Univ of California Los Angeles School of Medicine; Skin Research Found of California, Santa Monica)
Dermatol Surg 21:1017–1019, 1995   4–9

Introduction.—Carbon dioxide (CO_2) lasers have been used in the treatment of various skin conditions. However, conventional continuous-wave CO_2 lasers can cause thermal injury and scarring in the underlying skin.

This thermal damage can be avoided by the use of pulsed lasers or scanning skin lasers. An experience with laser skin resurfacing therapy was reviewed, including guidelines for pretreatment and posttreatment regimens to optimize the response to treatment.

Methods.—The experience included 30 patients with photodamaged skin. All underwent ultrapulsed CO_2 laser resurfacing with the UltraPulse 5000 Series CO_2 laser. The patients were managed with different pretreatment and posttreatment regimens. The results were assessed by physician evaluation and, in some cases, by skin biopsy and cutaneous patch testing.

Results.—Improvement was rated good to excellent in 80% of patients. Sixty-five percent of patients receiving a topical treatment regimen including Polysporin and Desowen ointment had a painful vesicular eruption in the treated area. Results of cutaneous patch tests were negative in every patient, suggesting contact irritant dermatitis in the laser-treated skin. The most prominent side effects in the short and intermediate term were hyperpigmentation and erythema. The most effective pretreatment regimen included topical retinoids and skin-lightening agents, with oral anti–herpes simplex medication and oral antibiotics given immediately before laser treatment. The posttreatment regimen included facial soaks with dilute acetic acid to minimize the need for topical therapy. Treatment with oral anti–herpes simplex medications and broad-spectrum antibiotics continued for 7 days after laser treatment.

Conclusions.—Carbon dioxide laser resurfacing is an effective treatment for photodamaged skin, but appropriate pretreatment and posttreatment care is essential. Topical medications may cause contact dermatitis, so steps must be taken to minimize this risk. This complication is apparently related to the temporary removal of an effective skin barrier by laser therapy.

▶ A burn is a burn is a burn.

P.W. McKinney, M.D.

UltraPulse Carbon Dioxide Laser With CPG Scanner For Full-face Resurfacing For Rhytids, Photoaging, and Acne Scars
Apfelberg DB (Atherton Plastic Surgery Ctr, Calif)
Plast Reconstr Surg 99:1817–1825, 1997   4–10

Background.—Carbon dioxide laser resurfacing is an accepted cosmetic treatment for rhytids, scars, and photoaging. Because of its precise control and excellent visualization, the author now uses UltraPulse carbon dioxide laser resurfacing instead of chemical peeling and dermabrasion. The results of full-face UltraPulse carbon dioxide laser resurfacing for rhytids, photoaging, and acne scars in 11 patients are reported.

Methods.—The patients were all women, average age 51 years. The indication for treatment was cosmetic rhytids in 4 patients, residual acne scars in 5, and photoaging in 2. All patients were treated with the Ultra-

Pulse carbon dioxide laser, with a computerized pattern generator scanner for rapid, uniform laserbrasion. The laser sequence consisted of closely applied adjacent squares at 60 W, 200 to 300 mJ, and moderate density. Wound healing was enhanced by preparing the skin with Retin-A and bleaching agents. A moist dressing was applied after treatment, and Zovirax was given to prevent repeated oral herpes simplex infections. The patients were followed up for an average of 4 months.

Results.—None of the patients had any complications or side effects. Re-epithelialization took an average of 9.3 days, while redness and/or erythema resolved in an average of 8.9 weeks. All patients had good to excellent results.

Conclusions.—Very good cosmetic results are reported with the use of the UltraPulse carbon dioxide laser for full-face resurfacing in patients with rhytids, photoaging, and acne scars. The procedure rejuvenates the facial skin without side effects and complications. Good patient selection and preparation are essential. The use of a computerized pattern generator scanner permits rapid, repeatable, precise, and safe treatment parameters with uniform desurfacing.

▶ The results with resurfacing can be very impressive, but what of the changes which occur in the mechanics of the skin? A deep second-degree burn is what is required for deep lines, yet we see such skin in old thermal burns and it is not attractive particularly in animation. I am not suggesting we don't resurface, but I am suggesting that the future is unclear as to the biomechanics of the skin after resurfacing.

P. W. McKinney, M.D.

Effects of Dermabrasion on Acne Scarring

Aronsson A, Eriksson T, Jacobsson S, et al (Lund Univ, Sweden; Royal Inst of Technology, Stockholm; Univ Hosp MAS, Malmö, Sweden)
Acta Derm Venereol 77:39–42, 1997   4–11

Background.—The benefits of dermabrasion for acne scarring are traditionally demonstrated with photographs taken before and after the procedure. In the group of patients currently presented, the outcomes of dermabrasion were assessed by a variety of methods.

Methods.—Twenty-five patients were assessed before and up to 1 year after dermabrasion for acne scarring. Outcomes were determined based on the patients' and physicians' overall impressions, by counting and measuring lesions in specified areas, and by photographic documentation.

Findings.—The number of superficial scars was significantly reduced at 3 and 12 months. Deep scars were also reduced at 3 and 12 months, though the 12-month values had begun to revert toward preoperative values. Small scars and wide scars were also decreased significantly at 3 and 12 months, but the significance lessened with time. The physicians thought that superficial scars were definitely improved, whereas deep scarring became more pronounced after dermabrasion. Small scars showed an unmistakable tendency for a net improvement. However, wide scars seemed to get worse. Nine patients were satisfied with the outcomes, 12 said they were content, and 4 were clearly dissatisfied. Overall, the patients were happier with the results than the investigators were.

Conclusions.—Dermabrasion appears to be most effective for superficial scars. The outcomes for more severe forms of scarring were less predictable.

▶ Note the comments that in comparison to results at 3 months, at 6 months, as the edema subsides in the junction between the epidermis and the dermis, the wrinkles reappear. This happens in any "resurfacing" technique.

P.W. McKinney, M.D.

Tumescent Dermasanding With Cryospraying

Chiarello SE (Univ of South Florida, Tampa)
Dermatol Surg 22:601–610, 1996

4–12

Background.—Renewed interest in the art of dermasanding has been sparked by the new carbon dioxide resurfacing lasers. A detailed description and pictorial display of tumescent dermasanding with cryospraying was presented.

Technique.—After proper patient selection, the surgeon prepares the patient in a standard fashion. Approximately 30 cc of tumescent anesthesia is then injected into the upper lip with a 21- or 22-gauge needle. The blebs created by the previous injection of 1% xylocaine with epinephrine are injected. Approximately 30 cc is also needed for the lower lip and chin. The lips must be blown up until the tissue is tense. However, injections must be even and undulations avoided. Excellent overhead lighting and stereoscopic magnifying lenses enable the surgeon to see the "hills and valleys" of the wrinkles to the end of the treatment. The extreme turgor produced by the tumescence enables the surgeon to effectively sand over a flat, rigid surface, devoid of waves and undulations. Finger pressure is not necessary. The field is nearly bloodless. The appropriate sterile carbide sandpaper, wet with Aquanil or Cetaphil, is then used. The surgeon applies gentle, even pressure and avoids excessive drag on the skin. At the end of the procedure, a dressing is applied. The patient returns in 24–36 hours for a change of dressing and reassessment. Approximately 5 days after the procedure, the patient is checked again for slow-healing, crusted areas. By this time, most of the physiologic dressing is gone, and only a few crusts remain.

Conclusions.—Tumescent dermasanding with cryospraying is simple, effective, safe, and inexpensive in the removal of wrinkles. Strict attention to detail is needed to maximize outcomes and minimize complications.

▶ Proved techniques should not be abandoned in the stampede for the "new." Dermasanding is more controllable than acid, less prone to danger than the laser, and should be less expensive in that it does not require such a massive investment. However, it may take longer, and on a volume basis, perhaps the laser may be cost-effective (see Reference 1).

P.W. McKinney, M.D.

Reference

1. Waldorf H: Skin resurfacing of fine to deep rhytides using a char-free carbon dioxide laser in 47 patients. *J Dermatol Surg Oncol* 21:940–946, 1995.

Prevention of Facial Herpetic Infections After Chemical Peel and Dermabrasion: New Treatment Strategies in the Prophylaxis of Patients Undergoing Procedures of the Perioral Area
Perkins SW, Sklarew EC (Indiana Univ, Indianapolis; Univ of Maryland, Baltimore)
Plast Reconstr Surg 98:427–433, 1996   4–13

Background.—Widespread herpes simplex virus infection of the face can occur after chemical peel and dermabrasion procedures. Latent herpes simplex virus of the perioral area can be activated by chemical, inflammatory, or mechanical trauma, and may result in severe, widespread infection. Such infections have been observed in patients with severe burn injuries to the face and in immunocompromised individuals. Perioral herpes simplex virus activation is predictable in individuals who have had chemical peel or dermabrasion of this area and who have a positive history of oral-labial herpes simplex virus infection. Acyclovir is a synthetic purine nucleoside analogue that is active against herpes simplex virus-1 and herpes simplex virus-2. Prophylactic acyclovir has become part of the standard care for individuals with a positive history of oral herpetic infection, but there are no uniform recommendations for dosage for individuals undergoing chemical peel or dermabrasion of the perioral area. Outcomes in individuals who had chemical peel or dermabrasion procedures of the perioral area before and after acyclovir was commercially available were evaluated.

Methods.—The cases of 181 consecutive patients who had chemical peel or dermabrasion procedures of the perioral area during a period of 7 years were evaluated retrospectively. Patients who had a past episode of oral herpetic infection were given prophylactic treatment with oral acyclovir 600 mg/day in the early study years, or 2,400 mg/day in later study years. Active infection was treated with acyclovir 4,000 mg/day, then 2,400 mg/day. A subset of 12 patients underwent procedures before acyclovir was commercially available and formed a comparison group. The minimum follow-up was 6–24 months.

Results.—No patients were lost to follow-up. Overall, postoperative herpetic outbreaks of the perioral and facial areas occurred in 18 patients. Individuals who had chemical peel were more likely to have infection than those who had dermabrasion. Although it is generally believed that only individuals with a positive history of oral herpes simplex virus infection are at risk for infection after these procedures, 8 of 121 patients with a negative history of such infections had perioral or widespread facial outbreak. A high rate of infection was seen in individuals who had a positive history of oral herpetic infection, but who were not pretreated with acyclovir. There was an 8.3% incidence of infection in individuals with a positive history of oral herpes simplex virus infection who were pretreated with acyclovir. All these patients had smaller dosages of 600 mg/day in the early study years. After higher dosage protocols were begun, there were no further outbreaks. Individuals pretreated with smaller doses of acyclovir had milder symptoms than those who had no pretreatment. Patients who had no pretreatment had more lesions over a much broader facial area.

Discussion.—The effectiveness and optimal therapeutic dosage of acyclovir needs to be determined in a randomized, prospective study. Withholding acyclovir prophylaxis in a control group may not be ethically acceptable. Prophylactic acyclovir is recommended for all individuals regardless of history who are undergoing chemical peel or dermabrasion of the perioral area. Treatment should continue for a full 2 weeks after the procedure. Such pretreatment can minimize postoperative infection with herpes simplex virus.

▶ Note the dosage used and the fact that it includes all patients regardless of history, which is prudent. Often patients won't know they have had an infection or they will have forgotten.

P.W. McKinney, M.D.

Obagi's Modified Trichloroacetic Acid (TCA)-controlled Variable-depth Peel: A Study of Clinical Signs Correlating With Histological Findings
Johnson JB, Ichinose H, Obagi ZE, et al (Louisiana State Univ, New Orleans; Pendleton Mem Methodist Hosp, New Orleans, La; Stanford Univ, Calif)
Ann Plast Surg 36:225–237, 1996   4–14

Background.—Trichloroacetic acid (TCA) has been increasingly used recently in chemosurgical superficial dermatologic peels. Obagi has developed a modified TCA solution designed to slow the procedure and has identified clinical signs that indicate the depth of solution penetration. At the 50:1 level, epidermal sliding is observed. A uniform solid white frosting appears at the 50:2 level. At the 50:3 level, all background pink disappears and the skin appears grayish. The validity of these clinical signs was investigated using sequential biopsy findings.

Methods.—Twenty patients underwent at least 4 weeks of skin preparation with intensive application of Retin-A tretinoin, hydroquinone, and lactic acid before undergoing the chemical peel with a solution of 41.7% TCA in a 10% glycerin diluent. The mechanisms of the acute signs were investigated in 4 patients with 3-mm punch biopsy specimens taken 5 minutes after the clinical sign appeared. The biopsy material was examined with light microscopy and with electron microscopy in 2 patients. The longer term correlation between histologic findings and clinical signs of the depth of peel was evaluated with punch biopsy specimens obtained at 48 hours and 6 weeks after the chemical peel in 4 patients. In the other 12 patients, the thickness of the new dermis was assessed, using punch biopsy material obtained before and 6 weeks after chemical peel to a 50:2 level.

Results.—Histologic specimens of tissue at the acute 50:1 level revealed only mild changes with a thinner stratum corneum (Fig 1). Electron microscopy revealed nuclear leaching of the epidermal cells with chromatin concentration on the nuclear membranes. There was irregular cytoplasmic organelle coagulation and intercellular space edema. There was also nuclear leaching and shrunken mesenchymal cells in the papillary

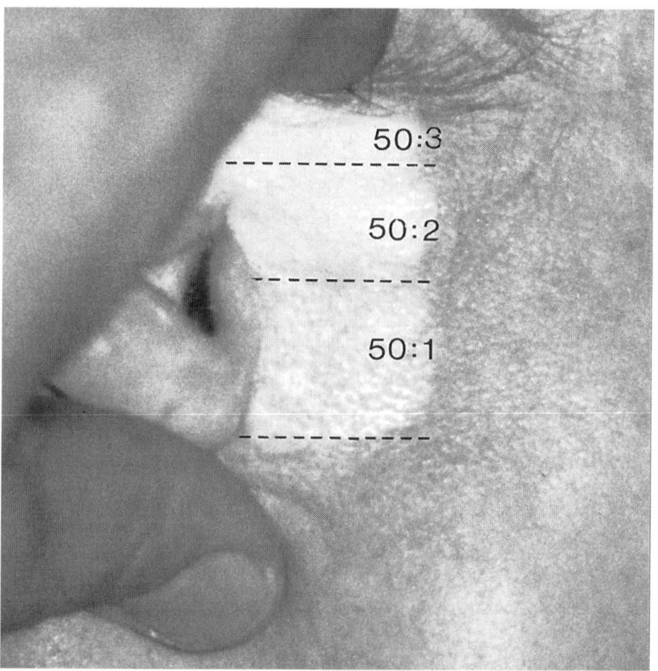

FIGURE 1.—Comparison of 3 levels of chemical peel. Appearance at 10 minutes of peel depth 50:1 is solid white with strong pink background and epidermal sliding. At 50:2 the appearance is solid white with no pink/very faint pink background and no epidermal sliding and at 50:3 the appearance is solid white with a grayish hue and total loss of pink. These are positioned from bottom to top, respectively. (Reprinted with permission from Johnson JB, Ichinose H, Obagi ZE, et al: Obagi's modified trichloroacetic acid (TCA)-controlled variable-depth peel: A study of clinical signs correlating with histological findings. *Ann Plast Surg* 36:225–237, 1996.)

dermis. Specimens of the acute 50:2 level had complete loss of the stratum corneum and near total loss of the stratum granulosum. Ultrastructural changes included more severe cytoplasmic organelle coagulation, intercellular swelling, and coagulative shrinkage of mesenchymal cells. The specimens of the acute 50:3 level revealed condensed squamous epithelium with nuclei arranged in parallel. Coagulation extended to the deep vascular dermal plexus. Collagen fibers had interfibrillar granules and microvesicular swelling.

The dermal changes were progressive, as shown by the biopsy specimens at 48 hours and 6 weeks. By 6 weeks, chemical peel at the 50:2 level resulted in a new layer of fibrillar collagen in a laminar pattern replacing the upper reticular dermis. This new dermal layer was almost the full thickness of the reticular layer in patients undergoing 50:3-level peel. After a 50:2-level peel, the new dermis accounted for an average of 33% of the full thickness of the dermis.

Conclusions.—The validity of Obagi's clinical signs was supported by the histologic and electron microscopic findings.

▶ In "resurfacing" techniques or whatever method is used (mechanical, chemical, heat), the operator must have a guide with which to gauge the depth of the burn; all of them could go too deep or be too superficial. Resurfacing could probably be done with a blow torch or cigarette lighter.

P.W. McKinney, M.D.

Utilizing the Ultraviolet (UV Detect) Camera to Enhance the Appearance of Photodamage and Other Skin Conditions

Fulton JE Jr (Newport Beach, Calif)
Dermatol Surg 23:163–169, 1997

4–15

Background.—The development of standard ultraviolet (UV) photographic techniques has improved outcome monitoring and patient education. The incorporation of standardized UV photography into one cosmetic dermatology practice was described.

Methods.—Patients with Fitzpatrick skin types I to III were photographed with visible and UV light. The UV "detect" camera was a 35 mm single lens reflex camera with Ultra 1200 electronic flash, a 90 mm macro lens, and a 315 to 390 mm UV filter. Follow-up photographs were taken to document changes after treatment.

Findings.—The UV camera proved very useful in documenting sun damage to the skin's pigment system. In children, the UV camera detected damage that was not readily apparent (Figs 2 and 3). The UV detect camera also helped document changes in patients with melasma, vitiligo, and posttraumatic or postoperative hypopigmentation. The camera was also used to monitor treatment programs designed to redistribute the pigment.

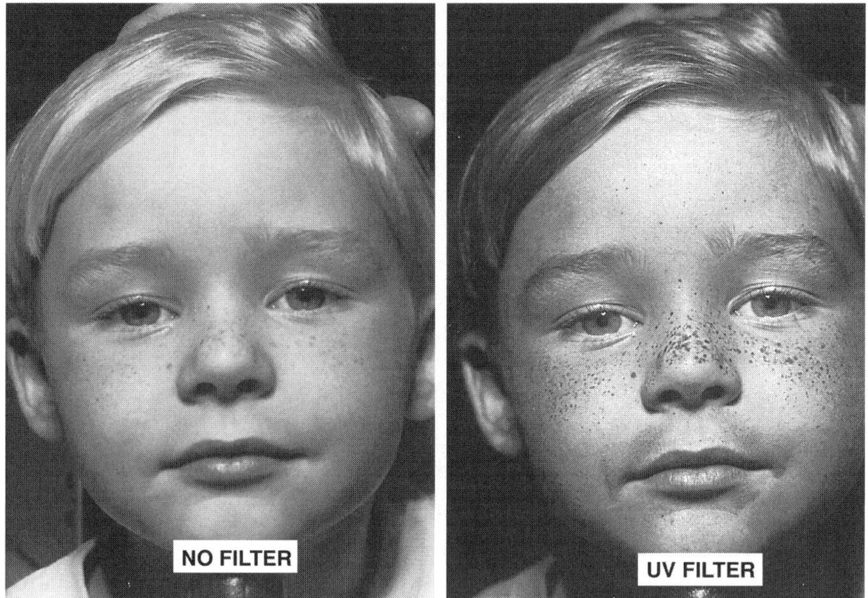

FIGURE 2.—A 4-year-old patient demonstrating with the UV photograph the increased clumping of melanin following sun damage. (Courtesy of Fulton JE, Jr: Utilizing the ultraviolet (UV detect) camera to enhance the appearance of photodamage and other skin conditions. *Dermatologic Surg* 23:163–169, 1997.)

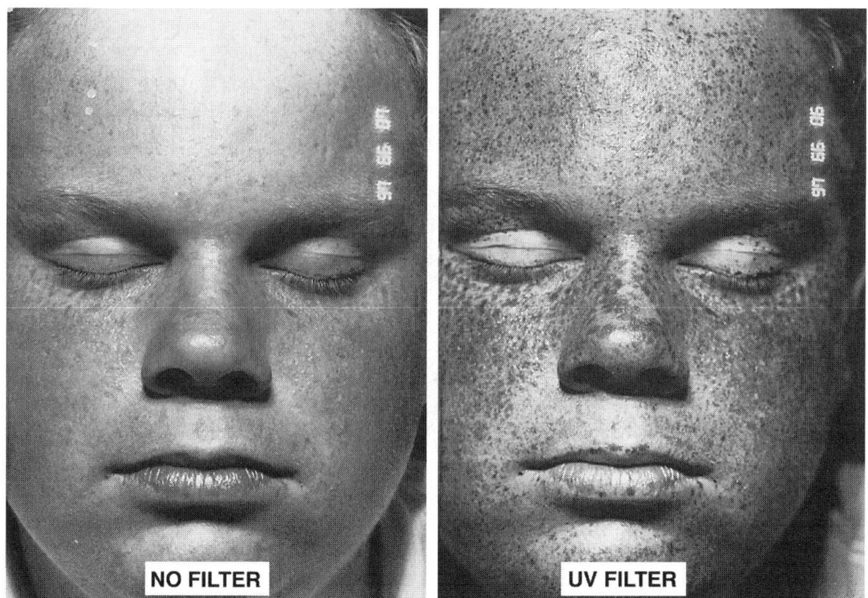

FIGURE 3.—A 16-year-old patient demonstrating extensive sun damage everywhere except in the middle of the upper eyelids. Note the complete loss of pigment on the bridge of the nose. This may be where skin cancers will develop in the future. (Courtesy of Fulton JE, Jr: Utilizing the ultraviolet (UV detect) camera to enhance the appearance of photodamage and other skin conditions. *Dermatologic Surg* 23:163–169, 1997.)

Conclusions.—The UV camera should be an integral part of sun damage detection. This camera documents pigmentary changes and demonstrates improvement after treatment.

▶ The ultraviolet filter accentuates the changes in a dramatic fashion (see Figure 2).

P.W. McKinney, M.D.

Skeletal

Angle-splitting Ostectomy for Reducing the Width of the Lower Face
Deguchi M, Iio Y, Kobayashi K, et al (Osaka Shirakabe Inst, Japan)
Plast Reconstr Surg 99:1831–1839, 1997   4–16

Background.—Mandibular contouring surgery to reduce the width of the lower face can be done in patients who wish to have their large, square-shaped, or broad face made small, round, or slender. Conventional angle ostectomy can successfully correct the prominent mandibular angle. However, it is usually necessary to resect lateral protrusions of both the mandibular angle and part of the anterior mandibular body. An experience with angle-splitting ostectomy to reduce the width of the lower face is reported.

Methods.—The experience included 76 patients — 67 women and 9 men, mean age 31 years — who underwent surgery to reduce the width of the lower face. In the early part of this 5-year experience, the authors combined shaving of the lateral cortex with multistaged, curved cuts of the mandibular angle. However, this was a complex and time consuming technique with some important drawbacks: the resulting mandibular angle tended to lack individuality, and the width of the lower face was sometimes not fully reduced.

The authors therefore modified their approach by performing an angle-splitting ostectomy (Fig 1). This procedure was designed to remove the excessive bone affecting the width of the lower face in the frontal view. The ostectomy was performed in the area posterior to the inferior alveolar nerve in the mandible. This procedure was performed in 29 patients.

Results.—All 29 patients undergoing angle-splitting ostectomy had good results, both subjectively and objectively. The procedure achieved maximal reduction in the width of the lower face, because bone was resected flat on the sagittal plane (Fig 3). The result was a natural relief of the mandibular angle. The postoperative contour was highly predictable. There was no need for masseter muscle resection, and there were no cases of hematoma. Postoperatively, the patients had only mild trismus, mental nerve paralysis, and swelling. Postoperative recovery was quick.

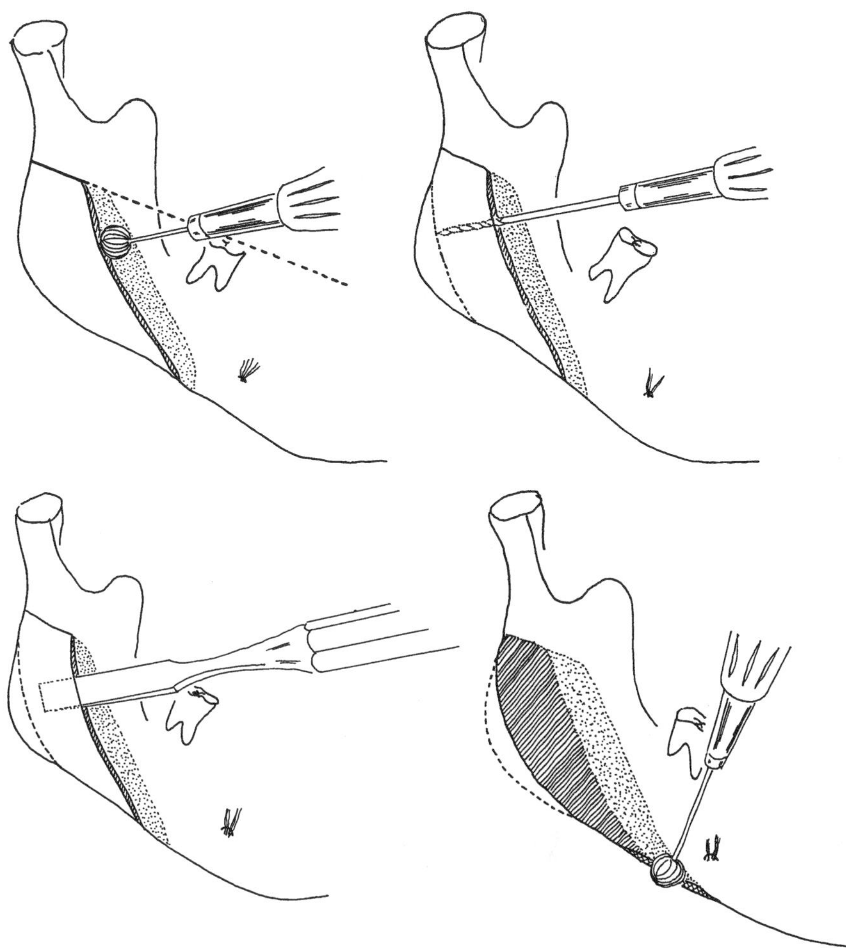

FIGURE 1.—Illustrations showing the procedure. Above left, the dotted area is shaved with a round burr, and a deep groove is hollowed out along the line extending from the occlusal plane with a drill burr. This groove serves as the upper boundary of the splitting ostectomy. Above right, using the drill burr, perforations are opened at 2- to 3-mm intervals. All layers including the medial cortex are resected in case the posterior or inferior margin protrudes outward. Below left, splitting is done with a chisel about 10 mm in width along the perforations created with the drill burr. Below right, bone projections are trimmed with a round burr at the edge of the ostectomized area near the mental foramen. (Courtesy of Deguchi M, Iio Y, Kobayashi K, et al: Angle-splitting ostectomy for reducing the width of the lower face. *Plast Reconstr Surg* 99:1831–1839, 1997.)

Discussion.—Angle-splitting ostectomy is an effective and safe alternative to conventional procedures for narrowing the lower face. It minimizes damage to the masseter muscle and other soft tissues, and carries few complications. The aesthetic results are good, even in patients with facial asymmetry.

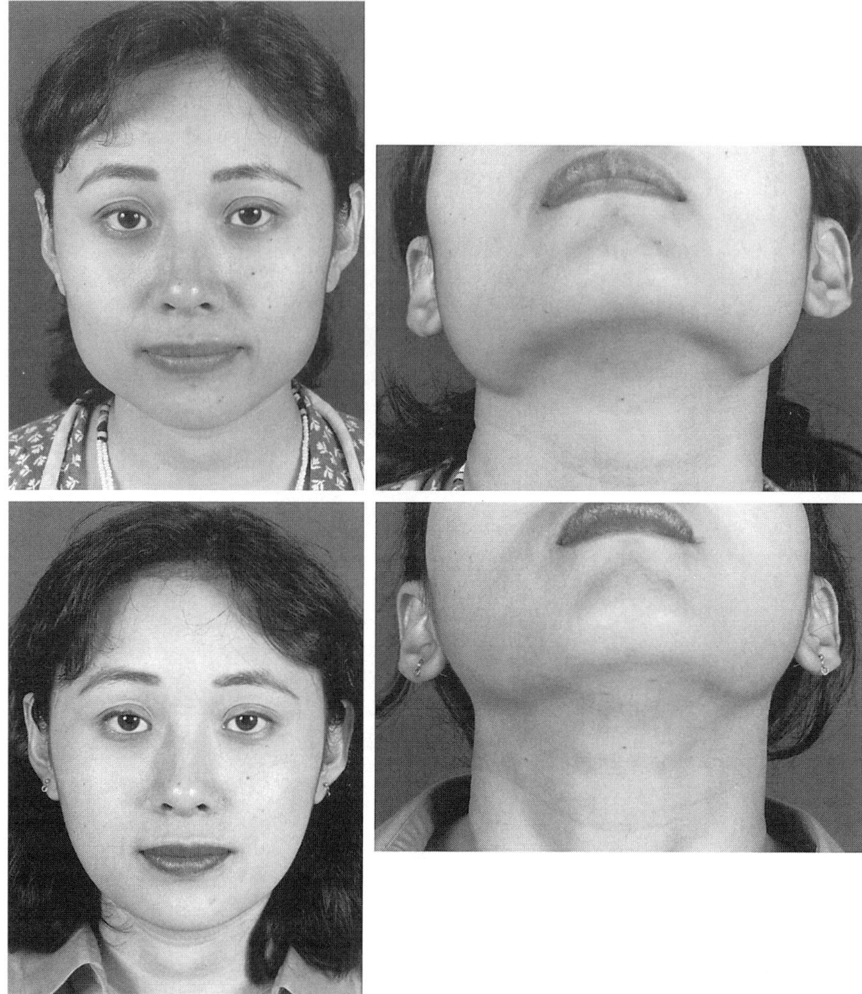

FIGURE 3.—Case 2 (a 27-year-old woman). Angle-splitting ostectomy was performed to meet the patient's desire to have her lower facial asymmetry corrected and to have a slender face. As a result, her face regained symmetry, and its contour was satisfactorily improved. The upper panels (above) are photographs taken before the operation, and the lower ones (below) are photographs taken 3 months postoperatively. (Courtesy of Deguchi M, Iio Y, Kobayashi K, et al: Angle-splitting ostectomy for reducing the width of the lower face. *Plast Reconstr Surg* 99:1831–1839, 1997.)

▶ An important "Jeminizing" technique, the skeleton is the foundation of the soft tissue and we should consider its modifications when we consider facial rejuvenation.

P.W. McKinney, M.D.

Simultaneous Osseous Genioplasty and Meloplasty

Wider TM, Spiro SA, Wolfe SA (Univ of Miami, Fla)
Plast Reconstr Surg 99:1273–1281, 1997   4–17

Introduction.—Fifty patients who had combined meloplasty and osseous genioplasty between 1975 and 1995 were studied to determine whether this procedural combination has advantages or disadvantages.

Study Group.—The charts and operative reports of 50 patients who underwent combined meloplasty and genioplasty with a single surgeon were reviewed. There were 5 male and 45 female patients, with an average age of 50 years. The average follow-up available was 2.23 years. This series included 40 sliding advancement genioplasties, 7 genioplasties with interpositional bone grafts, and 3 reduction genioplasties.

Technique.—The combined operation is usually performed with the use of general anesthesia, but can be performed using local anesthesia with sedation. The genioplasty precedes the meloplasty. The lower buccal sulcus is infiltrated with a vasoconstrictive solution. An incision is made on the labial side and subperiosteal dissection is performed over the lower border of the symphysis. The midline of the symphysis is marked and the horizontal osteotomy is marked perpendicularly for symmetry. The inferior segment is advanced. The anterior cortex of the superior segment should be juxtaposed to the posterior cortex of the inferior segment. The osteosynthesis is achieved by 3 wires. The total horizontal advancement is usually 6–8 mm. Meloplasty is performed (Fig 2) with wide subcutaneous dissection in the face and neck connecting with the submental dissection. The platysma is plicated laterally to the anterior border of the sternocleidomastoid fascia. Incisions are closed with nylon and silk. Other procedures can then be performed. A lightly compressive padded dressing is applied for 1 day. The patient eats only a soft diet for several days.

Complications.—There were 10 complications in this series. There were 2 small hematomas. There were 2 hypertrophic postauricular scars and 2 hypertrophic submental scars that were revised. There was 1 wound infection that resolved with antibiotics. One patient had a prolapsed submandibular gland that was excised. One patient experienced transient weakness of the marginal mandibular nerve and 1 patient had transient numbness of the unilateral lower lip. There were no cases of permanent paralysis or paresthesia. From 1 month to 3 years postoperatively, 8 patients complained that their chins were "too strong" and 6 underwent revisional surgery. At 5–7 years postoperatively, 1 male and 1 female patient complained that their chins were too short.

Conclusions.—Osseous genioplasty can be performed simultaneously with meloplasty, and this combination procedure is safe and reliable. Complications tend to be minor and patient satisfaction is high.

▶ The number of complications with osseous genioplasty in skilled hands is the same as that of foreign implants.

P.W. McKinney, M.D.

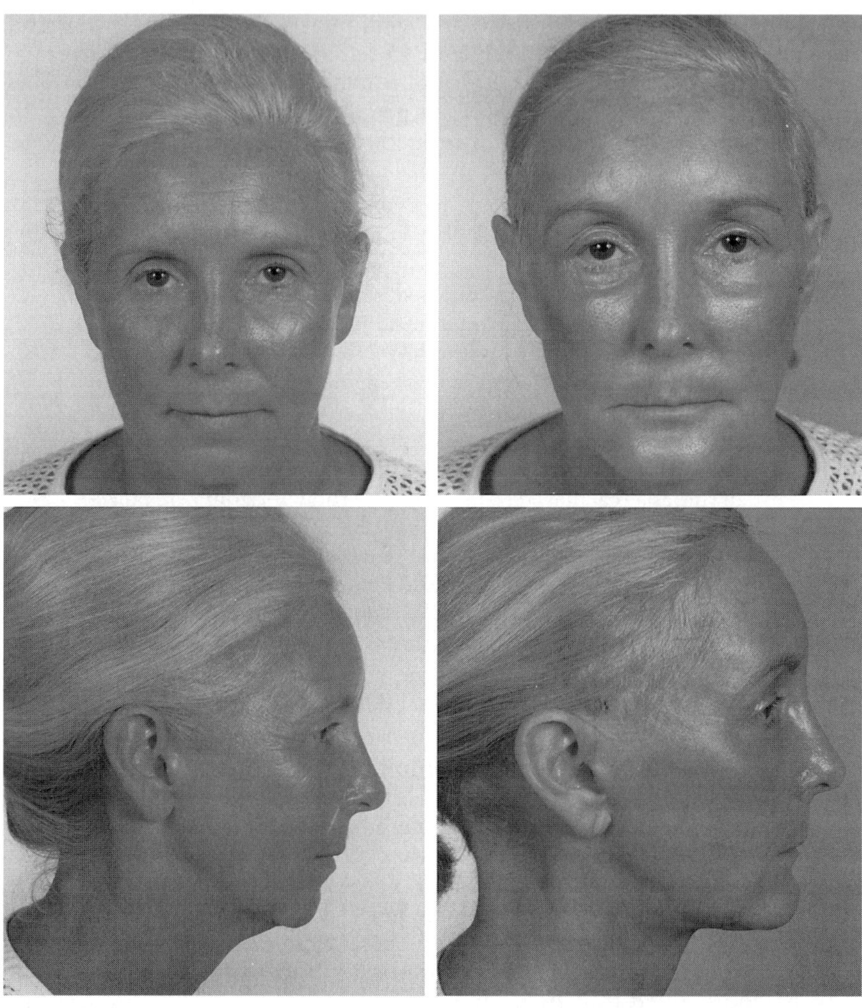

FIGURE 2.—A 54-year-old woman before and 6 weeks after meloplasty, submental lipectomy, lower lid blepharoplasty, and sliding genioplasty. The tightening in the neck is obtained both by the forward pull of the advanced segment and the posterior plication of the platysma. (Courtesy of Wuder TM, Spiro SA, Wolfe SA: Simultaneous osseous genioplasty and meloplasty *Plast Reconstr Surg* 99:1273–1281, 1997.)

(*Continued*)

FIGURE 2 (cont.)

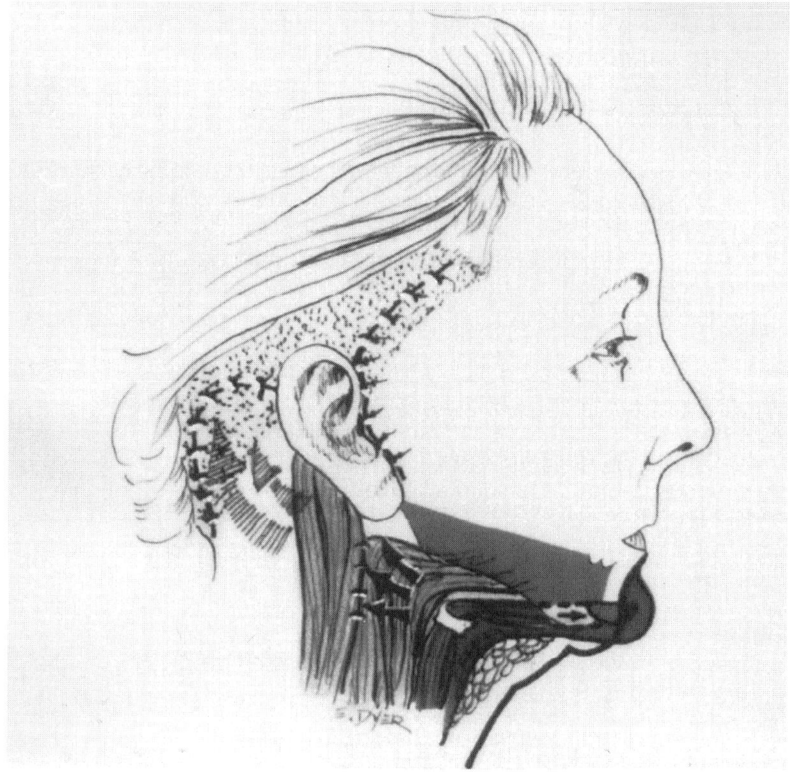

Labial Incompetence: A Marker for Progressive Bone Resorption in Silastic Chin Augmentation

Matarasso A, Elias AC, Elias RL (Manhattan Eye, Ear, and Throat Hosp, New York; Massachusetts Gen Hosp, Boston)
Plast Reconstr Surg 98:1007–1014, 1996   4–18

Background.—Bone erosion below silicone rubber implants occurs in most patients undergoing augmentation genioplasty. Although such erosion generally is thought to be self-limiting with minimal adverse consequences, the implant needs to be removed if the teeth are jeopardized or the sensibility of the mental nerve changes. Osteoplastic genioplasty may be needed to restore aesthetic contour to the chin and avoid functional problems. Several factors contributing to this phenomenon have been identified, but the functional aberration of a tensed mentalis muscle has not been addressed.

Methods and Findings.—The records of patients undergoing orthognathic surgery with silicone chin implants were reviewed. Six patients needed implant removal because of significant bony erosion. All had received appropriately sized Silastic implants. Progressive bony erosion was found to be correlated with preoperative baseline labial incompetence and mentalis muscle hyperactivity. Erosions were grade II in 1 patient and grade III in 4, 1 of whom had dental root exposure. Severe resorption also occurred in the 6th patient, with mentalis muscle strain after attempts to contain the lower denture.

Conclusions.—Labial incompetence seems to be a reliable marker for ongoing mandibular resorption after Silastic augmentation. Thus, an alternative approach should be considered in patients with microgenia and lip strain. Routine follow-up assessment and radiographs may be warranted for patients with labial incompetence who already have had Silastic chin implants.

▶ As a rule of thumb, an implant with a projection greater than 5 mm is at risk of shifting or eroding, and a bone advancement chin should be considered instead with a wide-based anatomical implant. Greater projections occasionally can be accomplished safely without these problems, but one must be alert to the potential dangers. The older concept of enough to do the job is fallacious.

P.W. McKinney, M.D.

A Simple Method of Reduction Malarplasty
Hwang YJ, Jeon JY, Lee MS (Konkuk Univ, Seoul, Korea)
Plast Reconstr Surg 99:348–355, 1997   4–19

Background.—Because the Oriental face is generally short and wide, a prominent zygoma in relation to a flat nose makes the face seem flatter. In Korea, a prominent zygoma is viewed unfavorably. Outcomes of a simple, effective technique for decreasing the prominent zygoma were assessed.

Methods and Outcomes.—Twenty-six patients aged 19–47 years underwent reduction of the prominent zygoma. All but 1 were women. The zygoma body was shaved, and the zygomatic arch was displaced inwardly after 2-point fracturing, green-stick fracture anteriorly, and complete osteotomy posteriorly through a small preauricular and upper buccal sulcus incision. At a mean follow-up of 8 months, the postoperative results were satisfactory to all patients. Complications included seroma in 2 patients, transient facial nerve paresis in 1, and mild zygoma asymmetry in the early postoperative period in 1. All complications completely resolved with conservative treatment (Figs 3 and 4).

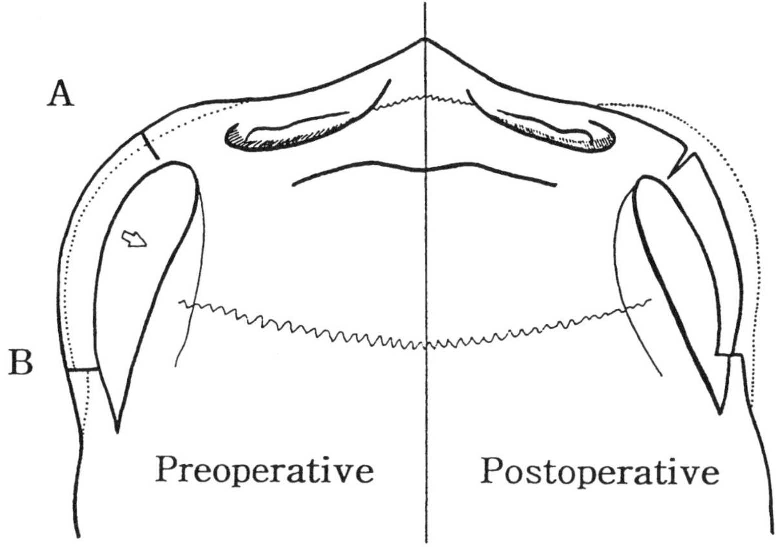

FIGURE 3.—Preoperative left-side view shows partial- (**A**) and full-thickness (**B**) osteotomy and shaving area (outer side from dotted line) and postoperative right-side view shows reduction not only of anterolateral protrusion but also of width of the face by inward displacement of arch. (Courtesy of Hwang YJ, Jeon JY, Lee MS: A simple method of reduction malarplasty. *Plast Reconstr Surg* 99:348–355, 1997.)

Conclusions.—This simple technique for reducing the prominent zygoma has several advantages. The skin incision is small, resulting in an inconspicuous scar. No foreign bodies, such as wires or miniplates, are used. Also, postoperative discomfort is reduced compared to that with other procedures. Finally, satisfactory outcomes are achieved.

▶ Shaving has led to thickening of bone in some patients and has to be exaggerated.

P.W. McKinney, M.D.

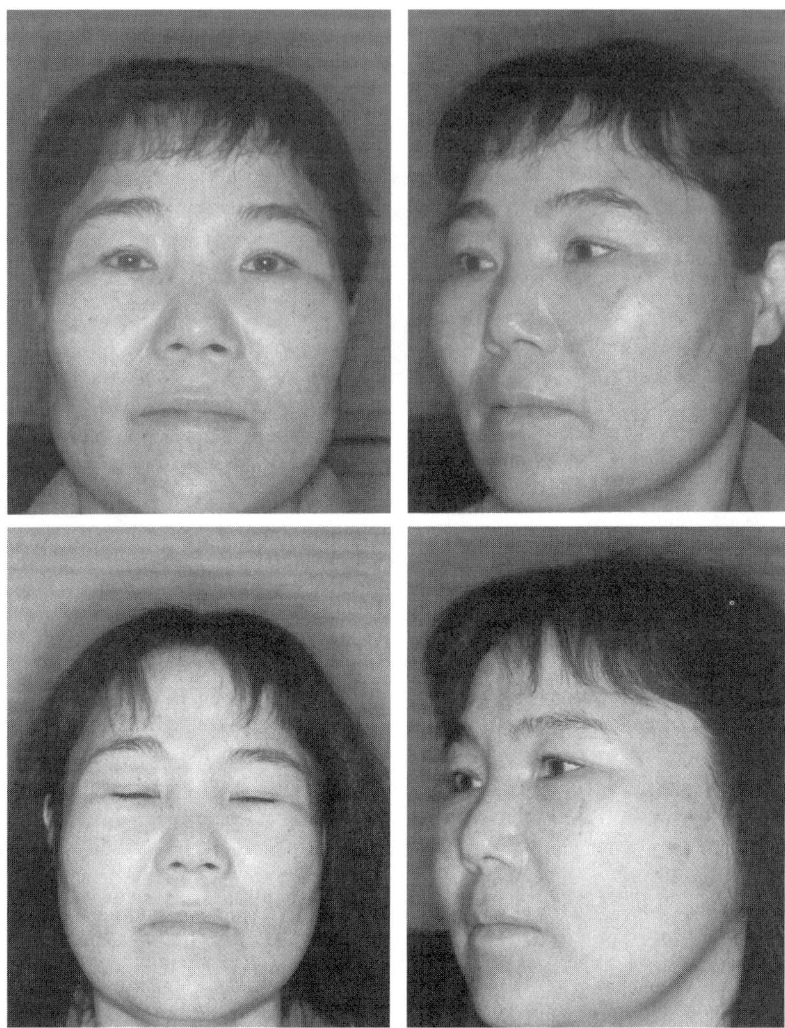

FIGURE 4.—A 50-year-old woman with malar prominence. Preoperative (**top**) and 1-month postoperative views (**bottom**). (Courtesy of Hwang YJ, Jeon JY, Lee MS: A simple method of reduction malarplasty. *Plast Reconstr Surg* 99:348–355, 1997.)

Face, Neck, and Brow

Value of Liposuction in Improvement of Cervicofacial Contours (French)
Mole B (Paris)
Ann Chir Plast Esthet 41:299–307, 1996

4–20

Background.—The author reports his 10-year experience with liposuction of the cervicofacial region.

Methods.—Seventy-five cervicofacial liposuction procedures were performed, mainly in women between 41 and 45 years of age. The procedure was isolated in 81% of cases and in 19% of cases was combined with other procedures such as a facelift. Patients were selected on the basis of age, skin quality, and weight. When these variables were not ideal, patients were counseled that a secondary intervention would probably be needed. Liposuction was performed in a systematic manner (Fig 4), typically with microcannula attached to a syringe. Between 6 and 70 cc (average, 20 cc) of fat were removed with 2- and 1.5-mm cannulas.

Findings.—About one third of the results were excellent, one third were good but not quite up to expectations, and one third introduced side effects without improving the appearance. The most significant side effects were facial paralysis, cutaneous irregularities, and small wattles. The first

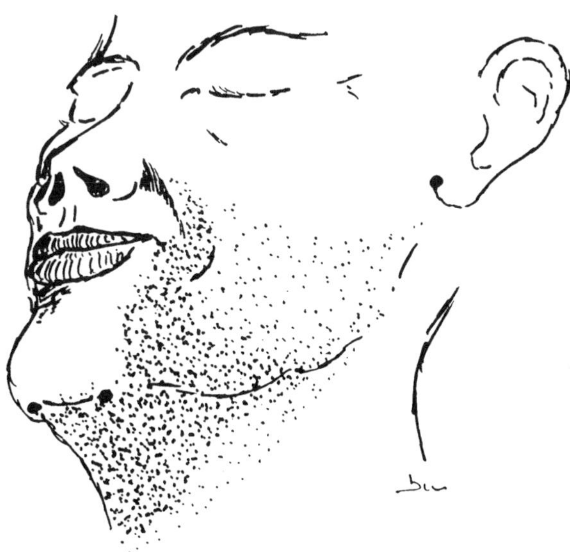

FIGURE 4.—Distribution of cervicofacial liposuction and sites of penetration (*solid circles*). (Courtesy of Mole B. Value of liposuction in improvement of cervicofacial contours (French). *Ann Chir Plast Esthét* 41:299–307, 1996.)

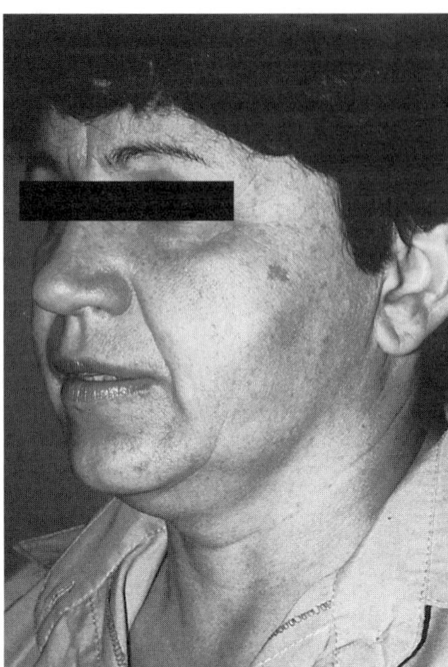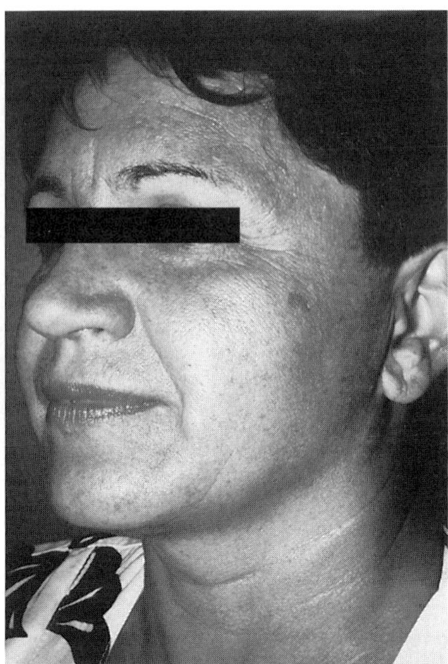

FIGURE 2.—**B**, 43-year-old woman. **D**, result 3 months after simple liposuction of the chin. (Courtesy of Mole B. Value of liposuction in improvement of cervicofacial contours (French). *Ann Chir Plast Esthét* 41:299–307, 1996.)

2 effects have not recurred since the author began using microcannulas attached to a syringe. The best results were under the chin (Fig 2). Three patients required a second operation for best results.

Conclusion.—Cervicofacial liposuction with microcannulas attached to a syringe — so-called "liposculpture" — is an integral part of the plastic surgeon's armamentarium when performing procedures in the cervicofacial region. Results, however, depend on skin elasticity and skin retraction, which are variable. Thus, surgeons should use prudence when promising results to patients and should consider other procedures that might improve results over liposuction alone.

▶ As Figs 1 and 2 show, patient selection and technique are very important. Small puncture wounds through the dermis with a 1.5-mm catheter will avoid trouble and should extract only vapors, i.e., wisps of fat. This avoids the corn row look caused by excessive removal. This is particularly true if an open technique through the flaps is used because edema sets in and one may remove too much fat. I prefer to tighten the face first and then do the suction, both open and through separate stab incisions.

P.W. McKinney, M.D.

Isolated Cervicofacial Liposuction Applied to the Treatment of Aging (French)
Flageul G, Illouz Y-G (Paris)
Ann Chir Plast Esthet 41:620–630, 1996   4–21

Background.—Liposuction has been used for almost 20 years in rejuvenating the face. Liposuction's strengths are its ability to correct a fatty contour and to arrest sagging skin caused by skin retraction. This report focuses on the use of isolated liposuction in treating the cervicofacial region.

> *Technique.*—Three incisions, each 3 mm long, are made in the middle of the submental region and in the right and left retrolobular areas. A solution is injected to magnify the thickness of the fatty tissue, after which sequentially thinner cannulas (3 and 2 mm) are used to create tunnels for removing the subcutaneous fat. After the procedure, Elastoplast is applied for 72 hours.

Findings.—No hemorrhagic or neurologic complications have been encountered by these authors. Nonetheless, complications such as irregularities, adhesions, and local depressions have occurred. Generally, however, results have been excellent and lasting (Figs 7 and 8). Results are best when the skin is elastic, when little excess skin is present, and when sufficient subcutaneous tissue is present.

Conclusion.—Isolated liposuction can be used to combat the effects of aging, particularly when the patient does not want a facelift. Positioning the liposuction tunnels along the lines of skin tension encourages skin retraction along those lines. The benefits of liposuction are particularly complimentary when combined with chemical peeling, endoscopic surgery, and laser surgery.

▶ There are slight differences in doing a facial suction, but one has to be very careful of dents and if anything is done, I use 1½–2 mm catheter maximum with just vapors and slight aspirations removed.

P.W. McKinney, M.D.

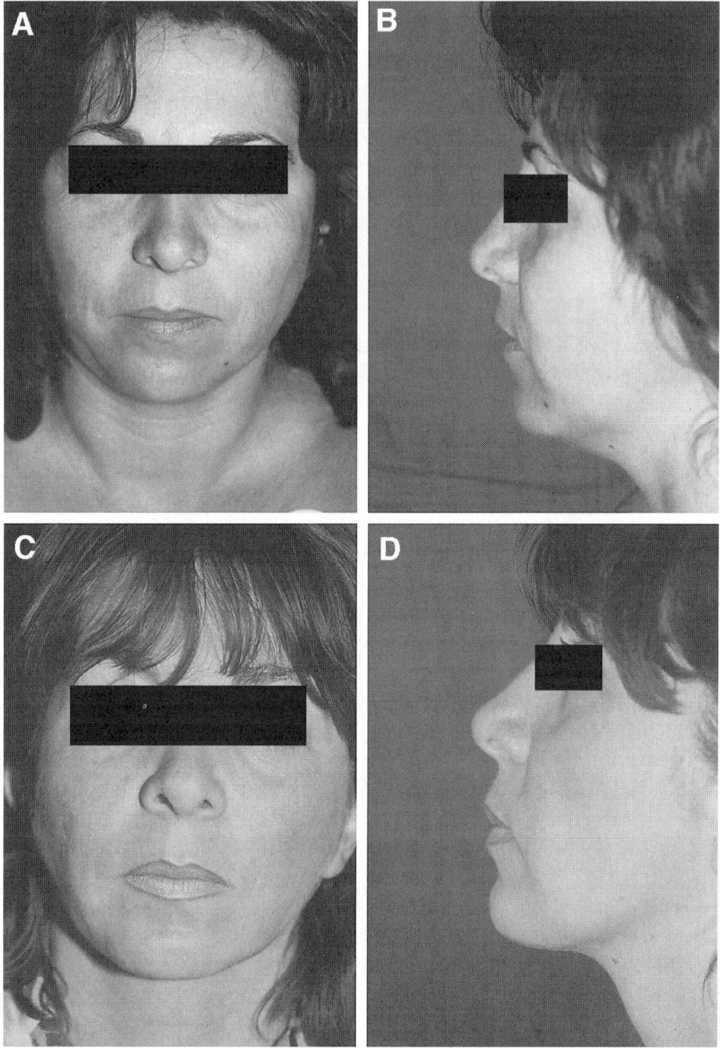

FIGURE 7.—A 41-year-old patient, showing a typical aspect of a "tired face." Liposuction of the chin, of the inferior third of the face extended up to the middle third, allowing a good modeling of the malar pad contour. **A** and **B**, preoperative views. **C** and **D**, 6-month result. The term "lifting effect" is here quite legitimately used. On the profile view, besides the correction of the neck and jowl, one can observe a remodeling of the middle third of the face. (Courtesy of Flageul G, Illouz Y-G. Isolated cervicofacial liposuction applied to the treatment of aging (French). *Ann Chir Plast Esthét* 41:620–630, 1996.)

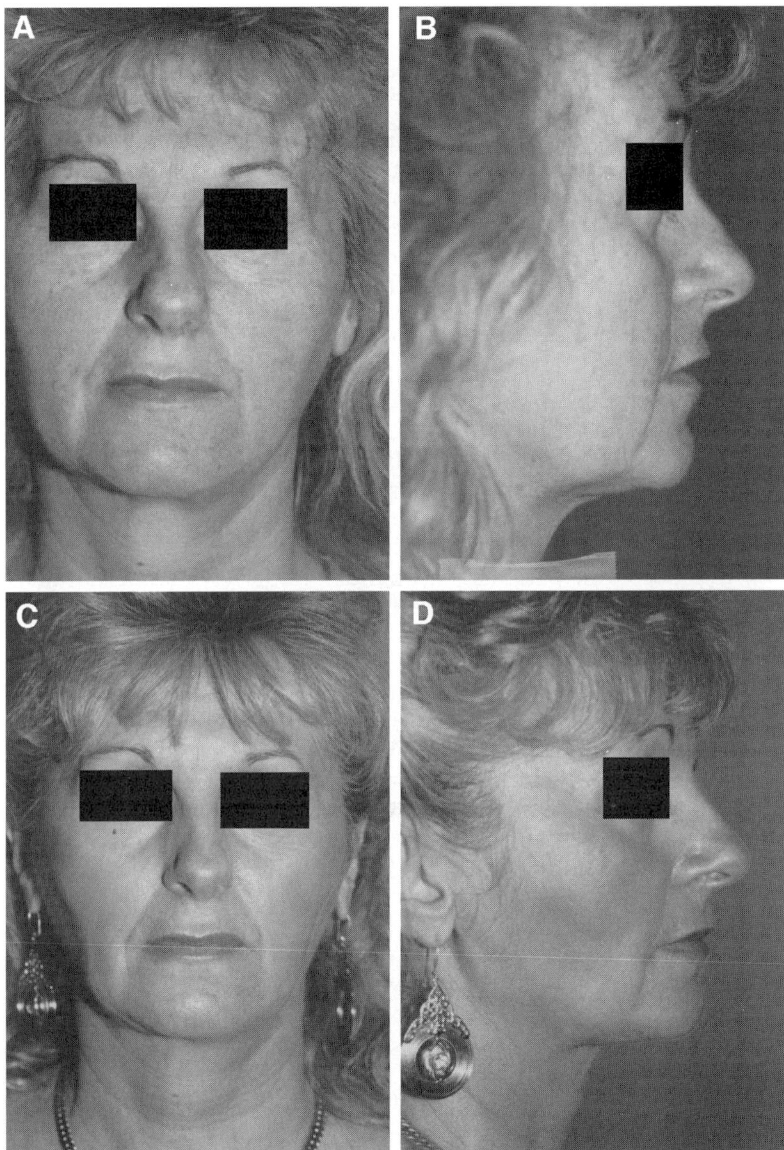

FIGURE 8.—Borderline indication. A 55-year-old woman had liposuction of the mental region and the inferior and middle thirds of the face. **A** and **B**, preoperative view. **C** and **D**, 6-month result. (Courtesy of Flageul G, Illouz Y-G. Isolated cervicofacial liposuction applied to the treatment of aging (French). *Ann Chir Plast Esthét* 41:620–630, 1996.)

The Management of Platysma Bands

McKinney P (Chicago)
Plast Reconstr Surg 98:999–1006, 1996

4–22

Introduction.—Addition of the midline approach in reduction of platysma bands can lead to complications including hematoma, infection, and a temporary "leatherneck" appearance. With the lateral approach alone, however, the bands may be persistent. The records of 200 consecutive patients who underwent correction of platysma bands were reviewed to determine the best method of treatment and identify those patients in whom the extra risk of midline work is justified.

Methods.—Platysma bands were classified into 4 types according to the required operative treatment. Bands I are barely visible in the neck and are handled by a lateral submucosal aponeurotic system flap alone without midline work. Bands II through IV are moderate bands that are visible in the neck and differ in the type of surgery indicated. Bands II need only midline suturing of the platysma muscle, whereas Bands III require resection of redundant edges of the muscle and midline suturing. Patients with bands IV need a lateral pull as well as midline work.

Results.—Sixty-one patients with bands I underwent a lateral pull only. Complications in this group included leather skin (6%), hematoma (6%), scar revision (3%), and infection (3%); reoperation was required in 3% of patients. The remaining 138 patients with bands II, III, or IV had midline work. A complete platysma flap, as described by Connell, was performed in 3 patients; 13 had a Z-plasty as described by Weisman; and 14 had a corset as described by Feldman. Leather skin occurred in 10% of patients with midline work; hematoma, scar revision, infection, and the need for reoperation each occurred at a rate of 3%. Creation of a muscle sling by suturing the edge of the muscle in the midline proved more effective than Z-plasty, plications, and/or excisions for correction of prominent platysma bands.

▶ The technique of platysma bands suturing the midline is well known so I have not repeated that information here, but those who do not have a clear understanding of the technique can look at the original article. The point is that when the midline is entered through a submental incision, the morbidity increases. A patient would be back in circulation sooner with a lateral pull alone. However, for a subset of patients—those whose bands are noticeable in the neutral position—a lateral pull of the submucosal aponeurotic system flap alone will probably be insufficient; therefore, the surgeon must make the call as to when the extra morbidity is worth the amount of improvement that can be obtained.

P.W. McKinney, M.D.

A Comparison Between Parallel Hairline Incisions and Perpendicular Incisions When Performing a Face Lift

Camirand A, Doucet J (Aesthetic Plastic Surgery, Montreal)
Plast Reconstr Surg 99:10–15, 1997   4–23

Introduction.—It is unclear what is the best type of incision to make when performing a face lift: parallel or at a perpendicular angle to the hair follicles. In one technique, flaps of hair follicles with their associated papillae are advanced under the distal flap of the face lift to get hair to grow through and anterior to the scar. This technique was described, and a double-blind study comparing incisions made parallel and perpendicular to the hair follicles was reported.

Technique.—To preserve deep papillae and the deep part of the follicles, incisions are made with a scalpel beveled 30 to 45 degrees to the surface of the scalp (Fig 2). Micro W incisions are used to avoid tension, with the proximal flap incised in micro W fashion and the distal flap excised in a straight line. Imbrication of these 2 incisions produces minimal pleating with a virtually invisible scar.

Study Findings.—Parallel and perpendicular incisions were compared in the same patient—the incision was made parallel in 1 patient and perpendicular to the hair follicles on the other side. The results were compared in double-blind fashion. Based on the absence of hypopigmentation, the non-linearity of the scar, and the abundance of hair into and in front of the scar, the aesthetic results were judged to be better with the incision made parallel to the hair follicles.

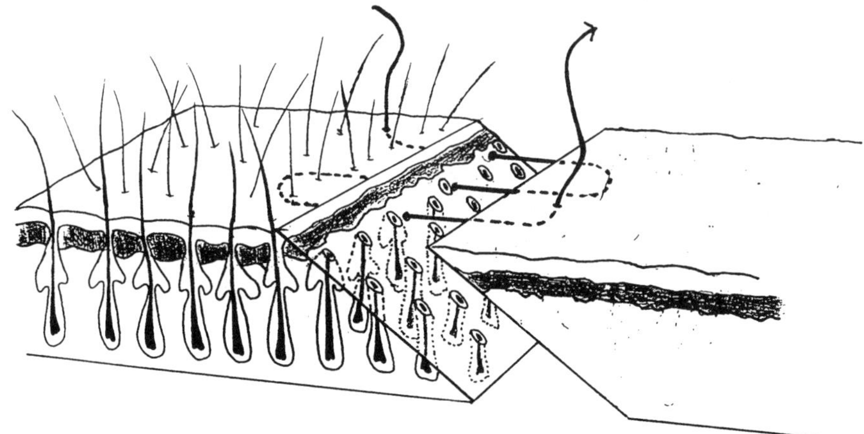

FIGURE 2.—Beveled list incision: the proximal flap (on the left) contains deep hair follicles, and the distal flap (on the right) will serve as a biological dressing, allowing the hair follicles to grow into and anterior to the scar. (Courtesy of Camirand A, Doucet J: A comparison between parallel hairline incisions and perpendicular incisions when performing a face lift. *Plast Reconstr Surg* 99:10–15, 1997.)

Conclusions.—When performing face lifts, making the incision perpendicular to the hair shaft provides better aesthetic results. Beveling the incision as described preserves the deeper part of the hair follicle in the proximal flap, permitting hair to grow into and in front of the scars. The technique requires meticulous closure with no tension.

▶ I love it when authors challenge dogma. This technique has worked very well and does help to hide scars. It has been confirmed by other authors as well.[1]

P.W. McKinney, M.D.

Reference

1. Kerth JD, Toriumi DM: Management of the aging forehead. *Arch Otolaryngol Head Neck Surg* 116:1137–1142, 1990.

A Dynamic Analysis of Changes in the Nasolabial Fold Using Magnetic Resonance Imaging: Implications for Facial Rejuvenation and Facial Animation Surgery
Gosain AK, Amarante MTJ, Hyde JS, et al (Med College of Wisconsin, Milwaukee)
Plast Reconstr Surg 98:622–636, 1996 4–24

Background.—Surgical reduction of the nasolabial fold in aging patients continues to be challenging. In addition, re-creating a natural nasolabial fold is 1 of the most difficult aspects of facial reanimation surgery. Magnetic resonance imaging was used in young and elderly women to determine the relative contribution of skin, subcutaneous tissue, and muscle to dynamic changes in the nasolabial fold during facial animation and aging.

Methods.—The 16 healthy volunteers, half aged 16–30 years and half aged 60 years and older, underwent imaging with their faces in repose and while smiling. Anatomical landmarks were observed, and measurements were obtained on the MRI console.

Findings.—Image resolution of the facial tissue planes was excellent. With the face in repose, comparisons between age groups showed progressive thickening of the dependent part of the cheek fat pad and overlying skin, with no evident change in the muscle plane comprising the levators of the upper lip. This resulted in a deeper, more acute nasolabial fold in the older women. Both age groups had a significant shortening of the mimetic muscles with smiling, with the lateral mimetic muscles drawn closer to the underlying facial bones. This occurred through redistribution of the cheek fat pad. Projection of surface landmarks in the cheek mass in young women was maintained with smiling.

Conclusions.—To reduce the nasolabial fold, surgery should be directed to the skin and subcutaneous tissue planes superficial to the mimetic muscles to the upper lip. To re-create a natural nasolabial fold, contraction of the levator muscles to the upper lip should result in redistribution of the cheek fat pad without changing the surface projection of the cheek mass or upper lip. This can be achieved only if the reconstructed levator muscle is positioned deep to the cheek fat pad, with its insertion toward the deep surface of the upper lip.

▶ This resurrects the argument of periosteal vs. deep-plane face lifts. It does not consider the fact that the subperiosteals shred the periosteum and splay it out over the cheek. This may be why subperiosteal dissections appear to rejuvenate as well as more superficial dissections. Without the "splaying" effect, the deeper dissections theoretically will not smooth the surface.

P.W. McKinney, M.D.

Pathogenesis and Treatment of the Nasolabial Fat Pad: Nasolabial Dermolipopexy (French)
Trepsat F (Lyon, France)
Ann Chir Plast Esthet 41:613–619, 1996

4–25

Background.—After plastic surgery to the perioral or nasolabial regions, the nasolabial fat pad can tubulize into a tube continuous with the jowl. Other surgeons have treated this problem with extensive liposuction of the nasolabial fat pad, with a "super submucosal aponeurotic system" flap, and with thinning of the fat pad, among other techniques. This author reports his experience with a subadipose facelift and internal fixation of the nasolabial fat pad to the inferior orbital margin, anchored by an external plastic plate.

> *Technique.*—First, the least possible nasolabial fat is left connected to the skin. The fat is separated from the fibromuscular plane via SACS. Subadipose detachment is extended from the side of the nose to the top of the lip and down to the jowls. The nasolabial fat pad is opened by 2 or 3 incisions, and a 2.5 × 1-cm plate of semirigid material, such as radiographic film, is applied to the external skin (which also helps prevent tubulization of the fat pad). The fat pad is then internally suspended to the inferior orbit via Prolene sutures from the top of the fat pad to right below the lip, and the sutures are tied off externally. Lifting typically occurs in about 8 days, after which the plastic plate and sutures are removed.

Conclusion.—Based on 2 years of experience, this technique of external plate dermolipopexy has shown good results for patients with marked nasolabial fat pads, particularly when the rest of the cheek is not fatty. The piece of external plastic provides extra support for lifting during the postoperative period.

▶ I prefer a subperiosteal lift when elevating the malar regions. When limited to the malar elevation, I believe this accomplishes the same thing without leaving the synthetic material in place.

P.W. McKinney, M.D.

Facial Rejuvenation: A Combined Conventional and Endoscopic Assisted Lift

de la Fuente A, Santamaría AB (Madrid)
Aesthetic Plast Surg 20:471–479, 1996   4–26

Background.—The introduction of endoscopic techniques has benefited facial rejuvenation procedures, especially in the upper face and midface. An approach to facial rejuvenation that combines conventional and endoscopic procedures was presented.

A Combined Conventional and Endoscopic Assisted Lift for Facial Rejuvenation.—An endoscopic assisted method is used for a forehead lift. For the face and neck, however, the conventional lift is still preferred. Young and middle-aged patients with midface ptosis and pronounced nasolabial/nasoyugal folds without significant skin excess are good candidates for subperiosteal endoscopic midface lifts with no skin resection. Another good indication for subcutaneous endoscopic assisted lifts is ptosis of the temporomalar or facial area. This minimally invasive technique is less traumatic and time-consuming, and permits a greater range of possibilities for individual needs because it limits the incision and dissection and is better accepted by patients (Fig 17).

Conclusions.—The combination of conventional and endoscopic techniques provides more possibilities for individual needs, limits the extension of the excision, and reduces morbidity. This approach also meets with better patient acceptance.

▶ For younger patients, this approach avoids the peri-auricular scar altogether and makes moot the polemic question of pre-tragal or post-tragal incisions.

P.W. McKinney, M.D.

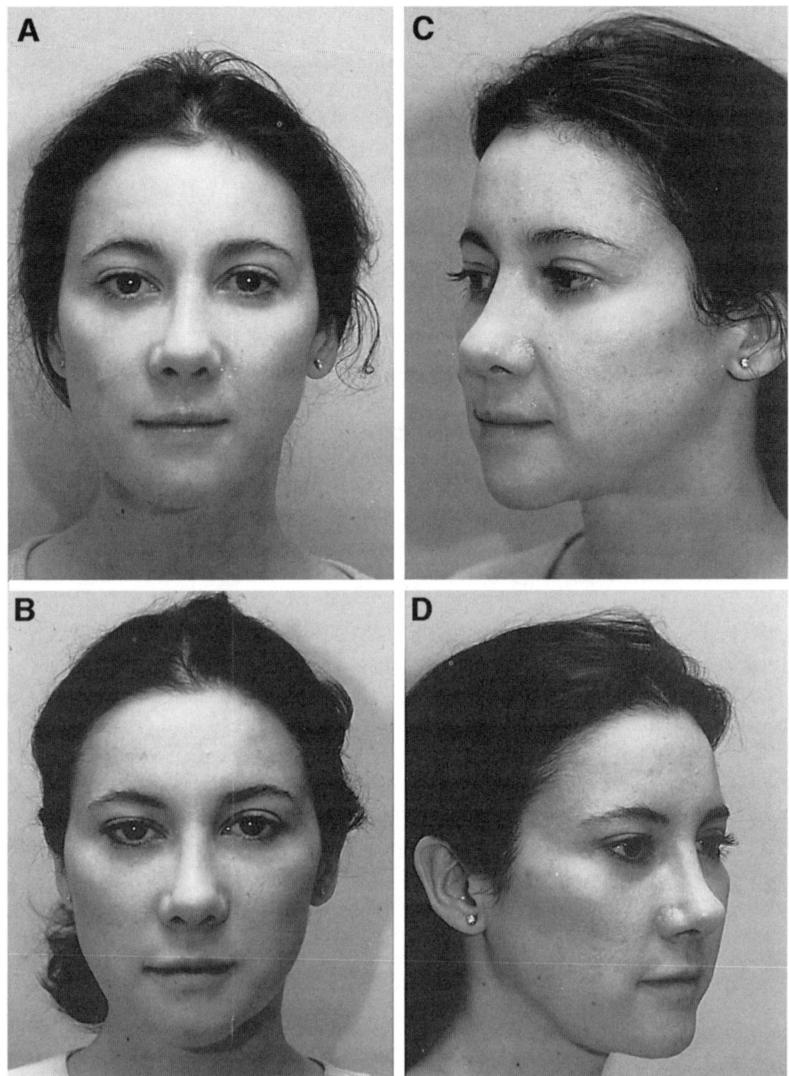

FIGURE 17.—Preoperative frontal (**A**) and oblique (**C**) views of a 35-year-old patient. She had already had a malar shell implant. Six months postoperative (**B** and **D**) views after only an endoscopic midface lift. Observe the improvement of the superior part of the nasolabial fold and the malar area. (Courtesy of de la Fuente A, Santamaría AB: Facial rejuvenation: A combined conventional and endoscopic assisted lift. *Aesth Plast Surg* 20:471–479, 1996. ©1996 Springer-Verlag New York Inc.)

Results of Biplane Facelifts With Maximal Skin Underlining and Vertical SMAS Flap (French)

Mitz V, Leblanc P, Maladry D, et al (Hôpital Boucicaut, Paris)
Ann Chir Plast Esthet 41:603–612, 1996   4–27

Background.—Evaluating the results of plastic surgery is difficult because many patients will not return for consultation unless they are unhappy. These authors used a questionnaire and follow-up visits to determine patient satisfaction after face lifts involving a submucosal aponeurotic system (SMAS) flap.

Methods.—Questionnaires were sent to 148 patients who had undergone a facelift between 1989 and 1994. Patients used a 10-point scale (0 = no improvement, 9 = maximum improvement) to rate their satisfaction with the results in 3 areas: the nasolabial folds, the jowls, and the neck. Only 54 patients (36%) who filled out a questionnaire returned for consultation (mean follow-up, 26.8 months after surgery), and results for these patients are reported.

Findings.—Overall, 70% of patients reported satisfactory results. Almost 75% of patients reported improvement (scores of 5 or higher on the 10–point scale) for the nasolabial folds, 77% for the jowls, and 60% for the neck. Conversely, almost 16% of patients reported no improvement (score of 0) for the nasolabial folds, 17% for the jowls, and 32% for the neck. After 2 years, degradation of results was reported by 29% of patients for the nasolabial folds, by 32% of patients for the jowls, and by 11% of patients for the neck. Complaints regarding wrinkles were common: 9% of patients complained about "lion's wrinkles," and 15% about perioral wrinkles. Finally, almost one third of patients claimed that, before surgery, they had not been sufficiently informed regarding the recuperation period.

Conclusion.—Although the majority of patients were satisfied with the results, there is room for improvement. Patients reporting the worst results for the nasolabial folds often had thick, fatty skin, and greater resection may be helpful in these cases. Those reporting the worst results for the jowls tended to be patients for whom the jowls were the most important aspect of the facelift. Regarding those reporting the worst results for the neck, many procedures had not given great enough attention to the platysma. Wrinkle complaints could be lessened by greater attention to dermabrasion during the facelift. Overall, however, use of the SMAS flap was associated with patient satisfaction.

▶ I respect the fact that an experienced author indicates a 10% dissatisfaction rate. Much of this depends upon what picture the surgeon paints as to what the patient can anticipate in terms of changes. It is still amazing to me that in spite of the fact that we emphasize reduction rather than elimination of the patient's problems, patients return to complain about the very thing you cautioned them about. This "selective hearing difficulty" probably relates to multiple consultations and the patients' perceptions of what you said to them.

P.W. McKinney, M.D.

Subperiosteal Minimally Invasive Laser Endoscopic Rhytidectomy: The SMILE Facelift
Ramirez OM, Pozner JN (Plastic and Aesthetic Surgical Ctr, Lutherville, Md)
Aesthetic Plast Surg 20:463–470, 1996   4–28

Objective.—Total facial rejuvenation requires an integrated approach to achieve an aesthetic balance. Minimally invasive procedures involving subperiosteal minimally invasive laser endoscopic (SMILE) rhytidectomy were performed on 11 patients to reposition lip elevators and correct oral frowning without risk of flap necrosis.

Technique.—With the patient in the sitting position, 3 to 5 incisions are made in the scalp, 2 temporal, 1 central, and/or 2 paramedian. The temporal line is freed, large veins are preserved, and the upper forehead and scalp are dissected to the vertex and the superior orbital rim is exposed. A subperiosteal midface lift is performed. Cervicoplasty, if necessary, is accomplished through a submental incision. After closure, laser resurfacing is performed with a Coherent Ultrapulse 5000C laser.

Results.—No patients had flap necrosis. Patients were followed up for up to 8 months. Recovery was uneventful with the exception of 1 patient who had a herpes simplex infection.

Case 1.—Woman, 47, with upper and lower blepharoplasty, had an endoscopic forehead lift, midface lift, and full facial laser resurfacing.
Case 2.—Woman, 48, with dermabrasion and mini-facelift, had a forehead lift, midface lift, and full facial laser resurfacing.
Case 3.—Woman, 39, with acne scarring and asymmetric malar area, had a forehead lift, midface lift, cheek implants, and full facial laser resurfacing.

Conclusion.—The subperiosteal approach to total facial rejuvenation combined with laser resurfacing results in excellent flap vascularity and uneventful postoperative recovery.

▶ A subperiosteal approach offers the best vascularity of the flap and, therefore, combining it with a peel is safe. Some authors combine peels with a sub-SMAS approach, but this is extremely risky and the peel has to be very light.

P.W. McKinney, M.D.

Is There a Difference? A Prospective Study Comparing Lateral and Standard SMAS Face Lifts With Extended SMAS and Composite Rhytidectomies
Ivy EJ, Lorenc ZP, Aston SJ (Manhattan Eye, Ear, and Throat Hosp, New York)
Plast Reconstr Surg 98:1135–1143, 1996   4–29

Background.—Extended submucosal aponeurotic system (SMAS) and composite rhytidectomies involve extensive dissection with increased soft-tissue reaction and postoperative recovery time. The risk of nerve injury is increased because the necessary dissection is close to the facial nerve. Limited SMAS, conventional SMAS, extended SMAS, and composite rhytidectomies were compared in a prospective study.

Methods.—Twenty-one patients, aged 47 to 70 years, were randomly assigned to undergo a limited or conventional SMAS face lift on 1 side and an extended SMAS or composite rhytidectomy on the other. The minimum follow-up period was 1 year.

Findings.—At the completion of the operation, more improvement was observed in the reversal of midfacial ptosis and flattening of the nasolabial folds with extended SMAS and composite rhytidectomies. The nasolabial folds and oral commissure were improved most dramatically with the composite flap. After 24 hours, however, the differences in the midface and nasolabial folds were no longer apparent. There were no differences between sides at the 6- and 12-month assessments.

Conclusions.—Limited and conventional SMAS face lifts yield outcomes just as good as those achieved with extended SMAS and composite rhytidectomies at 6 and 12 months after operation. None of these procedures improve midface ptosis and the nasolabial folds. Thus, the increased surgical risk, morbidity, and convalescence associated with the more extensive procedures do not seem justified in average patients.

▶ This is a provocative study that ended the original presentations at the American Society of Aesthetic and Plastic Surgeons meeting. It was very convincing when the audience had a chance to see more examples of results than are shown in this article. Although one can find limitless criticism of the scientific methodology of the authors' approach, their question is valid. Intellectually, I believe strongly that not all patients need the same operation, and that determining whether a ptotic fat pad, a ptotic jowl, or a bad neck is present can lead the surgeon to the right therapy (i.e., a midface procedure in a younger patient with a ptotic fat pad and a slight jowl, but a good neck, would avoid a pre-auricular incision altogether, whereas an older patient with a previous lift, a minor jowl, and mainly a neck problem without ptosis of the cheek pad could benefit from subcutaneous lift with less risk and considerably less expense). The concept of "one size fits all" is something most surgeons have abandoned in rhinoplasty, and I think we will find the same to be true of rhytidectomy.

P.W. McKinney, M.D.

▶ The authors are to be congratulated for trying to determine whether "more or new" is better. My bias suggests that they are correct in their assessment, but I would feel better if I knew that they had presented accurate photos of consecutive patients to a panel of experts who were unaware of what procedure had been performed. That should have been provided with criteria with which to judge the results, then their assessments could be compared to determine interrater reliability. Moreover, in keeping with the authors' suggestion, longitudinal studies using similar evaluators (unaware of the procedure performed) could address the issue of longevity of these procedures.

S.H. Miller M.D.

Aesthetic and Safety Considerations in Composite Rhytidectomy: A Review of 145 Patients Over a 3-Year Period

Pina DP (Clinica Pompêo de Pina, Goiânia, Brazil)
Plast Reconstr Surg 99:670–678, 1997   4–30

Introduction.—Many surgeons have been using the technique of composite rhytidectomy described by Hamra in 1990. The author of this study presents his experience with composite rhytidectomy and describes a contribution to the original technique that includes cheek fat undermining through the upper approach instead of the lateral approach.

Methods.—The study population underwent 145 composite rhytidectomies from September 1992 through October 1995. There were 133 primary, 8 secondary, and 4 tertiary procedures, all performed by the same surgeon and with local and block anesthesia. Patients ranged in age from 40 to 70 years. Upper blepharoplasty is performed using a conventional technique. For inferior blepharoplasty, the orbicularis dissection is extended to the inferior and lateral border of the orbicularis. In contrast to Hamra's technique, cheek fat is undermined through the upper approach—a variation that is easier to perform and reduces the anxiety of getting under the zygomaticus muscle. As the suborbicularis dissection reaches the inferior and lateral border of this muscle, the orbicularis flap is kept under strong upper traction. Undermining then continues down to the nasolabial fold and upper lip.

Other variations to Hamra's technique take place during cervical undermining. If a cervical fat sculpture is needed, sharp dissection is used to get the flap as thin as 0.5 cm. When no fat sculpture is needed, blunt dissection is used and all fat is left in the cutaneous flap. Systematized surgical steps and a "second look" before closing each anatomical area help to prevent bleeding and postoperative hematoma.

Results.—Complications have included motor nerve injury in 3 patients. In each case, however, eyelid function was completely recovered within 4 weeks. There was a single sensory nerve injury (retroauricular with spontaneous return). No instances of expanding hematoma, skin slough, seroma, hypertrophic scar, or scar revision have been noted. Although only 4 patients received antibiotics postoperatively, no infections developed. In addition to good aesthetic outcome, the modified technique offers a quicker and easier recovery period.

► Approach through the eyelid is safer than going "over the horizon" from the standard lateral approach. I prefer the subperiosteal approach when I am going through the lower lids as it is bloodless. One can elevate the cheek pad and hide the orbital rim; this is an important diagnostic point because if one feels the puff of the lower lid and the infraorbital rim is just beneath this, it is not orbital fat but swelling over the infraorbital rim. Elevation of the malar fat pad is the correct treatment for this condition. Elevation of the cheek pad by itself also connects the infraorbital fat herniation in many cases.

P.W. McKinney, M.D.

Management of Parotid Leakage Following Rhytidectomy

McKinney P, Zuckerbraun BS, Smith JW, et al (Northwestern Univ, Chicago; Univ of California, Los Angeles)
Plast Reconstr Surg 98:795–797, 1996   4–31

Introduction.—The surgical treatment of aging deformities of the lower face and midface has gone through various phases. Techniques that use deeper planes of dissection have been developed to improve the results of rhytidectomy. These techniques often result in aggressive undermining of the superficial muscular aponeurotic system, and have a higher risk of complications. For example, damage to the parotid gland parenchyma can occur and result in subcutaneous salivary collections that may appear as parotid pseudocysts and progress to fistulas. Prolonged collections can cause thinning of the overlying skin and external rupture. A salivary collection can interfere with healing. Treatment to allow drainage and quick resolution of the pseudocyst is necessary. Repeated aspiration only prolongs the course, whereas insertion of a suction drain aids resolution. Two cases that illustrate the difference were described.

Case 1.—Woman, 73, had redundant tissues of the head and neck. An endoscopic subperiosteal brow lift, lower blepharoplasty, dermabrasion, and a lower face lift were performed. A sub-superficial muscular aponeurotic system dissection was done to the mid-cheek into the cheek line and neck. A parotid gland parenchymal laceration was noted during dissection of the superficial muscular aponeurotic system on the left side. A hematoma developed on the left side of the face 7 days after surgery. The hematoma was drained. A fluctuant swelling developed over the left masseter 9 days and 11 days after surgery. Needle aspiration was performed each time. When the swelling again reappeared, the rhytidectomy incision was opened and a suction drain was inserted. Drainage stopped after 5 days and the drain was removed. There were no further complications.

Case 2.—Woman, 56, sought rejuvenative surgery of the head and neck, and a sub-superficial muscular aponeurotic system rhytidectomy was performed. Pain and swelling developed on the right side of the jaw in the area overlying the parotid gland 3 days after surgery. On day 10, aspiration was performed, but the swelling reappeared the next day. The fluid was aspirated and the patient was started on propantheline. During the next 2 weeks, aspirations were done daily, but the swelling reappeared within hours each time. On day 38, nearly 3 weeks of aspirations alone and 10 days of pressure with aspirations had been performed. The cheek was flat and the pseudocyst seemed to resolve. For another 3 months, the patient had minor swelling with a sensation of fullness.

Discussion.—Parotid pseudocysts can occur after trauma or as a postparotidectomy complication. Suction drainage is recommended for postrhytidectomy pseudocysts or fistulas. Suction drainage allows more complete drainage and allows the skin flaps to adhere more quickly, preventing recurrent fluid collection. Pseudocysts usually resolve within 1 week when suction drains are used. This treatment is inconvenient to the patient, although this may be outweighed by the quick resolution.

▶ I will try aspiration 1–2 times, but if there is no improvement and it is a 2- or 3-cm tense mass, the placement of a drain will offer the patient more rapid healing.

P.W. McKinney, M.D.

New Use for the Temporalis Superficialis Fascia in the Facial Contour: Lip Sculpture
Diniz VM (Belo Horizonte, Minas Gerais, Brazil)
Aesthetic Plast Surg 20:519–526, 1996   4–32

Background.—After adolescence, the face begins to atrophy, resulting in flaccidity, loss of elasticity, hypotonia, muscular relaxation, and skin dehydration. The sunken places in the centripetal areas of the face cannot be corrected by conventional rhytidoplasty, even with good musculocutaneous stretching. The use of autologous grafting of the temporalis superficialis fascia was described.

New Use for the Temporalis Superficialis Fascia in the Facial Contour.— One surgeon has grafted 303 areas since 1989. These grafts are easy to obtain, resulting in no donor area problems. The grafts eliminate peribuccal wrinkles, contributing to the filling in and increase of the turgidity of the lips by hardening them. The cutaneous vermillion line is projected. The fasciae are interposed between the skin and muscles by dominating the skin action and having exceptional integration with no absorption. Place-

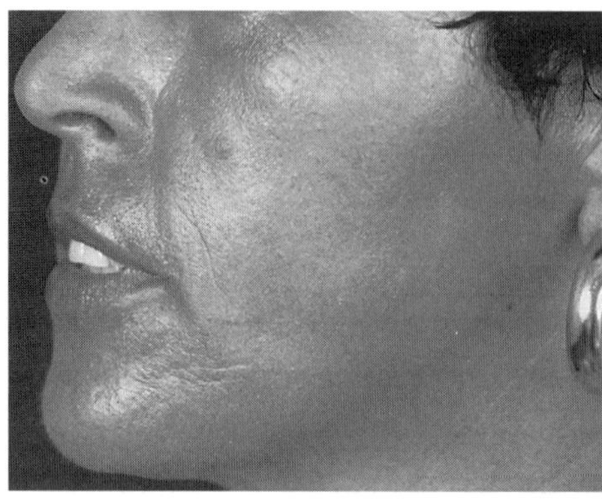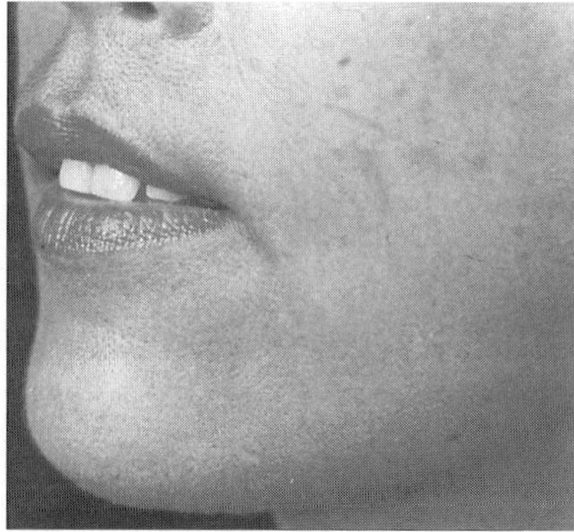

FIGURE 5.—Preoperative (A) and postoperative (B) views associating facelifting with fascial pieces, erasing labial wrinkles. Eight months postoperative. (Courtesy of Diniz VM: New use for the temporalis superficialis fascia in the facial contour: Lip sculpture. *Aesthetic Plast Surg* 20:519–526, 1996. © Springer-Verlag New York Inc.)

ment of the pieces of fascia is visualized with the assistance of a Reverdin needle. The same material is used to correct rhinoplasty sequelae and the increase of volume in the congenital or acquired sunken face (Fig 5).

Conclusions.—Autologous temporalis superficialis fascia grafts contribute positively to facial rejuvenation techniques. The fascia grafts smooth out the radial folds of the mouth, yielding definitive outcomes.

▶ Conventional wisdom teaches us to fill out the vermilion, but as the authors have shown in Figure 5, correcting the anatomical defect (an overriding principle of aesthetic surgery) gives a very sophisticated result in these patients, and the authors have placed this along the white roll in this case.

P.W. McKinney, M.D.

Wide Polytef (Gore-Tex) Implants in Lip Augmentation and Nasolabial Groove Correction

Conrad K, MacDonald MR (Univ of Toronto)
Arch Otolaryngol Head Neck Surg 122:664–670, 1996   4–33

Introduction.—Aging often makes the lips appear more narrow and exaggerates the natural nasolabial groove. Surgical improvement of these signs of aging may include attempts at lip augmentation and nasolabial groove correction. In the new technique described here, polytef was used for implantation along the upper and lower red lips and medial to the nasolabial skin crease.

Methods.—Polytef implantations were performed in 33 patients (all women) who wanted improved lip contour and 62 patients (52 women and 10 men) who sought correction of pronounced nasolabial grooves. Forty-four of 54 lip implants were made to the upper lip and 10 to the lower lip. A total of 134 implants were used to correct nasolabial grooves. Polytef was implanted via a new technique in which a subcutaneous tunnel is created. The shaped implants are usually 4 mm in thickness. Patients were followed for 12 to 54 months to assess outcome and satisfaction with cosmetic improvement.

Results.—No patient complained of sensory loss in the area of augmentation. Implants were most often described as being detectable as a "firmness." Preoperative and postoperative photographs documented improvement in the upper and lower lips and the nasolabial groove. The revision rate was initially high, and in most cases, additional polytef was added to increase volume or to reposition the original implant. Only 4 patients, 2 in each group, were not pleased with the final outcome.

Discussion.—Polytef has not been recommended for cosmetic lip augmentation or the removal of wrinkles, but the patients in this series were generally satisfied with results. The wide polytef implants were placed by means of subcutaneous tunneling, a technique that proved safe, simple, and effective.

▶ I have been leery of foreign material in a mobile thin area such as the lip, but others have reported good results.

P.W. McKinney, M.D.

Upper and Lower Lip Augmentation by Buried, Deepithelialized Local Flaps: An Alternative to the Use of Foreign Material Implants When Shortening the Lips
Kostianovsky AS (Buenos Aires, Argentina)
Aesthetic Plast Surg 20:433–437, 1996   4–34

Background.—Requests for lip augmentation are increasing, perhaps because of the simplicity of synthetic material injection. However, synthetic materials can have a short duration and yield bizarre results. Upper and lower lip augmentation by buried, deepithelialized local flaps was discussed.

> *Technique.*—A subnasal "moustache" is tailored in the upper third of the lip and left attached to its bed. If the surgeon intends to fill in the upper lip vertically in the central part only, as well as the nasolabial sulci, the original flap is divided horizontally into 4 secondary flaps. These include 2 inferior flaps based laterally, which will be buried in the crease after being freed from medial to lateral, and 2 superior ones, based at the very center of the lip, which are undermined from lateral to medial and buried under the filtral ridges and to the vermilion. A single stitch grasping the tip of the flap is used to secure the flaps to the skin for a few days. The entire original flap could be used in halves for filling in each side of the central lip if they are not needed for the nasolabial sulci.

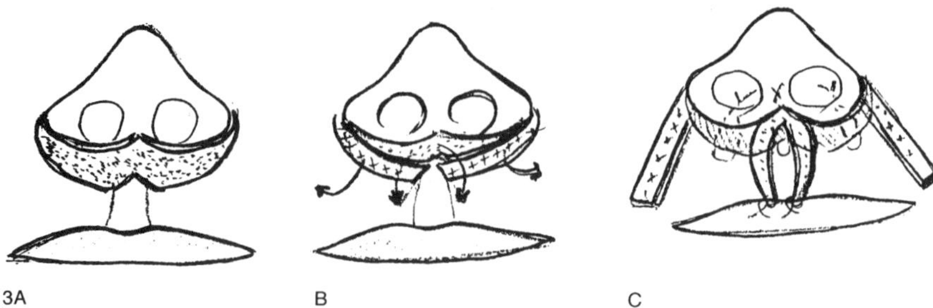

FIGURE 3.—**A,** for upper lip augmentation; a "moustache"-like flap is decorticated. **B,** the flap is horizontally divided into 4 flaps. **C,** 2 lower flaps for nasolabial sulci and 2 upper flaps for filling in filtral ridges and central vermilion. (Courtesy of Kostianovsky AS: Upper and lower lip augmentation by buried, deepithelialized local flaps: An alternative to the use of foreign material implants when shortening the lips. *Aesthetic Plast Surg* 20:433–437, 1996. Copyright 1996 Springer-Verlag New York Inc.)

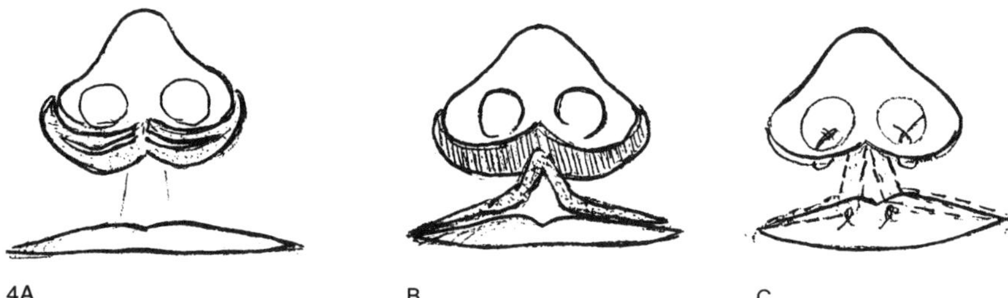

FIGURE 4.—**A,** the same decorticated flap could be tailored as a spiral. **B,** the flap is unrolled, allowing it to reach filtral ridges and vermilion down to the labial commissures. **C,** original "moustache" wound is closed by horizontal stitches; the knot at the nasal floor. Two stitches from the vermilion at the Cupid's bow peak and 2 from labial commissures grasping the flaps secure their position. (Courtesy of Kostianovsky AS: Upper and lower lip augmentation by buried, deepithelialized local flaps: An alternative to the use of foreign material implants when shortening the lips. *Aesthetic Plast Surg* 20:433–437, 1996. Copyright 1996 Springer-Verlag New York Inc.)

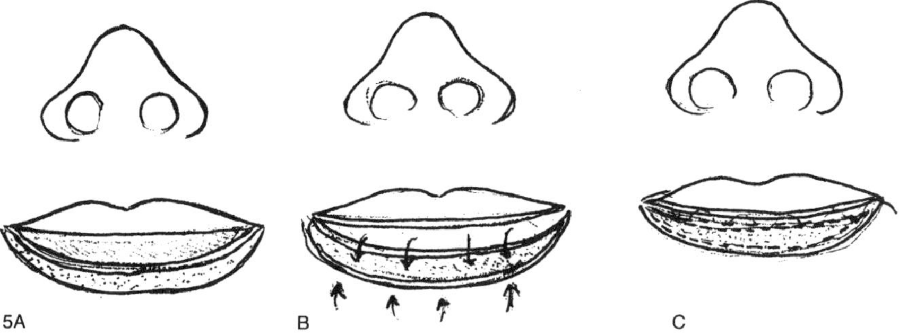

FIGURE 5.—**A,** for lower lip augmentation, a 3-mm decorticated flap is tailored below and following the mucocutaneous junction. **B,** The flap is left in situ and is covered by the slightly undermined vermilion and inferior skin, which is (**C**) sewn by an intracuticular running suture. (Courtesy of Kostianovsky AS: Upper and lower lip augmentation by buried, deepithelialized local flaps: An alternative to the use of foreign material implants when shortening the lips. *Aesthetic Plast Surg* 20:433–437, 1996. Copyright 1996 Springer-Verlag New York.)

However, in such cases, the flap can also be tailored as a spiral and based at its very center. For each side, the flap is left attached at the lower part of its center, and the surgeon cuts it as a narrow strip, beginning from the upper medial part. This strip is unrolled, then buried under the filtral ridges and vermilion border subdermally from Cupid's bow peaks to commissure. One stitch at the commissure and one at the level of Cupid's bow peak ensure flap position for a few days. The original wound is closed with several horizontal mattress sutures.

For vermilion augmentation, a narrow 3-mm deepithelialized flap is tailored below and following the mucocutaneous junction. With this flap left in situ, the superior semimucous and inferior cutaneous margins are undermined slightly to advance over the decorticated flap. The wound is closed with an intradermal running suture and a few single stitches (Figs 3–5).

Conclusions.—Lips augmented with dermofat flaps remain enlarged, with barely noticeable scars. This technique should be considered for patients seeking lip enhancement.

▶ This is a useful procedure but only in those older patients who will scar kindly (i.e., with dry, weathered skin), as the authors have illustrated. In young patients with oilier skin, this scar could be very troublesome.

P.W. McKinney, M.D.

Galea and Subgalea Graft for Lip Augmentation Revision
de Benito J, Fernández-Sanza I (Barcelona)
Aesthetic Plast Surg 20:243–248, 1996   4–35

Purpose.—More and more women are seeking aesthetic surgery to increase lip thickness. Lip augmentation procedures can be done as local plasties or as implants of heterogeneous or autogenous materials. Sometimes, different plasty and implant techniques are combined. An experience with the use of aponeurotic galea and subgalea grafts for lip augmentation was reviewed.

Methods.—The experience included 42 patients in whom the aponeurotic galea and subgalea grafts were used for lip augmentation. Augmentation of senile lips was done in 9 patients, upper lips in 7, and both upper and lower lips in 26. Unless concomitant surgical procedures were being done, all augmentations were done with the use of local anesthesia. The surgical technique introduced aponeurotic galea and subgalea into the space between the orbicular lip muscle and vestibular mucus, just behind the vermillion (Fig 1). The aponeurotic galea grafts ranged in length from 10 to 12 cm, and in width from 1 to 2 cm. The exact dimensions depended on the previous lip volume and the distance between the 2 buccal com-

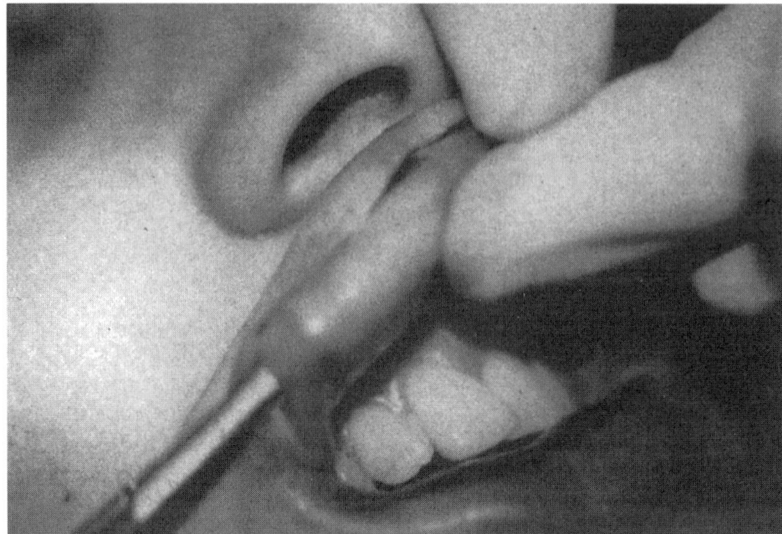

FIGURE 1.—Tunnel dissection through small incisions in the upper lip. The *inkline* shows the limit between the dry mucus and the gland vestibular mucus. (Courtesy of de Benito J, Fernández-Sana I: Galea and subgalea graft for lip augmentation revision. *Aesthetic Plast Surg* 20:243–248, 1996. Copyright 1996, Springer-Verlag New York Inc.)

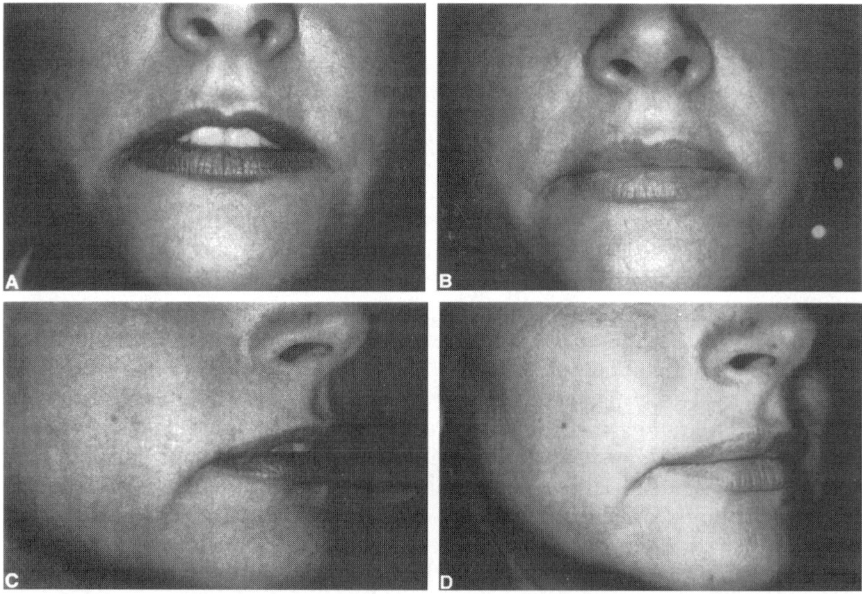

FIGURE 2.—Preoperative front (**A**) and profile (**C**) views of 35-year-old patient. One-year postoperative front (**B**) and profile (**D**) views. (Courtesy of de Benito J, Fernández-Sana I: Galea and subgalea graft for lip augmentation revision. *Aesthetic Plast Surg* 20:243–248, 1996. Copyright 1996, Springer-Verlag New York Inc.)

missures in "smile position." Thirty-one patients were available for 2-year follow-up.

Results.—Thirty-two percent achieved a moderate but persistent increase in the vermillion, 42% had a somewhat smaller lip volume than hoped for, and 26% were left with the same lip thickness. All lips were correctly shaped from an aesthetic viewpoint (Fig 2). The grafts were noticeably hardened on palpation; two thirds of the patients had tightness or even pain when smiling. Two patients required a second operation. Discomfort appeared to be less for patients with greater projection of their lips.

Conclusions.—Aponeurotic galea and subgalea grafts appear to be a useful material for moderate lip enlargement. This is an easily obtained, soft, and stretchable autologous material. The extent of enlargement of the labial mucus appears to be largely determined by its elasticity. This technique should make a useful addition to the available options for lip augmentation.

▶ I had always placed grafts between the white roll and the mucosa, but the placement behind the red line (wet mucosa) plumps the lip forward in a nice manner. See Figure 2.

P.W. McKinney, M.D.

Expanded Polytetrafluoroethylene Augmentation of the Lower Face

Sherris DA, Larrabee WF Jr (Mayo Clinic, Rochester, Minn; Univ of Washington, Seattle)
Laryngoscope 106:658–663, 1996　　　　　　　　　　　　　4–36

Objective.—Deep wrinkles and creases around the mouth are an aesthetic problem in the aging face. Soft-tissue augmentation can result in tissue antigenicity and rapid absorption. A retrospective review of lower face augmentation studies using expanded polytetrafluoroethylene (E-PTFE) in its microporous form has demonstrated safe and reliable augmentation, high biocompatibility, low tissue antigenicity, and increasing stability.

Methods.—Between January 1991 and January 1993, lower face E-PTFE augmentation was performed on 41 patients. Augmented sites included lips (21 patients, 63 sites), melolabial folds (18 patients, 36 sites), marionette lines (6 patients, 12 sites), the chin (2 patients, 2 sites), and the lower cheek (2 patients, 2 sites). Patients were followed up after surgery and interviewed within 4 weeks of surgery about loss of sensation.

> *Technique.*—Care is taken not to stretch the implant, and its size is individualized to the patient. The implant is vacuum impregnated with kanamycin before insertion into the melolabial crease at the superior and inferior ends of the crease. Subcutaneous tunnels are

constructed at points that are one third of the distance above the crease and two thirds of the distance below the crease. Triangular augmentation pockets are elevated inferiorly and laterally first with tenotomy scissors, then with the sharp end of a Cottle elevator, and finally with the blunt end of the elevator. The implant is placed using alligator forceps, and the incision is closed.

Results.—Complications included 1 seroma necessitating implant removal and 1 secondary procedure to increase insufficient augmentation and to correct a minor contour abnormality. The overall complication rate was 9.8%, and the complication rate per site was 5.2%. No extrusion, rejection, sustained foreign-body reaction, or systemic autoimmune disorder has been observed. Lip sensation is normal in all patients. The external melolabial-crease incision left no scar.

Conclusion.—Short-term use of E-PTFE for lower face augmentation is safe and effective. Additional studies are needed to establish long-term results.

▶ I have used this material for nasal dorsal augmentation (2 mm). I have seen 1 patient with lip augmentation who objected to its firmness, perhaps because this was too large an implant or because of unfavorable capsule formation. I still have concerns about foreign material.

P.W. McKinney, M.D.

Aesthetic Analysis of the Eyebrows
Gunter JP, Antrobus SD (Univ of Texas, Dallas)
Plast Reconstr Surg 99:1808–1816, 1997   4–37

Objective.—The possibility of achieving the perfect brow after browlift has been enhanced by new techniques and instrumentation. For the purpose of defining the ideal brow, brow aesthetics were evaluated by reviewing photographs of a group of fashion models and before and after photographs of a group of patients who underwent facial rejuvenation.

Methods.—Computer imaging was used to alter the shape and position of models' eyebrows and to produce 4 different shapes. Aesthetic results were evaluated by groups of plastic surgeons attending a symposium. The shape and position of the eyebrows of 7 patients are discussed.

Results.—Brows need to be evaluated while considering the entire periorbital area, including the eyelids. Criteria for attractive eyes were developed. Common surgical mistakes include overelevating brows, placing the brow peak medially, creating too high a lateral peak, large asymmetric differences in brow height, overresection of the medial brow depressors, and unmasking deep hollowing in the eyes.

Conclusion.—Simply performing a brow lift will not necessarily improve the patient's appearance. The eyebrow must be repositioned or reshaped or both to suit the individual and to harmonize with the shape of the periorbital area.

▶ We have to measure the "glide" factor, that is, we can set the periosteum or galea but we can't control the superficial fat; hence, some patients are going to relapse not because of slippage or release but because of the glide of superficial fat.

P.W. McKinney, M.D.

Biodegradable Positive Fixation for the Endoscopic Brow Lift
Pakkanen M, Salisbury AV, Ersek RA (Tampere, Finland; Southwest Texas State Univ, Austin)
Plast Reconstr Surg 98:1087–1091, 1996   4–38

Background.—Although various modifications have been proposed over the years, brow lift usually entails a bicoronal incision with subgaleal dissection. In endoscopic brow lift, the periosteum of the orbital rims and zygomaxilla can be separated and repositioned without the need for skin excision. One technique of and experience with endoscopic brow lift was reported, including the use of biodegradable positive fixation.

Technique.—The technique uses 2 inconspicuously placed incisions near the midportion of the scalp, avoiding the need for bicoronal incision. Subperiosteal dissection then is performed to the orbital rims and zygomatic arch anteriorly and to the occipital base posteriorly. This dissection permits contracture of the occipitalis muscle to contribute to brow repositioning and lifting. Seven sutures of long-acting poly-L-lactide acid then are placed through the pericranium of the periosteum and frontalis, along the superior and lateral border of the orbital rim. The sutures are secured to 2 absorbable pins placed in the outer table of the cranium. The pins allow positive fixation for more than 6 weeks, maintaining precise positive positioning until there is complete wound healing and reattachment of the structures. The pins are barely palpable and are resorbed within 6 to 24 months.

Experience.—This technique has been used in 14 patients since 1993. The 24-month results are promising. There are a few weeks of postoperative puckering, but this problem is justified by the final results. There are few complications; swelling may occur, along with periorbital ecchymosis and temporarily reduced sensitivity to the forehead and scalp. There have been no recurrences of brow ptosis and no treatment failures.
Conclusions.—Promising results are achieved with this endoscopic technique of brow lift using biodegradable positive fixation. This technique provides precise, positive positioning without the need to remove percu-

taneous screws. Longer follow-up is needed to confirm the results achieved.

▶ Until we know the value of any type of fixation, I prefer the concept of something that does its job and leaves quietly.[1] Whether one uses suture to a drill hole on the outer plate or a pin that dissolves makes little difference.

P.W. McKinney, M.D.

Reference

1. McKinney P, Celetti S, Sweis I: An accurate technique for fixation in endoscopic browlift. *Plast Reconstr Surg* 97:824, 1996.

Endoscopic Forehead Lift: An Operative Technique
Daniel RK, Tirkanits B (Univ of California Irvine, Newport Beach, Calif)
Plast Reconstr Surg 98:1148–1157, 1996   4–39

Background.—The endoscopic forehead lift has been evolving in recent years. One group's experience with more than 100 such procedures was presented.

Methods and Findings.—After the first 60 procedures were performed, it was concluded that brow elevation could be maintained and the procedure done with acceptable morbidity. To further improve aesthetic outcomes, the procedure was modified significantly. Currently, several components appear to be critical. A subgaleal resection of muscle insertions should be used rather than a sub-periosteal approach to muscle origins. A complete periosteal release along the lateral orbital rim is needed. Vertical suspension is performed using screws and staples that are removed after 1 week. Finally, a lateral temporal expansion with absorbable sutures is performed.

Conclusions.—Effective eyebrow elevation between the intercanthal line and the top of the eyebrow is possible, with no significant expansion of forehead height. Refinements of the endoscopic forehead lift continue, with emphasis on how to change the shape of the eyebrow and reduce asymmetry.

▶ We are gaining experience with the endoscopic forehead lift and are grateful to the authors for adding some science to our quest. A factor that is not measured in browlift generally is the "glide" phenomenon (i.e., the extent of the superficial fat pads and how much the skin would glide under galeal periosteum), which may explain why it is difficult to permanently shape the brows or correct asymmetry by these methods. I am still amazed at the number of very fine surgeons who will not use an endoscopic approach, whereas I believe very strongly that it is the preferred method for the vast majority of patients.

P.W. McKinney, M.D.

Preventing Hairline Elevation in Endoscopic Browlifts
Hamas RS, Rohrich RJ (Univ of Texas, Dallas)
Plast Reconstr Surg 99:1018–1022, 1997   4–40

Introduction.—The open coronal browlift routinely results in a raised hairline. This elevation can be prevented by placing the incision along the hairline, but this solution is not ideal. An endoscopic-assisted method of brow elevation described here does not raise the hairline, nor is any skin or scalp resected.

Technique.—Problems that occur with existing methods of endoscopic browlifting are addressed by certain modifications: a single-plane endoscopic resection and direct suture fixation. Three 25- to 30-mm incisions are placed 15 mm behind and parallel to the hairline. Subgaleal dissection frees the back surface of the galea aponeurosis, and the front surface is freed from scalp and forehead skin along the hairline by dissecting inferior to each incision. Care is taken to dissect all fascia of the galea aponeurosis off the periosteum and the subcutaneous fat. To shorten the frontalis muscle–galea aponeurosis, it must be freed from adherent overlying skin and underlying periosteum. Plication sutures are placed with several interlocking distal bites, and the proximal suture is anchored into galea and dermis. The eyebrows are raised, leaving a temporary excess skin roll along the hairline. A modification of the technique allows the hairline to be raised in patients preferring this outcome.

Discussion.—Forty-seven patients, all women, have undergone this endoscopic browlift procedure. With an average follow-up of 9 months, satisfactory eyebrow elevation was maintained in all but 4 early cases. Eyebrow elevation ranged from 3 to 6 mm. Two patients chose to have the hairline raised and were pleased with the outcome; none of the other patients thought that the procedure resulted in hairline elevation. Complications were minor: 2 hematomas, 3 small seromas, and 2 very transient facial nerve paresis.

▶ I cannot measure much of a shift of the hairline in endoscopic browlift using a subperiosteal approach.

P.W. McKinney, M.D.

Endoscopic Forehead-Scalp Flap Fixation With K-Wire

Kim SK (Palo Alto, Calif)
Aesthetic Plast Surg 20:217–220, 1996

4–41

Objective.—Elevating the forehead and scalp can be accomplished by bone fixation or soft-tissue plication. Using Kirschner wire (K wire) to fix the forehead and scalp flap is less difficult and time consuming than bone fixation. New instrumentation that facilitates placement of the wires and the technique involved are discussed.

> *Technique.*—A cannula and trocar combination can be used to control depth of penetration into the bone. Alternatively, a special fixation pin with 2 different diameters so that it stops at a predetermined depth is under development. The forehead and scalp is elevated, and the temporal area is raised. After periosteal release, a 0.045 cannula-enclosed K wire is loaded on a driver in preparation for inserting it to a depth of 4 mm. The depth of insertion is controlled by a chuck that holds the wire in place in an acrylic guide until it is inserted through the scalp using a trocar. Once in place, the wire is driven into the skull and cut flush with the skin surface. The process is repeated with additional wires until the forehead is held suspended. Incisions are closed with staples. Staples and K wires are removed about 10 days later.

Results.—Satisfactory results have been obtained in 21 patients treated during a period of 18 months.

Conclusion.—Transcutaneous placement of K wires for endoscopic forehead–scalp flap fixation is a simple technique that does not require sutures. K wire placement, postoperative care, and K wire removal are simple and easy.

▶ If fixation is needed (and it seems that it is), K wire allows the placement of additional fixation without additional incisions. I still prefer drill holes through the bone because I feel comfortable with that and they are something I don't have to remove.

P. W. McKinney, M.D.

Transblepharoplasty Forehead Lift and Upper Face Rejuvenation

Ramirez OM (Johns Hopkins Univ, Baltimore, Md)
Ann Plast Surg 37:577–584, 1996

4–42

Background.—A brow lift and complete upper face rejuvenation can be done through upper blepharoplasty incisions. This procedure and its results in 14 patients were evaluated.

Technique.—The technique is indicated by male pattern bald-ness, a history of hair transplants, excessively high forehead, spas-tic frontalis syndrome, the need for periorbital or bicularis muscle repositioning, and when upper blepharoplasty is planned simulta-neously with the brow lift. The surgeon makes standard upper blepharoplasty incisions and dissects to the superior orbital rim. All soft tissues are elevated, but a cuff of periosteum and the overlying subgaleal fascia remains. The surgeon then dissects superiorly in the frontal area subgaleally or subperiosteally. If the dissection proceeds subperiosteally, the periosteum is entered about 1.5 cm above the orbital rim. In the temporal region, dissection is done in the subgaleal plane up to 1 cm above the zygomatic arch. With the endoscope introduced through the same incision, the surgeon can safely and accurately perform the dissection. Procerus and corru-gator muscle resection is done through the eyelid incision. The supratrochlear and supraorbital nerves are identified and pro-tected. The surgeon uses extra-fine-tip cautery for hemostasis. In

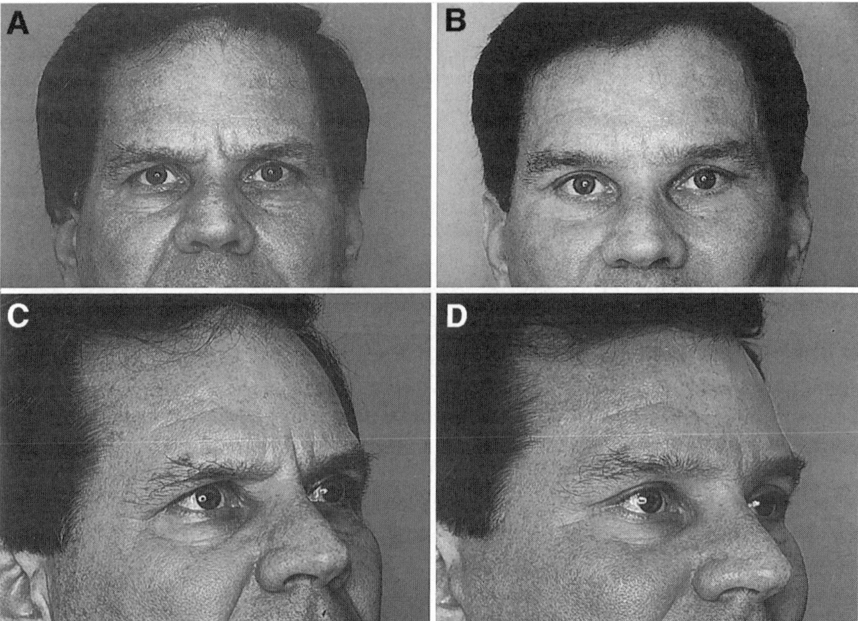

FIGURE 7.—**A,** preoperative frontal view of a 56-year-old patient with a high forehead, a stern look on his face, substantial brow ptosis, corrugator and procerus activity, and deep transverse forehead wrinkles. **B,** six-month postoperative frontal view after transblepharoplasty brow lift. Upper eyelid skin excision was minimal. Observe the elevation of the brow, the improvement of the transverse forehead wrinkles, the absence of the glabellar wrinkles, and improved aesthetics of his eyes. **C,** preoperative three-quarter view showing the patient with a high forehead, transverse forehead wrinkles, oblique deep glabellar creases, and substantial brow ptosis. **D,** postoperative three-quarter view. Observe the improve-ment in the aesthetics of the forehead, brow position, glabellar area, and upper eyelid. The improvement of the lower face results from the midface lift. (Reprinted from Ramirez OM: Transblepharoplasty forehead lift and upper face rejuvenation. *Ann Plast Surg* 37:577–584, 1996 by permission of Little, Brown and Company, Inc.)

the initial fixation, the retro-orbicularis oculi fat pad is sutured to the periosteum of the orbital rim. The surgeon sutures the tail of the brow to the temporal fascia and stabilizes the frontotemporal flap in an elevated position with an external tied-over dressing, percutaneous screws, or well-supportive contouring tape. The surgeon then closes the eyelids in a standard fashion.

Patients and Outcomes.—Fourteen patients have undergone this procedure. The endoscope was used in 12. Examination of the brow position, frontalis and corrugator activity, and upper face aesthetics showed outcomes similar to those of other techniques. Morbidity was also comparable. In addition, the new technique is more expeditious and results in fewer scars (Fig 7) than other techniques.

Conclusions.—Complete upper face rejuvenation can be performed through an endoscopic approach with several scalp slit incisions. The use of the endoscope makes the procedure more precise.

▶ This is a great technique for indications as described. It's hard to tell how much elevation you'll get with this, but Dr. Ramirez is certainly experienced in these techniques and feels it's similar to the endoscopic coronal.

P.W. McKinney, M.D.

Eyelids

The Surgical Anatomy of the Fat in the Upper Eyelid Medial Compartment

Ullmann Y, Levi Y, Ben-Izhak O, et al (Rambam Med Ctr, Garmish-Partenkirchen, Germany; Israel Inst of Technology, Haifa)
Plast Reconstr Surg 99:658–661, 1997   4–43

Background.—A previous clinical study of 55 consecutive patients found that although 56% had only 2 fat pads in the upper eyelids, 44% had 3 fat pads. The authors concluded that the third fat pad is anatomically and histologically an accessory medial extension of the lateral fat pad. This finding explained why some patients required secondary upper blepharoplasties, for the medial fat compartment had been left behind. The content of the medial compartment was investigated in 388 patients and 12 cadavers.

Methods.—The patients ranged in age from 39 to 75 years (mean, 56 years). All underwent primary aesthetic upper eyelid blepharoplasties. In addition, rhytidectomy was performed in 198 patients and lower blepharoplasty in 224. Careful attention was paid to the medial fat compartment of the upper eyelid. Histologic examination of fat was undertaken in samples from 5 cadavers and 5 patients.

Results.—The medial compartment of the upper eyelid was consistently found to contain 2 well-circumscribed fat pads. In 4 cadaver eyelids (16.7%), the medial compartment included 2 entirely separated fat pads, described according to location as the medial inferior pad and the medial superior pad. The fat pads in 11 cadaver eyelids (45.8%) were separated to only about half their length. In the remaining 9 eyelids, only the tips of the 2 fat pads were separated. Only the protruded part of the fat pads could be investigated in the patients. Most (59.8%) exhibited 2 separate fat pads in the medial compartment. In a single patient, the amount of resected fat and the extent of separation of the fat pads could differ between left and right eyelids. Histologic examination showed each of the medial fat pads to be circumscribed by a fibrous envelope. Adipose tissue within the fat pad was separated by fibrous septa.

Conclusion.—Surgeons who perform blepharoplasties should be aware of the possible existence of 2 different fat pads in each fat compartment of the upper eyelid. Residual fat in the medial compartments will result in fullness on the medial side of the upper eyelids after surgery.

▶ The medial and lateral fat pads are separate and of different colors in the upper lid and have different consistencies. Any fat excision should be conservative, otherwise the patient will have a hollow look.

P.W. McKinney, M.D.

Carbon Dioxide Laser Transconjunctival Lower Lid Blepharoplasty Complications
Trelles MA, Baker SS, Ting J, et al (Instituto Médico Vilafortuny, Cambrils, Spain; Cimarron Eye Ctr Inc, Oklahoma City; Day Laser Centre, Coogee, Australia; et al)
Ann Plast Surg 37:465–468, 1996   4–44

Objective.—Carbon dioxide laser lower eyelid blepharoplasty is a common cosmetic procedure. Complications associated with this procedure were reviewed.

Methods.—The retrospective study included 889 consecutive lower eyelid blepharoplasties. Seven hundred nine patients were women and 171 were men. All patients were followed up for at least 1 year to identify the intraoperative and early and late postoperative complications.

Results.—Complications were uncommon and usually not severe. The main intraoperative complication was corneal abrasion occurring when the upper eyelashes were trapped against the cornea by the Jaeger bone plate. This problem resolved with topical lubricants and short-term patching. All these complications occurred early in the series. Other intraoperative complications included lower eyelid perforation, eyelid burning, and hemorrhage. The hemorrhage sometimes was sufficient to produce ecchymosis, although there were no retrobulbar hematomas producing visual compromise. There were 2 cases of early postoperative conjunctivitis. Late complications included reoperation for removal of additional protruding fat, late hyperpigmentation in an area of hematoma formation, and granulomas.

Conclusions.—Complications of carbon dioxide laser lower lid blepharoplasty are uncommon and usually not serious. Most such complications are related to inexperience. The results suggest that carbon dioxide laser transconjunctival lower lid blepharoplasty is a safe and reliable procedure.

▶ It does not say this in the ads.

P.W. McKinney, M.D.

Periocular Skin Reshaping by CO_2 Laser Coagulation
Trelles MA, Kaplan I, Rigau J, et al (Instituto Médico Vilafortuny, Cambrils, Spain)
Aesthetic Plast Surg 20:327–331, 1996   4–45

Background.—In some patients undergoing blepharoplasty by the transconjunctival route, the excess of skin resulting from the overlaxness of the lower lid does not retract, and outcomes are disappointing. The results of a technique for controlled retraction of the eyelid by skin coagulation using the CO_2 laser were reported.

Methods.—Thirty-seven patients, aged 32 to 59 years, underwent transconjunctival lower lid blepharoplasty followed by coagulation of the skin area below both eyelids. After elimination of excess fat from the lower eyelids, the laser coagulation procedure was begun using CO_2 10 W defocused to 5 mm in diameter in 100-msec pulses. The Kaplan Pendulaser 115 with the optoguide was used with the focusing cone removed and the bare waveguide applied at about 2 to 3 mm from the skin surface.

Findings.—After 2 to 20 months of follow-up, outcomes were judged to be very good in 24 patients, good in 9, fair in 3, and bad in 1. In this last patient, a mild sclero-show developed. No other scarring or defects occurred after the scab was gone. Inflammation and edema resolved within about 3 weeks and erythema within 10 to 16 weeks after laser coagulation.

Conclusions.—Although the transconjunctival approach for blepharoplasty is safe for the treatment of lax skin on the lower eyelids, skin remodeling sometimes is needed. Laser reshape-coagulation may be an alternative method of choice for this purpose.

▶ Simultaneous conjunctival blepharoplasty with any resurfacing technique is safe as long as the blood supply is preserved to the flap. There is a small artery that comes in at the vertical of the mid-pupil but right at the infraorbital rim. If this is transected by any root, the flap is at risk.[1]

P.W. McKinney, M.D.

Reference

1. McKinney P, Zukowski M, Mossie R; The fourth option: A novel approach to lower lids blepharoplasty. *Aesthetic Plast Surg* 15:293, 1991.

Safety and Efficacy of Combined Upper Blepharoplasties and Open Coronal Browlift: A Consecutive Series of 600 Patients
Friedland JA, Jacobsen WM, TerKonda S (Phoenix, Ariz)
Aesthetic Plast Surg 20:453–462, 1996 4–46

Objective.—Upper facial rejuvenation usually involves a coronal forehead lift and blepharoplasty performed sequentially because of safety concerns. As laparoscopic procedures have become more common, endoscopic techniques have allowed complete upper facial rejuvenation to be performed as a combined procedure.

Technique.—An open foreheadplasty is performed using a bicoronal incision, with care taken not to injure hair follicles. The dissection is continued over the suborbital rim and over the radix area of the nose. The scalp and forehead are elevated, and the boundaries of the frontalis resection are marked. The frontalis muscle is cross-hatched and resected, and the procerus and corrugator supercilii muscles are dissected and divided. The forehead flap is re-draped, part is excised, and the excision is closed. The upper eyelid skin ellipse then is excised.

Results.—Between 1980 and 1995, 600 patients (96% women), aged 32 to 83, underwent concomitant procedures. Patients were followed up for an average of 5 years. More than 98% were satisfied with the appearance of their incisions and the lasting effects. Complications were rare and no adverse effects were reported. No patients required revision blepharoplasty, although 5 patients asked for secondary corrective procedures.

Conclusions.—The combined procedure was well tolerated with minimal morbidity. The convalescent period was short, the effect was lasting, and patient satisfaction was high.

▶ I support this technique of doing both procedures together unless there are ocular precautions, such as dry eye, contact lens wear, or a previous blepharoplasty, that raise the caution flag. I am pleased that the authors have documented this approach because one hears advice to do the blepharoplasty 3 months later, which adds considerably to the morbidity and expense, and in my view is unnecessary in most cases.

P.W. McKinney, M.D.

Use of a New Anchoring Device for Tendon Reinsertion in Medial Canthopexy

Antonyshyn OM, Weinberg MJ, Dagum AB (Univ of Toronto)
Plast Reconstr Surg 98:520–523, 1996

4–47

Background.—The Mitek Anchor System is a new device designed for ligament or tendon fixation to bone. Its use for medial canthal tendon reinsertion into bone was described.

Methods and Outcomes.—The Mitek Mini GII Anchor was used in a 22-year-old man with posttraumatic recurring isolated left telecanthus and a 62-year-old woman with recurrent basal cell carcinoma of the right cheek and medial canthal region. After the medial orbit was exposed subperiosteally and the preferred site for tendon reinsertion identified, a drill guide was introduced to protect the soft tissues, and an oblique 1.8-mm diameter drill hole was made at the exact location of tendon attachment. A 3-0 nonabsorbable suture was threaded through the hole in the anchor base. The anchor was then fitted into the inserter and inserted below the cortical surface. The medial canthal tendon was dissected through a 3-mm external incision just medial to the canthus, the tendon identified and mobilized, and the 2 ends of the suture were sewn to the tendon and snugged down flush to the bone at the anchor. The outcomes of this procedure were very satisfactory in the 2 patients described.

Conclusions.—The Mitek Mini GII Anchor System is simple and easy to use in tendon reinsertion in medial canthopexy. The system allows exact placement with minimal dissection.

▶ This technique is also used for forehead lifting as well as hand surgery. I am not sure how much time it saves compared with the drill hole technique.

P.W. McKinney, M.D.

Transconjunctival Blepharoplasty With Chemoexfoliation

Gilbert SE (Facial Plastic Surgery Ctr, Tulsa, Okla)
Ann Plast Surg 37:24–29, 1996

4–48

Background.—Transcutaneous blepharoplasty, the standard for aesthetic surgery of the lower eyelid, is associated with postoperative problems, including poor scarring, scleral show, and even frank ectropion. Although transconjunctival blepharoplasty (TCB) is a reliable technique for removing lower eyelid fat, it is not adequate in patients with excessive skin and may be responsible for increased lower lid wrinkling. The use of chemical peeling simultaneously with TCB was evaluated.

Patients and Outcomes.—One hundred forty-six patients underwent the 2 procedures at the same time. The minimum follow-up was 1 year. Seven different solutions were used, 6 of which were trichloroacetic acid–based. Subsequent peels were performed in all patients receiving a 15% to 35% solution. Overall, 27.4% of the patients undergoing the 2 procedures needed subsequent treatment. However, the use of solutions greater than 30% required a prolonged healing time that strained patient acceptance. A review of the first 50 patients indicated that a 25% solution was appropriate for most patients. Patients receiving solutions at this concentration were healed within 10 days, and only about 20% needed a repeat peel of 30% solution. Ninety-eight percent of the patients were satisfied with their final result.

Conclusions.—The simultaneous use of TCB and chemoexfoliation yielded excellent outcomes in lower eyelid appearance and pseudoherniated fat in most patients in the current series. No external lower eyelid scarring occurred.

▶ Our experience with this technique has been excellent.[1] Some have even used this with a skin muscle flap (but with a very limited undermining). However, I have had 1 patient out of 150 or so who came very close to a full-thickness burn when I used the Baker's formula phenol. Resurfacing is risky, and when combined with surgery, doubly so.

P.W. McKinney, M.D.

Reference

1. McKinney P, Zukowski M, Mossie R: The fourth option: A novel approach to the lower lid blepharoplasty. *Aesth Plas Surg* 15:293, 1991

Surgical Repair of Paralytic Lagophthalmos by Medial Tarsal Suspension of the Lower Lid
Castroviejo-Bolibar M, de Damborenea A, Fernández-Vega A (Conxo Hosp, Santiago de Compostela, Spain)
Br J Ophthalmol 80:708–712, 1996   4–49

Objective.—Seventh nerve palsy frequently results in lagophthalmos, sometimes leading to loss of Bell's phenomenon. A surgical procedure for improving palpebral closure was used in 11 patients.

Methods.—Ten patients with paralytic lagophthalmos and 1 with lagophthalmos associated with lateral lid retraction underwent the procedure to improve palpebral closure (Figs 1 and 2). Patients were examined monthly for 3 months, every 3–6 months for the first year, and every 6–12 months thereafter.

> *Case 1.*—Man, 72, with right facial palsy for 6 years and deformity from a previous tarsorrhaphy, had lagophthalmos of the right eye. After medial tarsal suspension (MTS), the patient's symptoms resolved and 6½ years later he is still symptom free.
>
> *Case 2.*—Woman, 82, with left lower lid tumor resected 7 years previously had the medial canthal and nasal lid areas restored and

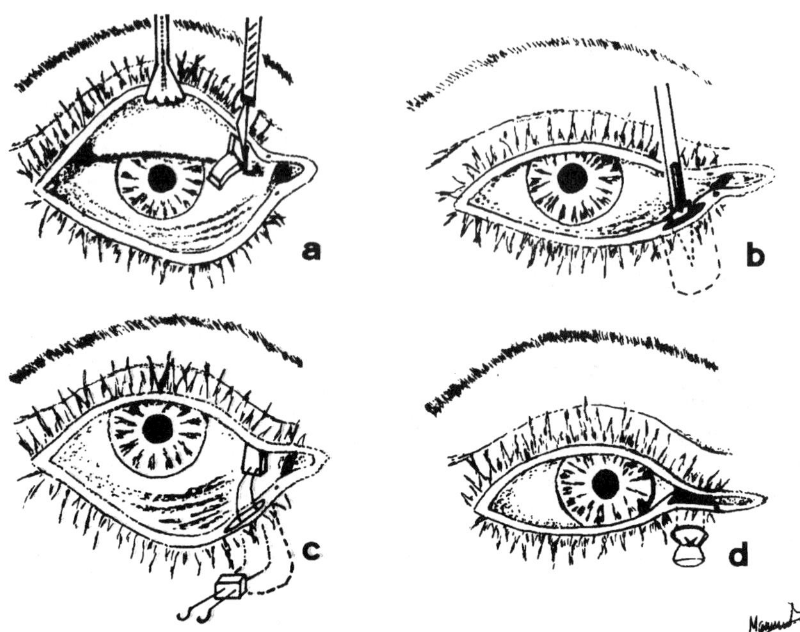

FIGURE 1.—Preparation of the upper lid tarsoconjunctival flap (TCF) and the lower lid pocket. A, the upper lid is averted and a nasal TCF is dissected. B, for the lower lid pocket a horizontal incision is made through the grey line of the lid margin. The pocket is deepened between the plane of the tarsus and the orbicularis. B, a 'U' suture, with the loop horizontal is passed through the tarsus of the tarsoconjunctival flap. The needles cross the pocket freely and then are pulled through the skin inserting the flap inside the pocket. D, the suture is knotted on a bolster. (Courtesy of Castroviejo-Bolibar M, de Damborenea A, Fernández-Vega A: Surgical repair of paralytic lagophthalmos by medial tarsal suspension of the lower lid. *Br J Ophthalmol* 80:708–712, 1996.)

a temporal tarsal suspension performed. No remaining defect or relapse is apparent 7 years later.

Results.—Medial tarsal suspension is safe and effective. The mean postoperative follow-up period was 5 years, 6 months. Medial tarsal suspension facilitated lid closure and lacrimal drainage, corrected ectropion, and decreased epiphora in patients with paralysis except for 1 patient. Three patients had slight lagophthalmos. All patients improved subjectively. Complications were minor and transient including 3 small hematomas.

Conclusion.—Medial tarsal suspension is safe and effective and is the only technique to provide long-term improvement for patients with lagophthalmos.

▶ This technique may be helpful for medial support in those rare cases where it is needed in aesthetic blepharoplasty; it is easily reversed.

P.W. McKinney, M.D.

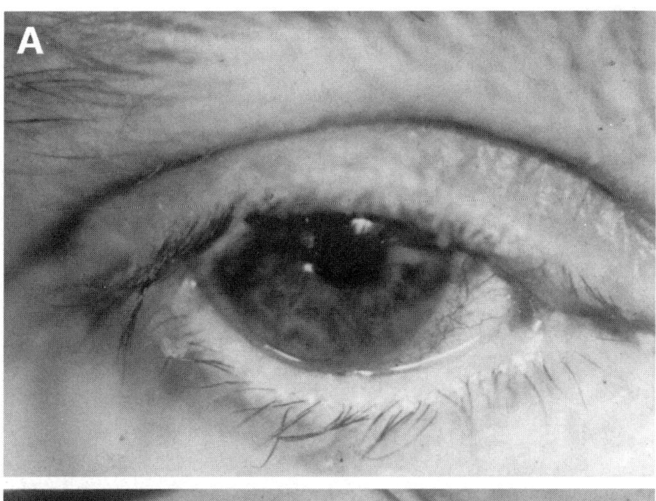

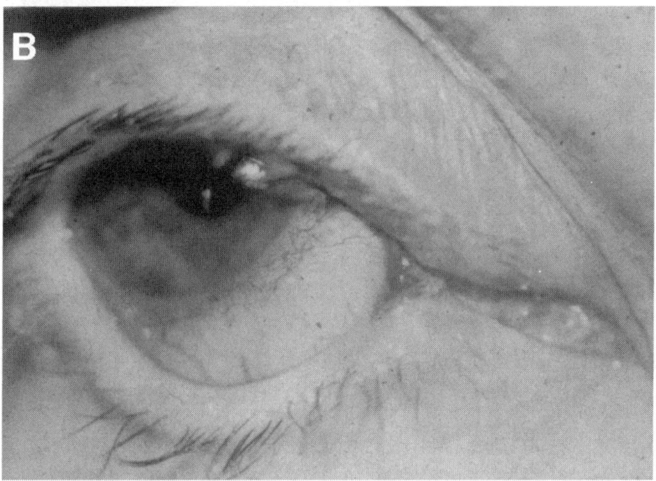

FIGURE 2.—A, appearance 2 weeks after the medial tarsal suspension of the lower lid. In normal conditions the flap is barely visible. **B,** it can be better seen when the lower lid is pulled down. (Courtesy of Castroviejo-Bolibar M, de Damborenea A, Fernández-Vega A: Surgical repair of paralytic lagophthalmos by medial tarsal suspension of the lower lid. *Br J Ophthalmol* 80:708–712, 1996.)

Management of Postblepharoplasty Lower Eyelid Retraction With Hard Palate Grafts and Lateral Tarsal Strip

Patel BCK, Patipa M, Anderson RL, et al (Univ of Utah, Salt Lake City)
Plast Reconstr Surg 99:1251–1260, 1997   4–50

Background.—The most common long-term complication after transcutaneous lower lid blepharoplasty is malposition of the lower eyelid. This is cosmetically unacceptable and is also associated with tearing, irritation, and exposure keratitis symptoms. Causes of lower eyelid malposition

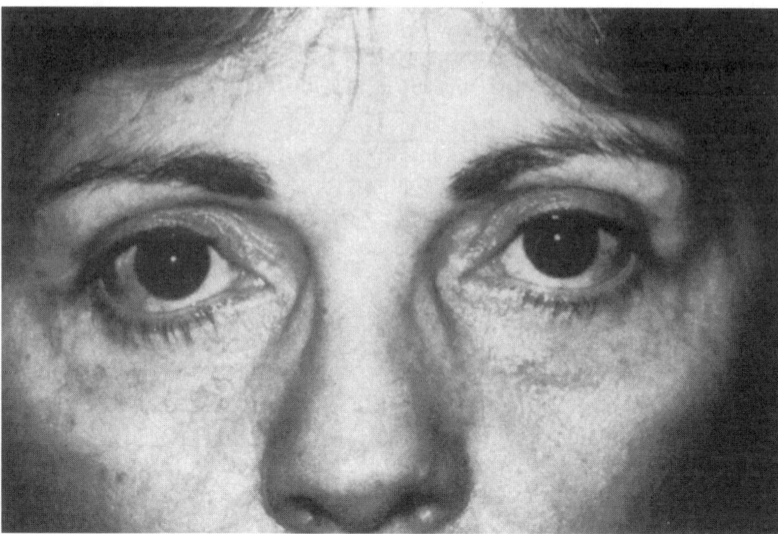

FIGURE 7.—Case 2. A 48-year-old woman 9 months after 4 eyelid blepharoplasties with lower eyelid retraction and severe ocular irritation. (Courtesy of Patel BCK, Patipa M, Anderson RL, et al: Management of postblepharoplasty lower eyelid retraction with hard palate grafts and lateral tarsal strip. *Plast Reconstr Surg* 99:1251–1260, 1997.)

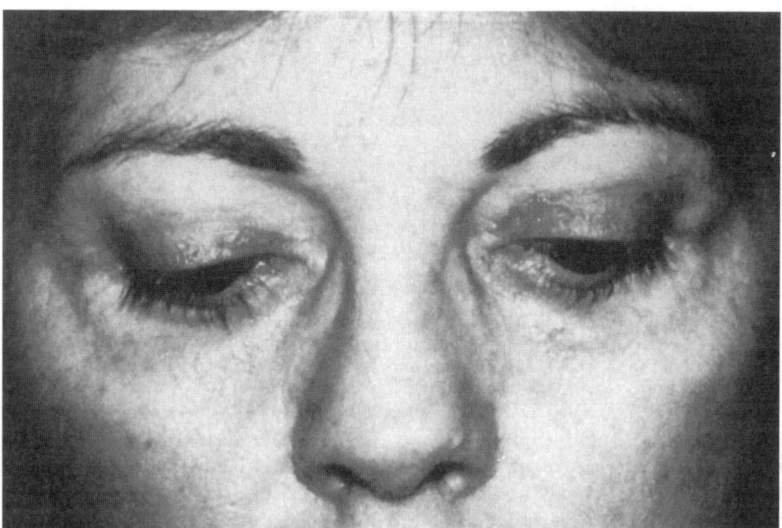

FIGURE 8.—Case 2. There is upper eyelid lag on downgaze with poor eyelid closure. Her eyes remain open while asleep because of lower eyelid retraction and insufficient upper eyelid skin, the latter presumably the result of her original blepharoplasty and secondary upper eyelid skin excision revision. (Courtesy of Patel BCK, Patipa M, Anderson RL, et al: Management of postblepharoplasty lower eyelid retraction with hard palate grafts and lateral tarsal strip. *Plast Reconstr Surg* 99:1251–1260, 1997.)

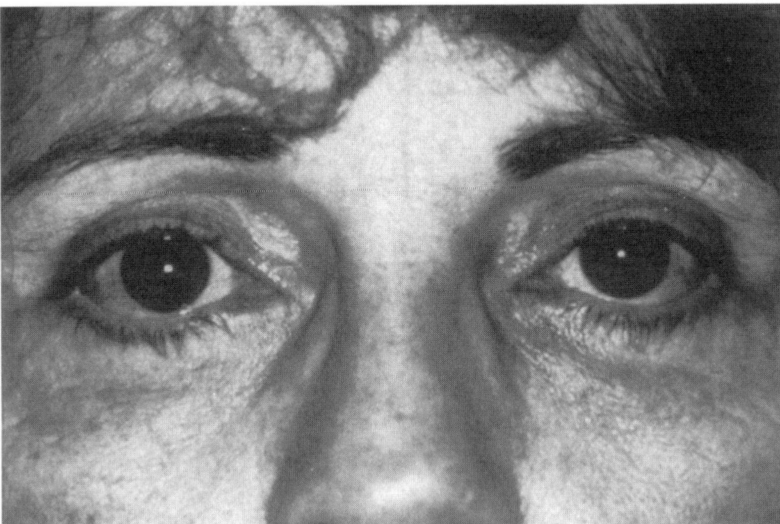

FIGURE 10.—Case 2. Two years after bilateral lower eyelid lateral tightening surgery (without grafts), the patient was referred with recurrent lower eyelid retraction, rounding of her lateral canthal angles, inferior scleral show, recurrent ocular discomfort, and a sad-eyed appearance. (Courtesy of Patel BCK, Patipa M, Anderson RL, et al: Management of postblepharoplasty lower eyelid retraction with hard palate grafts and lateral tarsal strip. *Plast Reconstr Surg* 99:1251–1260, 1997.)

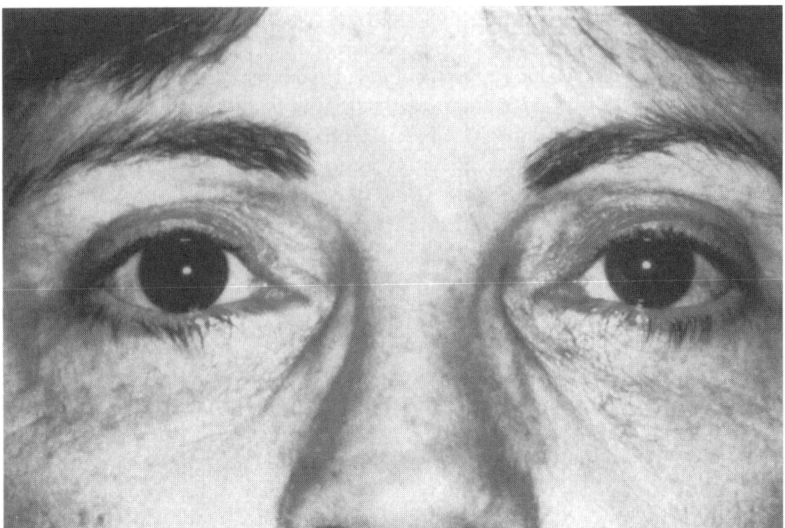

FIGURE 11.—Case 2. Nine months after bilateral lower eyelid retraction recession and insertion of hard palate mucosal grafts and lateral tarsal strips. The eyelids now cover the inferior cornea, and there is no scleral show and no more ocular discomfort. The patient is pleased with the cosmetic result. (Courtesy of Patel BCK, Patipa M, Anderson RL, et al: Management of postblepharoplasty lower eyelid retraction with hard palate grafts and lateral tarsal strip. *Plast Reconstr Surg* 99:1251–1260, 1997.)

include eyelid laxity, skin shortage, and scarring of the middle lamella. The use of hard palate mucosa grafts as spacers for the correction of lower eyelid retraction after transcutaneous blepharoplasty was evaluated in 29 eyelids of 17 patients.

Technique.—A detailed ocular examination is performed. Patients with severe middle lamella scarring undergo palate mucosal grafts using either general or local anesthesia. The 5-mm-wide and 20- to 25-mm-long hard palate graft is harvested between the gingiva and the midline. Traction is applied to the lower eyelid and all adhesions are divided. The graft is transferred to the bed and placed between the inferior border of the tarsus and the recessed conjunctiva and the lower eyelid retractors and sutured into place. A lateral tarsal strip is made and sutured as high as possible to the inner lateral orbital rim to correct laxity and provide support. Early overcorrection resolves over time. A bandage dissolvable collagen contact lens protects the cornea.

Results.—The follow-up ranged from 6 to 30 months. The lower eyelid position was within 0.5 mm of the inferior limbus in all eyes in this series. None of the patients had an ocular discharge. No patient complained of discomfort. The donor site healed within 1 month.

Case Report.—Woman, 48, had undergone upper and lower eyelid transcutaneous blepharoplasties in 1992. Following surgery, she had persistent ocular irritation, with bilateral lower eyelid retraction and nocturnal lagophthalmos (Fig 7 and Fig 8). She was referred in 1994 (Fig 10). She had bilateral eyelid laxity, lower eyelid retraction, tarsal flaccidity, and lagophthalmos. She had inferior punctate corneal erosions. She underwent bilateral eyelid tightening and hard palate grafting in 1995. The postoperative course was uneventful and the results were cosmetically pleasing, and there was a loss of discomfort (Fig 11).

Conclusions.—Lower eyelid malposition after blepharoplasty can be successfully managed with hard palate grafts and the creation of a lateral tarsal strip. The results are both cosmetically and functionally satisfactory.

▶ In severe cases, especially those patients with a "negative vector" eye, this procedure may be necessary. In milder cases with lax ligaments, the canthopexy (the strip, reefing, or repositioning) will suffice if the detrusors (middle lamella) scar is released.

P.W. McKinney, M.D.

A New Concept in Blepharoplasty
de la Plaza R, de la Cruz L (Madrid)
Aesthetic Plast Surg 20:221–233, 1996

Introduction.—The anatomy and function of the orbicularis oculi muscle are very complex, especially given the muscle's importance in facial expression. It is particularly prone to the undesirable effects that can occur with any type of aesthetic surgery, such as scar sequelae, normal regional dynamic disorders, edema, and iatrogenic acceleration of the aging pro-

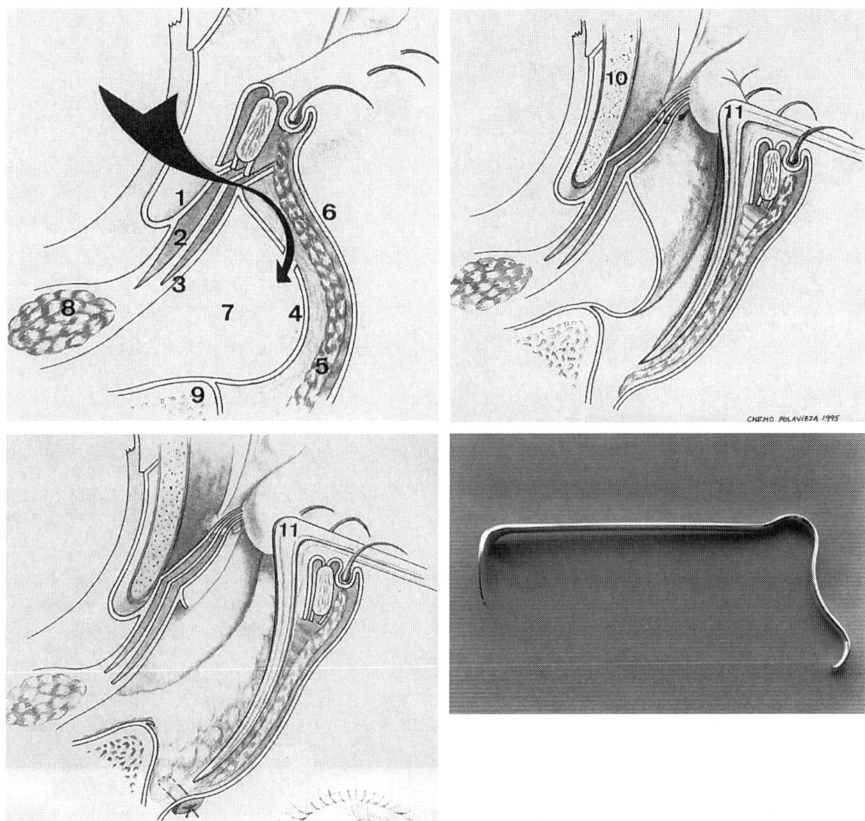

FIGURE 8.—**A**, transconjunctival approach. *1*, conjunctiva; *2*, Müller muscle; *3*, capsulopalpebral fascia; *4*, septum orbitale; *5*, orbicularis oculi muscle; *6*, skin; *7*, fat bags; *8*, inferior oblique muscle; *9*, orbital rim. **B**, as in **A** but with the transconjunctival retractor (*10*) and a specially designed instrument (*11*). **C**, through the transconjunctival route the septum orbitale was opened, the fat bags were dissected from the capsulopalpebral fascia, septum orbitale, and periosteum. The fat bags were everted and spread caudally beyond the nasojugal fold by pull-out transcutaneous stitches tied over small silicone pieces. **D**, Close-up of the instrument (*11*) shown in **B**. It was specially designed to separate the orbicularis oculi muscle and skin reaching 12–15 mm caudally to the arcus marginalis. The blade is longer than the normal Desmarres retractor and along the length of the blade runs a groove that serves as a guide for the needle which will fix the fat with 3 or 4 transcutaneous stitches, filling the palpebromalar sulcus. (From de la Plaza R, de la Cruz L: A new concept in blepharoplasty. *Aesthetic Plast Surg* 20:221–233, 1996. Copyright 1996, Springer-Verlag New York Inc.)

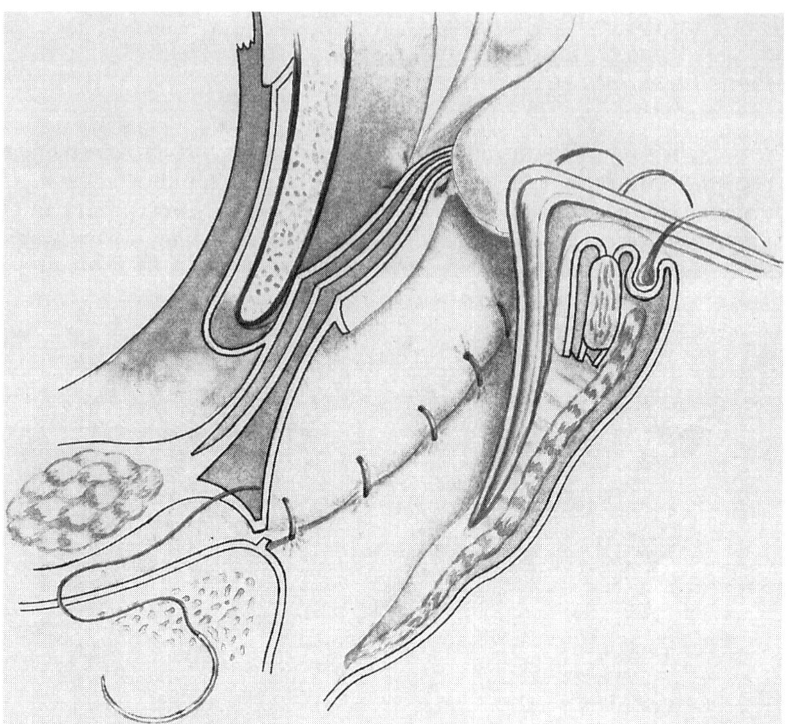

FIGURE 11.—Following the same steps illustrated in Figure 8, **A** and **B**, the fat bags are dissected from the capsulopalpebral fascia, the septum, and the periosteum. They retreat into the orbital cavity but are retained by suturing the lower edge of the capsulopalpebral fascia to the periosteum of the lower arcus marginalis. The suture is made with a nonresorbable 6/0 filament. (From de la Plaza R, de la Cruz L: A new concept in blepharoplasty. *Aesthetic Plast Surg* 20:221–233, 1996. Copyright 1996, Springer-Verlag New York Inc.)

cess. The causes of these undesirable effects in blepharoplasty were analyzed, and a new combination of techniques designed to achieve more natural and safer results was proposed.

Technique.—There is renewed interest in Loeb's "sliding pad" technique for the treatment of lower palpebral bags, in which the excess fat of the lower eyelids is used in pediculated fashion to correct depletion at the level of the suborbital sulcus. The modified technique uses a transconjunctival approach, avoiding cutaneous scarring and incision of the orbicularis oculi muscle (Fig 8). The fat from the palpebral bags is put back into the orbital cavity. The fat is retained in the cavity by suturing the capsulopalpebral fascia to the periosteum of the orbital rim. This prevents depletion of the orbita, provides a homogeneous and natural lower eyelid, and reduces the risk of intraorbital hematomas. In the transconjunctival approach, the lower edge of the capsulopalpebral fascia is sutured to the lower orbital rim (Fig 11). This prevents any secondary epithelialization of the conjunctival fornix and extension of the edema. It also permits natural correction of the palpebral fat bags and, if present, moderate skin excess. The technique is facilitated by using a transconjunctival retractor of the authors' design.

Discussion.—This approach to blepharoplasty can help to avoid the negative secondary effects of aesthetic surgery in this area. Keeping anatomical planes intact prevents scar adhesion and retraction, with their accompanying consequences. It also avoids the adverse effects that can result from sections and resections of the orbicularis oculi muscle. Although the procedure may seem complex, a well-selected combination of classic and modern blepharoplasty techniques can provide excellent results for the individual patient.

▶ I am pleasantly surprised that this technique does not cause a retraction of the detrusors or at least tethering with upper gaze. I like the concept for those with a tendency to have a hollow of the upper lid, where the conventional resection of fat may further skeletonize the structure. However, I have had some residual bulging with this technique, a few of which have led to revisions, so in severe cases I usually combine it with a partial resection of the fat and replacement of the remainder. We also need some studies on the reposition of fat into the palpebromalar sulcus as this is very much like removing fat in terms of my concept of the upper lid hollowing. However, when one studies the anatomy of the globe, there is a great deal of fibrous tissue in the orbital fat and surrounding muscles, and it may be that the hollowing of the upper lids we see is really from aging and/or resection of upper lid fat specifically, and perhaps not from lower lid fat resection.

P.W. McKinney, M.D.

Nose

Correction of the Hypoplastic Nasal Ala Using an Auricular Composite Graft

Kobayashi S, Haramoto U, Ohmori K (Tokyo Metropolitan Police Hosp)
Ann Plast Surg 37:490–494, 1996   4–52

Introduction.—Hypoplasia of the nasal ala is a deformity that becomes more apparent as the patient ages. The more challenging reconstructive procedures are those involving a mild deformity; there are few studies that address this problem. In the 8 cases reported here, auricular composite grafts were used to augment nasal alar size and thickness.

Methods.—Patients had a mean age of 22 years; 7 of 8 had a unilateral defect. In these patients, the hypoplastic nasal ala was the result of congenital or acquired deformities in childhood. With the patient under local or general anesthesia, the planned alar groove on the affected side is incised and the entire ala dissected subcutaneously up to the alar rim and nasal tip. Deformities are reconstructed using an auricular composite graft with large pieces of conchal cartilage that extend beyond the harvested skin and a small amount of elliptically shaped retroauricular skin. The total amount of harvested skin should be slightly wider than the defect itself and about one third the width of the harvested cartilage.

Results.—All grafts took perfectly, and in all but 1 case the postoperative shrinkage was minimal. A hematoma formed postoperatively in 1 patient, resulting in epidermal necrosis and hyperpigmentation of the graft. Four patients required minor scar revision along the inferior suture line of the skin.

Discussion.—A composite graft from the ear to the nose has a number of advantages: a small amount of skin and framework can be repaired simply in a 1-stage procedure, the donor skin matches the color and texture of the face, the cartilage maintains the alar shape, and donor site deformities are minimal. The ear composite graft may become a treatment of choice for minor nasal alar height and thickness deformities.

Suture Correction of Nasal Tip Cartilage Concavities

Neu BR (Univ of Toronto)
Plast Reconstr Surg 98:971–979, 1996   4–53

Objective.—Excessive concavity of the tip of the nose is difficult to treat by rhinoplasty. Using interlocking mattress sutures in a tension-control fashion can reverse concavities in a reliable way that maintains rim strip integrity.

> *Technique.*—The concave cartilage is exposed using the open approach, the cephalic alar cartilage is trimmed, and the concave cartilage is tented upward from the inside. The cartilage is sutured in position with a horizontal mattress suture placed at the apex parallel to the crus and tightened to hold the cartilage in the convex arch. Two or 3 miniature convex arches are linked to stabilize the convexity and 1 or 2 stitches are placed further from the apex of the concavity and interlocked. Nasal mucosa is not caught in the stitches. Patients have been followed up for 9 to 24 months with no loss of correction.

Conclusions.—The operation is versatile, reversible, and reliable. There has been no loss in correction for as long as 24 months. There is a learning curve for the technique.

▶ With a limited area such as the author described, perhaps the mucosa would be cooperative; however, I am concerned about the more extensive suture vector techniques. As Sheen has pointed out, every action has a reaction, and without mucosal undermining there may be some relapse. I favor the concept of anatomical correction before grafts whenever possible, and I like this concept.

P.W. McKinney, M.D.

Thick Skin and Cosmetic Surgery of the Nasal Tip: How to Avoid the Cutaneous Polly Beak
Botti G (Saló, Italy)
Aesthetic Plast Surg 20:421–427, 1996   4–54

Background.—Thick skin is usually considered a disadvantage in nasal tip cosmetic surgery. The supratip deformity known as "polly beak" and other aesthetic defects have been attributed to this feature. Guidelines for avoiding the occurrence of such problems were presented.

Avoiding the Cutaneous Polly Beak.—Avoiding excessive osteocartilaginous and mucosal excisions to which the skin would not be able to adapt may help prevent cutaneous polly beak. In addition, shaping the supporting framework and, if necessary, redistributing the osteocartilaginous fragments removed may be useful. Such grafts placed in the nose tip support the skin, which results in the tendency to accumulate less in the supratip region. Defatting the nasal tip may also help prevent polly beak. Also, application of an adhesive tape to the supratip area to create moderate pressure in the week after splint removal (with a nightly application for at least 1 month thereafter) may be beneficial. Procedures for correcting unwanted postoperative thickening of the skin in the supratip region also include injection of steroids or any other atrophy-inducing substance, dermabrasion, and, in exceptional cases, removal of a certain amount of cutis from the nasal dorsum (though unpredictable postoperative scarring will result).

Conclusions.—The characteristics of the skin over the nasal tip must be assessed very carefully when planning rhinoplasty. With such evaluation, steps can be taken to prevent iatrogenic deformities such as polly beak. The findings of such assessment are also useful in establishing realistic expectations of the surgical outcomes.

▶ As Dr. Constantian has shown us,[1] you must fill the skin sleeve rather than attempt to overreduce it, unless one is going to do external skin excisions and/or skin-shaving techniques to reduce the skin sleeve, both of which leave some scarring.

P.W. McKinney, M.D.

Reference

1. Constantian MB: Distant effects of dorsal and tip grafting in rhinoplasty. *Plast Reconstr Surg* 90:405–418, 1992.

The Quantification and Distribution of Nasal Sebaceous Glands Using Image Analysis

Michelson LN, Peck GC Jr, Kuo H-R, et al (Newark, NJ)
Aesthetic Plast Surg 20:303–309, 1996   4–55

Objective.—There are histologic differences between the skin of the distal and proximal nose. In patients with thick sebaceous skin, rhinoplasty is more difficult. External shaving for treating rhinophyma leaves little scarring and produces an aesthetic result particularly at the supratip. The points on the nose at which these differences in skin types become apparent were studied using cadaver nasal skins.

Methods.—Biopsy specimens of 24 locations of 2 nasal skins and 8 midline biopsy specimens of 7 nasal skins from 9 white cadavers were examined by a blinded dermatopathologist to determine the size, cross-sectional width, and depth of sebaceous glands.

Results.—The size, depth, and number of sebaceous glands were significantly larger in the distal nose. Two breakpoints were located between biopsy points that separated proximal nose, distal nose, and columella.

Conclusion.—The distal skin is thicker and has more, larger, and deeper sebaceous glands than does the skin of the proximal nose.

▶ This pattern also changes with age and acne. For example, a 15-year florid acne skin eventually thins and vice versa. For instance, acne develops in a 15-year-old with thin skin, the tip of the nose enlarges, and it is not the underlying cartilage that has caused this change.

P.W. McKinney, M.D.

The Use of the Labiocolumellar Crease Incision in Rhinoplasty

Spiro SA, Wolfe SA, Wider TM (Univ of Miami, Fla; Miami Children's Hosp, Fla)
Ann Plast Surg 37:569–576, 1996   4–56

Background.—Authorities continue to debate the criteria to be used in selecting patients for rhinoplasty. The outcomes of 100 consecutive rhinoplasties, the technique used, and the criteria for selection were reviewed.

Methods.—Sixty-three women and 37 men underwent rhinoplasty. Thirty-two procedures were primary; 45, secondary; 18, cleft; and 5, reconstructive. The open approach through the labiocolumellar crease incision was performed in 28% of the primary, 62% of the secondary, 78% of the cleft, and 80% of the reconstructive procedures.

Findings.—An open rhinoplasty was most likely to be done in patients with cleft nasal deformity, Binder's, or posttraumatic nasal deformities. The presence of a previous scar along the columellar base was an indication for labiocolumellar incision. Despite the significant amount of tip elevation in this patient subgroup, no circulatory compromise in the columellar base occurred. The most significant complication occurred in a patient undergoing secondary open rhinoplasty, in whom infection developed, followed by the spontaneous draining of a purulent collection through the supratip skin 4 days after surgery (Figs 2 and 4).

Conclusions.—Several myths about the labiocolumellar crease incision are currently circulating and should be dispelled. Adherence to the principles of aesthetic subunits will enable scar placement in a less noticeable position. The existence of a scar along the columella base should be an indication for open rhinoplasty.

▶ It's a longer flap. As the authors document, the circulation seems to be safe. I don't like scars in a sulcus, i.e., the labiocolumellar crease, alar wedges, or earlobes. However, other surgeons do this. The midcolumellar scar can be troublesome, particularly in the worm's view shown, whereas

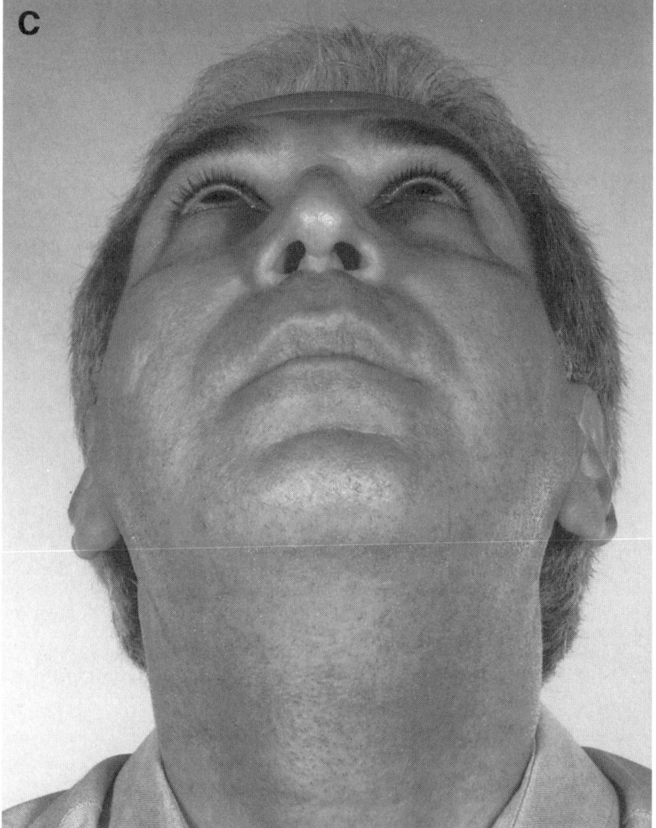

FIGURE 2C.—Preoperative view of a 52-year-old man dissatisfied with the result after a previous rhinoplasty. A V-shaped transverse columellar waist incision had been used, even though he had a deep labiocolumellar crease several millimeters below. A secondary rhinoplasty was performed through a traditional endonasal approach, with placement of crushed cartilage behind the previous columellar scar. (Reprinted from Spiro SA, Wolfe SA, Wider TM: The use of labiocolumellar crease incision in rhinoplasty. *Ann Plast Surg* 37:569–576, 1996, by permission of Little, Brown and Company, Inc.)

the columellar crease is not. Therefore, I think it has to be an individual selection. If it is an older patient with a marked crease such as shown in Figure 2C, the crease incision may be better.

P.W. McKinney, M.D.

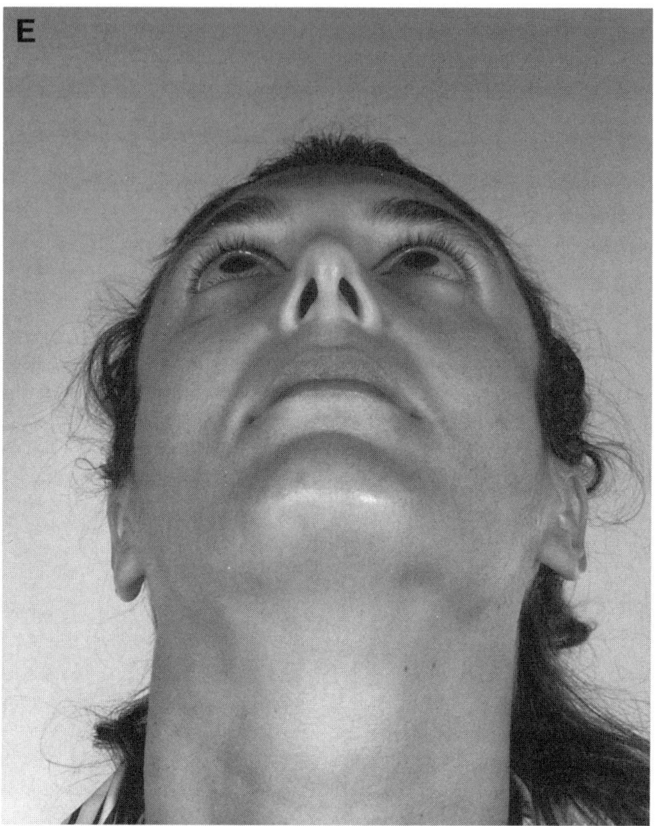

FIGURE 4E-F.—A 22-year-old woman dissatisfied with the result after previous rhinoplasty. She had difficulty breathing, with middle vault collapse on inspiration, secondary to overresection of the upper lateral cartilages. She was also unhappy with the prominent overprojecting tip. E, preoperative view; F, early postoperative view 6 months later. Note how well the labiocolumellar crease incision is camouflaged. (Reprinted from Spiro SA, Wolfe SA, Wider TM: The use of labiocolumellar crease incision in rhinoplasty. *Ann Plast Surg* 37:569–576, 1996, by permission of Little, Brown and Company, Inc.)

(Continued)

FIGURE 4 (cont.)

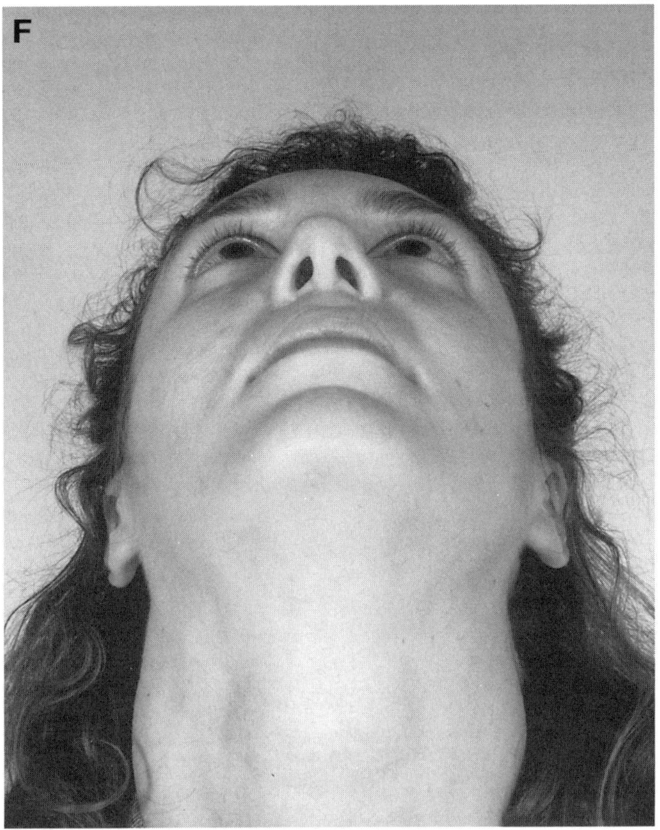

An Introduction of the Ultrasonic Scalpel: Utility in Treatment of Rhinophyma

Dufresne RG, Zienowicz RJ, Rozelle A, et al (Brown Univ, Providence, RI)
Plast Reconstr Surg 98:160–162, 1996   4–57

Background.—Many surgical approaches have been described for the treatment of rhinophyma. The UltraCision Harmonic Scalpel is a new instrument that enables rapid excision of rhinophymatous tissue while providing simultaneous hemostasis with minimal adjacent tissue damage. One experience with this new device was presented.

Methods.—Most patients were treated using local anesthesia in the tumescent manner. The scalpel was used in the higher amplification range, a setting that balanced ease of excision with optimal simultaneous hemostasis. To perform the excision, the surgeon used the enhanced cutting blade tip, applying slight pressure to the blade against hemorrhagic areas when needed. The surgeon was careful to keep the blade in the pilosebaceous zone of the nasal tissues.

Findings.—In most patients, initial healing was complete within 1 week. Even in patients needing the most aggressive treatment, full re-epithelialization occurred within 3 weeks. Postoperative pain was minimal. Narcotics were not needed. There was no conspicuous scarring or dyschromia. All patients were satisfied with their outcomes.

Conclusions.—The UltraCision Harmonic Scalpel consists of a surgically sharp scalpel blade with longitudinal US vibration of 50,000 Hz that causes coagulation of hemoglobin in small vessels at the moment of division, which results in hemostasis with little epidermal and dermal injury. This represents a significant advancement over other currently available techniques.

▶ Ultrasonic techniques are used for liposuction as well as dermabrasion, and it would be interesting to see if they cause less tissue damage than the heat of the laser.

P.W. McKinney, M.D.

Alar Reductions in Rhinoplasty
Gilbert SE (Univ of Oklahoma, Tulsa)
Arch Otolaryngol Head Neck Surg 122:781–784, 1996   4–58

Background.—The occurrence of notching prompts surgeons to limit the vestibular portion of alar narrowing procedures. In one surgeon's practice, cutaneous and vestibular resection was performed uniformly during alar reduction until 1993, at which time only the cutaneous part of the resection was done. The outcomes of each method were compared.

Methods and Findings.—Forty consecutive patients undergoing alar reduction during rhinoplasty were included in the study. Photographs taken 1 year after surgery were reviewed by 2 facial plastic surgeons and 3 plastic surgeons. The surgeons' ratings showed that notching and scarring were perceived significantly less in the patients who underwent alar reduction with only cutaneous excisions.

Conclusions.—Many different ways of narrowing the ala have been described, most of which do not cross the alar rim or sill to involve the vestibule. All can be revised to stop at the sill or rim. Doing so may yield better outcomes.

▶ Notice that the author placed the incision just above the groove. I prefer this technique also because once the incision is made in the groove, to my eye, it destroys the natural curve (which can never be re-created) and looks flat or stuck on.[1] However, there are fine authors who disagree with me on this.

P.W. McKinney, M.D.

Reference

1. McKinney P, Cunningham B: *Rhinoplasty.* New York, Churchill-Livingstone, 1989.

Surgery of the Naso-frontal Angle
Fontana AM, Muti E (Turin, Italy)
Aesthetic Plast Surg 20:319–322, 1996   4–59

Objective.—The nose is a prominent facial feature that defines the morphological features of the face and is characteristic of some racial differences. A balanced appearance is aesthetically important. A cranial or caudal shift affects the length of the dorsum with the caudal position determining a short nose and a cranial position determining a long nose. The rhinoplasty must bring the profile in harmony with the apex of the nose and must take into account the width of the nasofrontal angle. All that is necessary to correct a too narrow angle is to lower the dorsum more or less kyphotic and adjust its setting to the slope of the forehead. Treatment of an over-wide angle is more difficult.

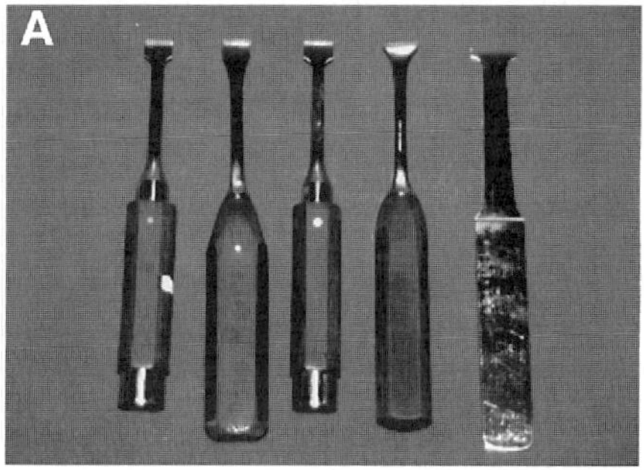

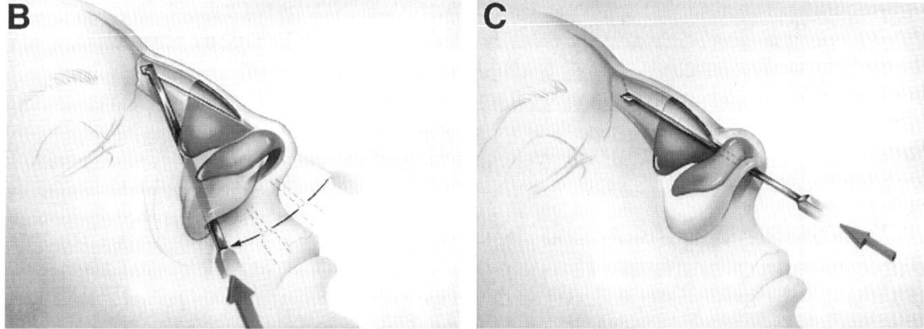

FIGURE 9.—**A,** a set of "Delta-shaped" chisels of different sizes. **B,** the "Delta-shaped" chisel cuts the dorsum following the normal technique. **C,** at 2–3 mm from the base of proper nasal bones, the tail of the chisel is shifted toward the base of the right nasal wall. In this position, the right wing of the chisel will resect the right proper nasal bone. The same maneuver will be repeated on the left side of the nose. (Courtesy of Fontana AM, Muti E: Surgery of the naso-frontal angle. *Aesthetic Plast Surg* 20:319–322, 1996. Copyright 1996 Springer-Verlag New York Inc.)

Methods.—Delta-shaped chisels were used to treat over-wide angles (Fig 9).

Conclusion.—Concepts of anatomy plus the surgeon's artistic sense are important in performing rhinoplasty to create an aesthetically pleasing outcome.

▶ I find it difficult to resect this area, as it swells because of the processus muscle and thicker skin. The decision has to be made before injection of the local anesthetic.

P.W. McKinney, M.D.

Paraffinoma Revisited: A Post-operative Condition Following Rhinoplasty Nasal Packing
Montgomery PQ, Khan JI, Feakins R, et al (St Bartholomew's Hosp, London)
J Laryngol Otol 110:785–786, 1996   4–60

Introduction.—Paraffin-impregnated tulle is commonly used in the packing of tissue cavities, as a dressing after surgical repair of wounds, and on skin-donor sites. Although paraffinoma is a well-known complication, nasal packing with paraffin gauze is still commonly done after rhinoplasty. A paraffinoma developed after elective rhinoplasty in 1 woman.

Case Report.—Woman, 40, had elective rhinoplasty. Nasal packs of paraffin gauze were applied after surgery and removed after 24 hours. Two months later, the patient was seen with a nontender swelling 0.5 cm in diameter in the glabellar region. There was no evidence of infection. The lesion was excised and a paraffinoma was diagnosed. Four months later, 4 separate swellings developed on both sides of the nose at the site of the infracture and local inflammation. Under histologic examination, the lesion had the appearance of an oleogranuloma, an inflammatory reaction to unabsorbable fatty material in tissue. The lesion is called a paraffinoma when the reaction is caused by paraffin oil. Electron microscopy showed large active macrophages with phagocytic vacuoles filled with flocculent material. Infrared spectrophotometry showed that the fat was nearly identical to paraffin oil. Microbiological analysis showed no bacterial, fungal, or parasitic infestation.

Discussion.—Paraffinoma is a characteristic granulomatous foreign body reaction to mineral oil that occurs slowly and reaches its maximum at about 3 months. Because there is no unique advantage to paraffin gauze in rhinoplasty, silicon mesh is recommended as a packing in nasal surgery to avoid this rare, but serious, complication after rhinoplasty.

▶ Res ipsa loquitor.

P.W. McKinney, M.D.

Subscribe to the related journal in your field!

Yes! Begin my one-year subscription to *Aesthetic Surgery Journal* (6 issues).

Name ___________________________________

Institution _______________________________

Address _________________________________

City _______________________ State ________

ZIP/PC __________ Country ________________

Specialty ________________________________
 (Students/residents, please list Institution)

Subscription prices (through 9/30/98)

		USA	Canada*	Int'l
Individuals	❏	$69.00	$90.95	$85.00
Institutions	❏	103.00	127.33	119.00
Students, residents	❏	46.00	66.34	62.00

Method of payment

Enclose payment (check or credit card number) and we'll send an extra issue FREE!

❏ **Check** (in U.S. dollars, drawn on a U.S. bank, and payable to *Aesthetic Surgery Journal*)

❏ VISA   ❏ MasterCard   ❏ Discover

❏ AmEx   ❏ Bill me   Exp. date__________

Card #________________________________

Signature ______________________________

*Includes Canadian GST

Individual/student subscriptions must be in the name of, billed to, and paid for by the individual.

Airmail rates available upon request.
Prices subject to change without notice.

J070983YA

Reservation Card for the Year Book

Yes! I would like my own copy of *Year Book of Plastic, Reconstructive and Aesthetic Surgery®* at the price of **$82.00** plus sales tax, postage, and handling. Please begin my subscription with the current edition according to the terms described below.* I understand that I will have 30 days to examine each annual edition.

Name ____

Address ____

City _______________________________ State _________ ZIP ________

Method of Payment

Check (in U.S. dollars, drawn on a U.S. bank, payable to *Year Book of Plastic, Reconstructive and Aesthetic Surgery®*)

❏ VISA   ❏ MasterCard   ❏ Discover   ❏ AmEx   ❏ Bill me

Card number _____________________________________ Exp. date: __________

Signature ____

Prices are subject to change without notice.

PMC-029

Your Year Book service guarantee:

When you subscribe to the *Year Book*, you will receive advance notice of future annual volumes about two months before publication. To receive the new edition, you need do nothing—we'll send you the new volume as soon as it is available. If you want to discontinue, the advance notice allows you time to notify us of your decision. If you are not completely satisfied, you have 30 days to return any *Year Book*.

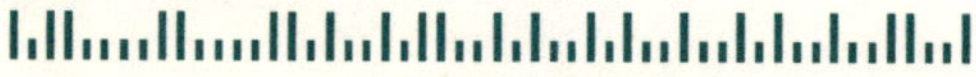

BUSINESS REPLY MAIL

FIRST-CLASS MAIL   PERMIT NO 135   ST LOUIS MO

POSTAGE WILL BE PAID BY ADDRESSEE

SUBSCRIPTION SERVICES
MOSBY–YEAR BOOK, INC.
11830 WESTLINE INDUSTRIAL DRIVE
ST. LOUIS   MO 63146-9988

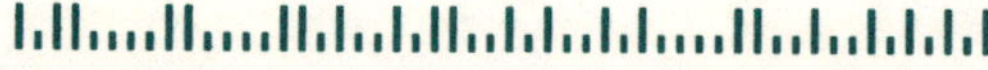

BUSINESS REPLY MAIL

FIRST-CLASS MAIL   PERMIT NO 135   ST LOUIS MO

POSTAGE WILL BE PAID BY ADDRESSEE

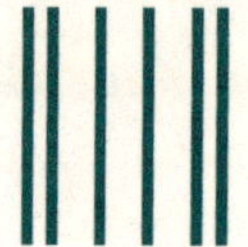 Mosby

PAT NEWMAN
11830 WESTLINE INDUSTRIAL DRIVE
PO BOX 46908
ST. LOUIS   MO 63146-9934

Want to speed up the process?

To order the *Year Book,*
you also may call 1-800-426-4545

To subscribe to the journal today,
call toll-free in the U.S.:
1-800-453-4351
or fax 314-432-1158
Outside the U.S., call: 314-453-4351

Visit us at:
www.mosby.com/Mosby/Periodicals

Mosby–Year Book, Inc.
Subscription Services
11830 Westline Industrial Drive
St. Louis, MO   63146 U.S.A.

Mosby

Comparison of Four Different Types of Osteotomes for Lateral Osteotomy: A Cadaver Study

Kuran I, Özcan H, Usta A, et al (Istanbul, Turkey)
Aesthetic Plast Surg 20:323–326, 1996   4–61

Background.—Several different instruments and techniques of lateral osteotomy for rhinoplasty have been described. Some of the key issues in this discussion are the site and type of the incision, the extent of periosteum dissection, and the direction of osteotomy. There are no research data about differences between the various types of osteotomes; rather, the selection is made according to the individual surgeon's preference. A cadaver study was performed to compare 4 different types of osteotomes used with the same surgical technique of lateral osteotomy.

Methods.—The study used 32 halves of 16 human cadavers. Four different instruments were compared: curved and narrow (Padgett P 1630 Silvers), curved and wide (Padgett P 4885 Neivert), straight and narrow (Padgett P 4761 Neivert), and straight and wide (Padgett P 7500 Forman). All instruments were used to perform the same osteotomy technique, one that included minimal periosteum dissection and low to high osteotomy. Significant differences between instruments in fracture line and mucosal injuries were evaluated.

Results.—The rate of mucosal laceration was significantly greater with wide osteotomes, 94% vs. 38%. The difference between straight and curved wide osteotomes was not significant. The rate of atypical fractures was 81% with straight and 44% with curved osteotomes; this difference was not significant. At no point did bone thickness on the osteotomy line exceed 3 mm.

Conclusions.—When used for lateral osteotomy, curved osteotomes produce more mucosal injuries and atypical fractures than straight osteotomes. Although the difference in atypical fractures is not statistically significant, curved osteotomes seem to produce a better osteotomy. A narrow, curved chisel is the best choice for low to high lateral osteotomy with minimal elevation of periosteum.

► I have always used the curved osteotome with a guard on the skin side to better feel where I was and, in fact, this probably tears less mucosa than having the guard internally, which was the way it was originally designed. Because it is so closely attached to the bone and periosteum that it is not easily separated, I blunt the side opposite to the guard with a sharpening stone to be less likely to tear the mucosa.

P.W. McKinney, M.D.

The Relative Importance of Septal and Nasal Valvular Surgery in Correcting Airway Obstruction in Primary and Secondary Rhinoplasty

Constantian MB, Clardy RB (Southern New Hampshire Regional Med Ctr, Nashua; Dartmouth Med School, Hanover, NH)
Plast Reconstr Surg 98:38–54, 1996   4–62

Objective.—Nasal airway obstruction can be the result not only of septal deviation or inferior turbinate hypertrophy or both but also of incompetence of the internal or external nasal valves. Unfortunately, patients' symptoms and clinical findings are not always correlated. Furthermore, the relation between valvular reconstruction and degree of improvement of the airway is not known. The relative importance of valvular and septal deformities in the hierarchy of causes of nasal airway obstruction was studied prospectively.

Methods.—Anterior active mask rhinomanometry was done in 160 patients (53 men), aged 14 to 72 years, before and 1 to 43 months after primary rhinoplasty (88 patients) or secondary rhinoplasty (72 patients). Patients were categorized depending on whether the obstruction was located in the external valves, internal valves, septum, or some combination.

Results.—There were 114 bilateral and 46 unilateral obstructions. Septal or valvular surgery or both corrected the problem for 152 patients, whereas 8 patients had some residual obstruction. Airflow improved rhinomanometrically in 140 patients, subjectively and clinically in 19. In 1 patient, obstruction remained. Correction of septum abnormalities alone did not have a significant effect on airflow. External valvular reconstruction increased airflow an average of 2.6 times over baseline values, and internal valvular reconstruction corrected airflow by an average of 2 times over baseline values. Patients receiving both corrections had an increased airflow of 3.8 times over baseline values. Spreader grafts and dorsal grafts approximately doubled airflow values over baseline measurements. Septum correction along with internal or external valvular reconstruction did not have a significant effect on airflow. However, septoplasty plus internal and external valvular reconstruction increased airflow 4.9 times over baseline values. For 110 patients with preoperative lateral obstruction, the septum was deviated toward the obstructed side in 46% but toward the contralateral side in 54%. Valvular reconstruction in 54 patients who had a previous rhinoplasty improved the airway in 49.

Conclusions.—Before rhinoplasty, a functional nasal examination should be conducted to determine the effect on airway obstruction of internal and external valves. Septum and turbinate assessments are not sufficient.

▶ The author has made a convincing case for evaluating and addressing several factors that may produce airway obstruction. However, the reader is appropriately cautioned by the author to avoid overinterpretation of the conclusions because the evaluative technique, rhinometry, is subject to significant variability. Furthermore, pretreatment of patients with phenylephrine before rhinomanometry excludes evaluation of a possible contribution of allergic rhinitis to airway obstruction.

S.H. Miller, M.D.

Early Secondary Corrections After Septorhinoplasty

Szalay L (Frankfurt, Germany)
Aesthetic Plast Surg 20:429–432, 1996   4–63

Objective.—Septorhinoplasty is a difficult procedure with a high rate of secondary correction, even in experienced hands. Most surgeons delay the secondary correction until at least 12 months after the primary rhinoplasty. At the study institution, it is thought that performing the secondary correction as soon as the need becomes apparent saves a lot of time and trouble for the patient and surgeon alike. Their experience with early secondary correction after septorhinoplasty was evaluated.

Technique.—The plaster of Paris splint is removed 12 days postoperatively. By this time, edema has usually resolved enough to see the need for secondary correction. The secondary correction is usually performed with local anesthetic only. The plaster must not be removed before the secondary correction, or else the newly developing edema could disguise the defect. Residual irregularities of the nasal dorsum can be corrected by careful undermining in the original plane of dissection. Preserved bone or cartilage from the initial operation can be used if needed. For insufficient tip projection, a portion of septal cartilage or lower lateral cartilage can be used as an onlay graft. Distortion of the nasal pyramid can usually be corrected by manual manipulation and pressure. Other early corrections may include correction of the nasal septum, secondary shortening of the nose, or secondary resection of the medial crura. All corrections are done under broad-spectrum antibiotic cover. In just 9 of 238 corrections was a further correction needed after early secondary correction.

Conclusions.—Early secondary correction, when needed, after septorhinoplasty is advocated. In a 15-year experience, no significant resorption of bony or cartilaginous fragments that had been replaced or readjusted have been seen. Early correction improves patient satisfaction, avoids the stress of a long waiting period, and prevents the misapprehension that the secondary procedure is needed to deal with a serious complication.

► This is an intriguing concept, one that saves the long period of dissatisfaction while awaiting a revision according to conventional wisdom. However, it will take a tremendous amount of experience to judge which is swelling and which is residual defect. I would have trouble judging this after 30 years of practice and several thousand rhinoplasties; however, other surgeons have done this and the tissues, as the author states, are a lot easier to work with.

P.W. McKinney, M.D.

Unilateral Osteotomies for External Bony Deviation of the Nose
Fanous N (McGill Univ, Montreal)
Plast Reconstr Surg 100:115–123, 1997   4–64

Background.—Correcting the externally deviated nose is a challenge. The recurrence rate of nasal deviation after surgery remains high. The current paper analyzes the mechanisms of unilateral osteotomies.

Unilateral Osteotomies for External Bony Deviation of the Nose.—Though most crooked noses seem well positioned in the midline at the end of regular rhinoplasty, the nasal pyramid may begin to migrate laterally several months later, partially reproducing the original deviation. The author emphasizes an approach to the externally deviated bony pyramid in which osteotomy is performed on only one side of the nose. During a regular rhinoplasty, the bilateral lateral osteotomies medially displace the lateral nasal walls. When only a unilateral osteotomy is performed, the nasal dorsum seems to deviate to the opposite side. The outcomes of unilateral vertical osteotomy, alone or combined with an additional diagonal osteotomy, have been predictable and satisfactory (Fig 3).

Conclusions.—Though the unilateral osteotomy technique is not new, it has not received the attention that it deserves. Little or no long-term change occurs in the satisfactory outcomes that are achieved.

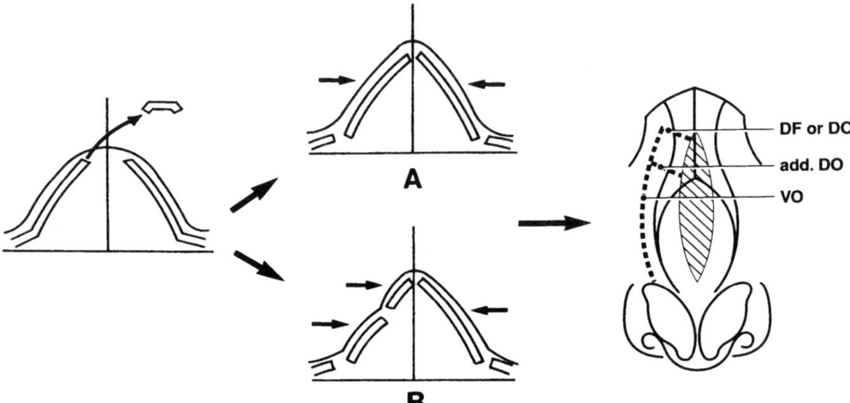

FIGURE 3.—Mechanisms of additional diagonal osteotomy. Routine rhinoplasty with hump resection, but the lateral walls are convex (VO, vertical osteotomy; DF or DO, diagonal fracture or diagnoal osteotomy; add. DO, additional diagonal osteotomy; A, bilateral vertical osteotomy). The lateral curvature persists, an additional diagonal osteomy (B) corrects the lateral convexity. (Courtesy of Fanous N: Unilateral osteotomies for external bony deviation of the nose. *Plast Reconstr Surg* 100:115–123, 1997.)

▶ An excellent analysis of how important it is to assess the individual shape of the bones to determine the fractures necessary to achieve changes. All osteotomies cannot be the same, but diagonal fractures with a 2 mm percutaneous osteotome is an accurate method. The percutaneous incision requires no suturing and, although it may initially dimple, it has never been a problem in 30 years of my practice. The danger of destabilizing the nose is a caution and a minimal undermining, and the diagonal osteotomy done before the vertical is a wise caution.

P.W. McKinney, M.D.

Modified Tragal Cartilage — Temporoparietal and Deep Temporal Fascia Sandwich Graft Technique for Repair of Nasal Septal Perforations
Hussain A, Murthy P (Aberdeen Royal Hosps NHS Trust, Scotland)
J Laryngol Otol 111:435–437, 1997   4–65

Background.—Repairing nasal septal perforations continues to be a challenge. The tragal cartilage inferior turbinate mucoperiosteal sandwich graft technique has been used for such repair. The outcomes of a modification of this technique were reported.

Methods and Findings.—Fifteen patients with nasal septal perforation were treated at 1 clinic during 2 years. Surgery consisted of a modified tragal cartilage-temporoparietal and deep temporal fascia sandwich technique. Follow-up ranged from 6 to 24 months. Repair was successful in 14 patients, with complete closure of the perforation and symptomatic relief. The remaining patients had undergone bilateral inferior turbinectomy, resulting in secondary bleeding necessitating intranasal packing and disruption of the septal repair. No early postoperative problems occurred. The appearance of the septum after splint removal was satisfactory in all patients.

Conclusions.—The modified tragal cartilage-temporalis fascia sandwich graft technique is successful in closing small- to medium-sized septal perforations. Its main limitation is the difficulty in closing perforations greater than 4 cm with 1 layer of tragal cartilage. The use of additional cartilage from the opposite tragus is recommended for perforations greater than 4 cm.

▶ Only 14 patients, but 100% success is impressive, especially with perforations of 1–3 cm size.

P.W. McKinney, M.D.

Extremities and Trunk

Penile Length in the Flaccid and Erect States: Guidelines for Penile Augmentation

Wessells H, Lue TF, McAninch JW (Univ of California, San Francisco; San Francisco Gen Hosp)
J Urol 156:995–997, 1996
4–66

Objective.—To provide a guide to urologists when advising patients on penile augmentation, a prospective study of flaccid and erect penile dimensions of 80 physically normal men was done.

Methods.—The study participants were being evaluated for sexual dysfunction but had no congenital or acquired abnormalities of the penis. None had a history of Peyronie's disease or penile surgery (except circumcision). A single examiner obtained tape measurements of the flaccid and the erect penis. To minimize the effects of temperature, flaccid length, circumference, depth of the prepubic fat pad, and stretched penile length were measured immediately after the men undressed. Penile length and circumference were determined after intracavernous injection of prostaglandin E1 for evaluation of erectile dysfunction. A mixture of phentolamine, papaverine, and prostaglandin E1 was injected if necessary to achieve full rigidity.

Results.—The 80 patients ranged in age from 21 to 82 years, with age distribution peaking in the third and sixth decades. Fifty-four were white, 16 were black, and 10 were Asian. The mean flaccid length of the penis was 8.85 cm and the mean erect length was 12.89 cm (Table 1). The mean erectile increase, the difference between these 2 measurements, was 4.04 cm. Shorter penises (9.5 cm or less) did not differ significantly from longer penises (10 cm or more) in erectile length increase (mean 3.98 vs. 4.06 cm). Penile volume increased an average of 40 cc with erection. Fat pad length was greater in men older than 40 years than in younger men, but these 2

TABLE 1.—Penile Dimensions in 80 Subjects

Dimension	Mean ± SD	(range)
Age (yrs.)	54 ± 14.37	(21–82)
Flaccid length (cm.)	8.85 ± 2.38	(5.0–15.5)
Flaccid circumference (cm.)	9.71 ± 1.17	(6.5–13.0)
Fat pad depth (cm.)	2.85 ± 1.59	(0.5–7.5)
Stretched length (cm.)	12.45 ± 2.71	(7.5–19.0)
Erect length (cm.)	12.89 ± 2.91	(7.5–19.0)
Erect circumference (cm.)	12.30 ± 1.31	(9.0–16.0)
Erect increase in length (cm.)	4.04 ± 1.65	(0.5–9.0)
Functional length (cm.)	15.74 ± 2.62	(9.0–21.0)
Flaccid vol. (cc)	43.62 ± 15.19	(21.25–87.0)
Erect vol. (cc)	80.16 ± 23.20	(33.75–152.0)

(Courtesy of Wessells H, Lue TF, McAninch JW: Penile length in the flaccid and erect states: Guidelines for penile augmentation. *J Urol* 156:995–997, 1996.)

age groups did not differ significantly in flaccid length of the penis, stretched length, or erectile length increase.

Discussion.—Information about the mean length and circumference of the flaccid and the erect penis may be of use to surgeons who are counseling patients considering penile augmentation. Any length within 2 standard deviations of the mean should be considered normal. Because depth of the pubic fat pad may significantly alter the perception of penile length, weight loss or suprapubic liposuction may be an alternative to penile lengthening.

▶ I am still waiting for the publication, in a peer-reviewed journal, of the technique and results of penile augmentation. All we have so far are reports of complications—no reports of results. Nevertheless, the procedure seems to be growing in popularity.

These authors present the most comprehensive study of penis size published to date. They include guidelines for selection of individuals who *should* undergo penile augmentation (although they do not tell their rationale for these guidelines), and recommendations for who *should not*. Will anyone listen?

R.L. Ruberg, M.D.

▶ Authors Wessells et al., are to be commended for their future assistance in defining norms for penile size. These guidelines should assist in preoperative counselling and planning in phallic reconstruction, including cases of trauma, intersex, micropenis, and gender reassignment using all of the current techniques available including free tissue transfer, corporal V-Y advancement as in cases of male exstrophy, and fat pad reduction using the technique of suction-assisted lipectomy and/or direct excision. Aesthetic penile surgery remains much more controversial and highly individualized, but the authors' data should be of assistance in preoperative planning during the consultation process. Much more remains to be learned and investigated in this expanding area of aesthetic surgery.

W.L. Funk, M.D.

Abdominoplasty With Two Fusiform Plications
Marques A, Brenda E, Pereira MD, et al (São Paulo, Brazil)
Aesthetic Plast Surg 20:249–251, 1996   4–67

Background.—Various procedures have been described for surgically managing the musculo-aponeurotic plane in abdominoplasty. Two important disadvantages have been associated with the classic xiphoid-pubic fusiform plication of the midline: the area becomes very flat in the first postoperative months, which then leads to bulging in the late postoperative period, probably because of tissue fraying. Surgery involving 2 fusiform plications outside the midline was recommended to avoid these disadvantages.

Methods.—Eleven patients, aged 26–57 years, underwent the procedure. A curved incision was made in the superior abdominal cavity in the suprapubic fold of the abdomen, with undermining at the level of the aponeurosis. Two vertical fusiform plications were created in the flanks with 0 cotton at the level of the transition of the sheaths of the rectus muscles with the external obliques. The patients were followed up for 8 months to 5 years.

Outcomes.—Surgery resulted in a slimmer waistline, which was maintained in the late postoperative period in 9 patients. The other 2 patients gained 6 to 8 kg, which almost completely destroyed the effect. None of the patients experienced complications.

Conclusions.—Two fusiform plications are recommended instead of the classic median xiphoid-pubic fusiform plication for abdominoplasty. The slimmer waistline produced intraoperatively was maintained in most patients in the late postoperative period without loss of the natural contour between the rectus muscles.

▶ According to some animal studies, excision and suturing is better than plication in terms of holding power.

P.W. McKinney, M.D.

Liposuction and Fat Grafting

The Liposhaver in Facial Plastic Surgery: A Multi-Institutional Experience
Becker DG, Weinberger MS, Miller PJ, et al (Tardy Facial Plastic Surgery Inst, Chicago; Oregon Health Sciences Univ, Portland; Univ of Virginia, Charlottesville)
Arch Otolaryngol Head Neck Surg 122:1161–1167, 1996   4–68

Introduction.—The various modifications of the original blunt liposuction cannulas have all retained the basic avulsion principle as the method of fat extraction. With soft-tissue shaving cannulas, fat removal is more precise and less traumatic. The results of the liposhaver in cosmetic facial surgery were reported for 19 patients who participated in a multicenter clinical trial of the device.

Methods.—A nonrandomized, nonblinded evaluation of the liposhaver was undertaken in patients having submental lipectomy, facelift with need for defatting beneath the facelift flap, and/or correction of deep nasolabial folds. The liposhaver was designed to cut fat preferentially but to be less efficient at cutting adjacent muscle and other soft tissue. Within the blunt, outer cannula lies a recessed oscillating blade that precisely cuts and extracts tissue as it is gently suctioned through the side port of the cannula. Surgeons at 3 centers reported details of each procedure and evaluated outcome. Preoperative and postoperative photographs were obtained.

Results.—The procedures were performed between August 1994 and April 1996. In all cases, the liposhaver was used successfully, and patients achieved the desired contour and profile result without any dimpling or asymmetry. There were no facial nerve injuries and no hematomas developed in the immediate postoperative period. All surgeons believed that the liposhaver was a precise, minimally traumatic, and efficient method of lipectomy. Some were able to rely on direct visualization to avoid cutting soft tissue other than fat, whereas other surgeons initially used precise surgical technique and knowledge of anatomy without direct visualization.

Discussion.—The liposhaver offers several advantages compared with conventional liposuction. Fat is removed precisely in a minimally traumatic manner, without potentially bruising back-and-forth motion. There is the potential, however, for injury to vital nerves or vessels in the head and neck area when the device is used in the power mode without direct visualization.

▶ This could also be effective for gynecomastia and perhaps less dangerous for ultrasonic liposuction.

P.W. McKinney, M.D.

Insulin-Induced Lipohypertrophy Treated by Liposuction
Barak A, Har-Shai Y, Ullmann Y, et al (Technion Israel Inst of Technology, Haifa)
Ann Plast Surg 37:415–417, 1996
4–69

Purpose.—Patients with diabetes may have insulin-induced lipohypertrophy develop as a complication of repeated subcutaneous insulin injection. Suction-assisted lipectomy (SAL) was used to treat this complication with good cosmetic and therapeutic results.

> *Case Report.*—Woman, 21, was evaluated for 2 large lipohypertrophic lumps in her lower abdomen (Figure). The lumps were associated with an insulin infusion pump that had been inserted in her lower abdomen, the needle location for which was changed every 2 days. The patient's blood sugar level was out of control. The pump was removed, and she began using other injection sites. However, the abdominal lumps persisted, and lipohypertrophy began developing at the other locations. Again, her blood sugar level was out of control. The abdominal masses, which measured about 8 × 5 cm, were treated by SAL. A total of 500 mL of aspirate was removed, mainly fibrofatty tissue. The aesthetic results were good, and the patient was able to resume insulin injections into her lower abdomen. The good insulin absorption at this location permitted better blood sugar control and avoided the need for painful and ineffective injections at the other sites.

Discussion.—The use of SAL to treat persistent insulin-induced lipohypertrophy in a patient with diabetes was reported. In this case, the liposuction offered not only aesthetic but also physiologic improvement by

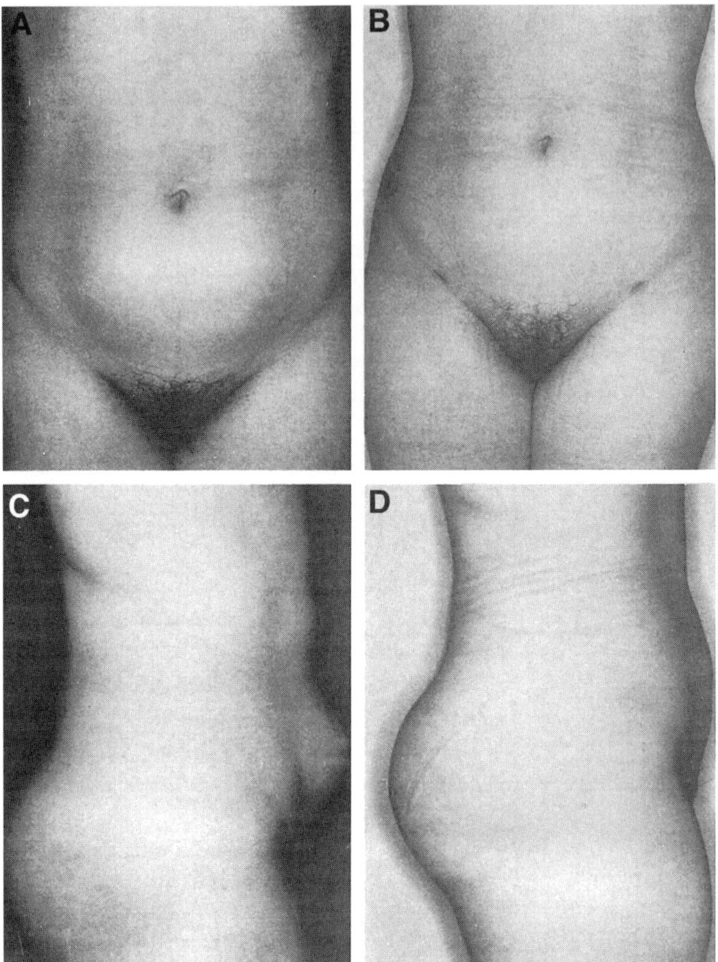

FIGURE.—A–D, preoperative anterior (**A**) and lateral (**C**) views of the lower abdominal area demonstrating the lipohypertrophic lumps. Postoperative anterior (**B**) and lateral (**D**) views of the lower abdominal area showing satisfactory results. (Reprinted from Barak A, Har-Shai Y, Ullman Y, et al: Insulin-induced lipohypertrophy treated by liposuction. *Ann Plast Surg* 37:415–417, 1996 by permission of Little, Brown and Company, Inc.)

permitting better insulin absorption at the treated site. Liposuction should be considered for diabetic patients with lipohypertrophy that does not respond to conservative treatment.

▶ I have used liposuction in 2 patients with lipohypertrophy from insulin injections. The results were comparable to those seen in this article. Both of my patients had significant localized fatty deposits in the lower abdomen. One also had started injecting her insulin in the hip areas because of the problem with the lower abdomen, and the lipohypertrophy had developed at this site as well. Liposuction was very successful in all treated areas, with great patient satisfaction.

R.L. Ruberg, M.D.

Standardization in Photography for Body Contour Surgery and Suction-Assisted Lipectomy
Gherardini G, Matarasso A, Serure AS, et al (Manhattan Eye, Ear and Throat Hosp, NY; MD Anderson Cancer Ctr, Houston; Univ of Miami, Fla; et al)
Plast Reconstr Surg 100:228–237, 1997   4–70

Background.—Specific guidelines for body contour photography have not been published. The current paper discusses further embellishments of conventional photographic standards and proposes new views for suction-assisted lipectomy and body contour methods. Standards for positioning the patient for photographing the arms, abdomen, hips, thighs, knees, calves, and ankles were also discussed, along with modifications of conventional views of the face and breast, where suction-assisted lipectomy is commonly performed.

Methods and Recommendations.—A model and professional photographic studio were used. In addition to the standard full-face frontal, oblique, and lateral views of the face undergoing liposuction, other views helpful in assessment and diagnosis are the close-up oblique view (for assessing bucal fat pads), a "grimace" view (for assessing platysmal bands), and a "reading view," with the neck flexed at about 50 degrees (for assessing submental fat). Arm views include the axilla with the upper arm perpendicular to the body, the elbow flexed at 90 degrees, the wrist neutral, and digits extended. For patients undergoing suction-assisted lipectomy of the abdomen, hips, thighs, and/or knees, a standard view is obtained with the feet 12 inches apart and hands folded above the breasts. Supplemental views of the abdomen include a close-up of the abdomen, the "diver's view," and a posterior view with gluteal muscles relaxed and tightened. Views of the knees, calves, and ankles should extend from the lower mid-thigh to the floor. A posterior view with the patient standing on tiptoe is also useful. For documenting skin tone and architecture, patients should be photographed in dark bikini underwear before and after surgery. This helps document the degree of skin flaccidity and tightening.

Conclusions.—Standard and supplemental views of patients undergoing suction-assisted lipectomy and body contour surgery were established in the current paper. These methods provide consistent photographic results for all practitioners.

▶ The most important thing we can do for our medical photography is standard pre-operative and post-operative lighting background and pose. Each surgeon has their own preference per views, type of flash, etc. I don't think that matters as much as, whatever is used, to have it the same before and after.

P.W. McKinney, M.D.

Body Sculpture: The Words Become Reality

Budo JA (Clinique St Joseph, Liège, Belgium)
Aesthetic Plast Surg 20:489–493, 1996   4–71

Purpose.—The results of liposuction have become more predictable in recent years. However, some areas remain difficult to treat by liposuction (i.e., the chin, the anterior and inner thigh, and the knee), especially when large amounts of fat are to be removed. Blood loss is another significant problem. An experience with ultrasonic (US) liposuction was presented.

Technique.—The US device consists of an electric generator, a handpiece, and cannulae for simultaneous aspiration and adipocytolysis. The apparatus functions in resonance mode, with low voltage and strong intensity settings. The use of US waves avoids the risk of perforation. Ultrasonic waves of alternating sinusoidal waves create a maximum of positive pressure to a maximum of negative pressure. The resulting suction is the source of cavitation, which resembles an implosion of the fatty cells. After being destroyed by the US waves, the fat is aspirated through the cannula.

Experience.—Fifty-six patients have been treated using the US liposuction device. Procedures were performed in the chin and neck, breast, waistline, abdomen, thighs, and knees. An average of 657 mL of fat was removed per procedure, in semiliquid and liquid form. Maximum perioperative blood loss was 50 mL.

Conclusions.—Ultrasonic liposuction permits very gentle and precise gestures, with the selectivity to permit superficial liposculpture. It can be used in areas previously rejected for liposuction, and reduces bleeding problems. Disadvantages include a longer operating time, more postoperative swelling, and a more complex setup.

▶ It would seem that US liposuction is easier and more precise than the conventional techniques. In addition, it can remove enormous amounts of fat in 1 procedure if one wishes to do that, although we have removed up to 9 L under local anesthesia with the tumescent technique, which I think is probably enough. There will be a learning curve with this technology and a danger of burn is not present in suction-assisted lipectomy. But for the world's most popular operation, it is a must-learn technique for truncal work. For the extremities and face, I doubt whether it is going to be a benefit.

P.W. McKinney, M.D.

Tumescent Liposuction Complicated by Pulmonary Edema

Gilliland MD, Coates N (Baylor College of Medicine, Houston)
Plast Reconstr Surg 99:215–219, 1997   4–72

Introduction.—The potential for fluid overload exists when rapid and high-volume hypodermoclysis is used in patients undergoing tumescent liposuction. In the case reported here, pulmonary edema developed shortly after the tumescent liposuction procedure was completed.

Case Report.—Man, 55, was an amateur bodybuilder who had undergone 3 previous liposuction procedures. To achieve more refinement in his abdomen and flanks, he sought further extraction of fat. The patient was placed under general anesthesia, then received an infusion of 7,900 cc of subcutaneous fluid into the area to be treated. During a 2.5-hour operation, 1,150 cc of supranatant fat and 2,750 cc of infranatant fluid were suctioned. Urine output was 450 cc. Except for difficulty in extracting fat from dense subcutaneous scar tissue, the operation was uneventful.

Twenty minutes postoperatively, however, the patient began to drop oxygen saturation to 84% to 92%. Right basilar rales without wheezes or rhonchi were noted at lung auscultation. Furosemide, 10 mg, was administered and resulted in immediate 350-cc urine output. The patient was transferred to the ICU because of persistent hypoxemia. Results of an ECG were normal and a chest x-ray study was nondiagnostic of pulmonary edema, pneumothorax, or fat emboli. Administration of furosemide produced 2,250 cc of urine over the next 4 hours, and oxygen saturation rose to 100% on 50% oxygen and 98% on room air. No further abnormalities were noted.

Discussion.—Large volumes of dilute lidocaine and epinephrine are infused subcutaneously in tumescent liposuction. In over 900 such procedures during which up to 15 liters were infused parenterally, this is the first case of pulmonary edema. In the patient reported here, IV fluid restriction and a larger diuretic dose near the end of the procedure might have prevented the complication. Patients with a history of intermittent fluid retention or other pulmonary problems might be treated more safely with serial liposuction.

▶ When liposuction originated, there were problems with hypovolemia because of the patient being NPO fluids of third space phenomena and blood loss. With the tumuscent technique (clyses), we have seen our first example of fluid overload. Why is it that as aesthetic surgeons, with time we lose sight of basic principles? For example, clyses is the way body fluids were replaced for many, many years. Imagine if this patient had been an older, nonathletic individual and had had 8 liters of fluid placed subcutaneously.

P.W. McKinney, M.D.

Intestinal Perforation After Suction Lipoplasty: A Case Report and Review of the Literature

Talmor M, Hoffman LA, Lieberman M (New York Hosp\Cornell Med Ctr)
Ann Plast Surg 38:169–172, 1997   4–73

Background.—Although relatively uncommon, intra-abdominal penetration with intestinal perforation is a potentially fatal complication of liposuction. More than half of the 7 patients reported to date have died. A patient with a perforated viscus after suction lipoplasty of the abdomen using the tumescent technique was seen.

Case Report.—A healthy woman, 50, underwent tumescent liposuction of the abdomen and rhytidectomy with no apparent complications. Within 24 hours of the procedure, however, the patient experienced nausea, vomiting, inability to tolerate oral intake, and diffuse abdominal pain. By the third day after surgery, fever and shaking chills had developed. She had not had a bowel movement or passed gas since her surgery. Her internist sent her to a local emergency department, where she was found to be tachycardic, hypotensive, and febrile, consistent with septic shock. Her abdomen was distended and diffusely tender to palpation with palpable crepitus. Bowel sounds were absent. A CT scan showed a large amount of free air and dilated loops of small bowel. Emergent exploratory laparotomy revealed an intense fibropurulent peritonitis in the peritoneal cavity. Six enterotomies were identified, affecting 5 feet of small bowel. A 30-cm segment of midjejunum was completely destroyed, necessitating small bowel resection. The remaining enterotomies were débrided, and the abdomen was irrigated. The operation lasted 4.5 hours. Cultures obtained during surgery grew *Klebsiella pneumoniae* and *Enterococcus faecalis*. The patient's postoperative course was complicated by new-onset atrial fibrillation, prolonged ileus necessitating total parenteral nutrition, and intrahepatic cholestasis. She was eventually discharged home 25 days after surgery.

Conclusions.—In this patient, multiple small-bowel enterotomies were made with the suction cannula during liposuction. This is a potentially fatal complication that requires early diagnosis and aggressive treatment. Patients must be instructed to seek medical care immediately if gastrointestinal problems develop in the early postoperative period after liposuction.

▶ The use of thin catheters, 1.5–3.5 mm, adds more finesse to our work, but at increased risk of perforation. I don't know that small catheters were used here, but I do know they are more dangerous in the suction techniques.

In addition, I would suspect the perforation probably occurred in the linea alba or at the costal margin which tends to flare when the patient is supine.

P.W. McKinney, M.D.

Small Intestinal Perforation and Peritonitis After Abdominal Suction Lipoplasty
Ovrebo KK, Grong K, Vindenes H (Haukeland Univ, Bergen Norway)
Ann Plast Surg 38:642–644, 1997   4–74

Purpose.—In patients with no history of abdominal surgery, suction lipoplasty for abdominal contouring is regarded as a safe procedure. However, the local complication rate increases when suction lipoplasty is combined with full abdominoplasty. Complications of abdominal suction lipoplasty in a patient with a history of abdominal surgery are reported.

Case.—Woman, 56, was hospitalized with signs of peritonitis. She had recently undergone 2 cosmetic abdominoplasties, with syringe-assisted liposuction performed the day before admission. She had had previous abdominal surgery, including abdominal hysterectomy and oophorectomy and resection of a colon adenoma, for a total of 4 laparotomies. Diffuse abdominal pain developed within 2 hours after the suction lipoplasty procedure. In addition to clinical signs of peritonitis, the patient had intraperitoneal gas on abdominal radiograph.

At laparotomy, the abdominal wall was stiff and fibrotic, with massive adhesions fixing it to the small intestine. Two small intestinal perforations were found which had caused leakage of bowel contents into the peritoneum. Surgery proceeded with resection and reconstruction of the perforated intestinal segment. The patient recovered uneventfully.

Discussion.—A history of abdominal surgery may raise the risk of complications in patients undergoing abdominal suction lipoplasty. In this case, intestinal perforation may have resulted from difficult handling of the liposuction instruments in the stiff subcutaneous skin. Closed suction could be used instead of repeated aspirations of seromas. In patients with a history of abdominal surgery, US or CT of the abdominal wall may be useful in detecting or ruling out underlying fascial defects or hernias.

▶ Suction with smaller catheters may penetrate the abdominal wall more often than we realize. One author (M. Zukowki, personal communication) found perforation of the abdominal wall in patients who had subsequent laparoscopy for other matters (perforations were identified in 4% of patients [2/50]). The smaller, sharper catheters are more accurate, but areas near the rib, intraabdominal scars, and the linea alba are vulnerable.

P.W. McKinney, M.D.

Lipoplasty in the Bulimic Patient

Willard SG, McDermott RE, Woodhouse LM (Tulane Univ, New Orleans, La)
Plast Reconstr Surg 98:276–278, 1996   4–75

Introduction.—Patients with bulimia nervosa seeking lipectomy may be exhibiting a variant of the purging behavior typical of these patients. Plastic surgeons must have a basic understanding of this disorder and the dangers of collaborating with the patient in a pathologic request for surgery. The number of suction-assisted lipectomy procedures performed in the United States is increasing, making it important for plastic surgeons to develop more sensitive screening policies. One study has shown that after lipectomy, only 76% of patients are satisfied, 30% believe that too little fat was removed, 29% claim that the fat recurred, and 50% report postoperative weight gain. In the United States, up to 20% of women may have symptoms of bulimia. These statistics suggest that many patients have unresolved issues relating to body image and weight. The plastic surgeon must be able to rule out patients with eating disorders, or must seek psychiatric consultation regarding the appropriateness of lipectomy in such patients. Individuals with bulimia often keep their symptoms a secret and are not physically identifiable because they often maintain normal weight. The cases of 2 women who were treated for bulimia nervosa and had surgical lipectomy were described.

Case Report.—Woman, 19, had a 4-year history of eating disorders and had been amenorrheic for the previous year. She was being treated for clinical depression with suicidal ideation. After 6 months of treatment at the Eating Disorders Clinic, she sought liposuction of her thighs and buttocks. Her weight was 122.5 lb and her body fat was 1% below normal range. The patient reported her bulimia to the plastic surgeon, who did not feel it was a medical risk that should preclude surgery, but when the surgeon was informed of the seriousness of the patient's psychiatric disorder, he decided not to perform the procedure. The patient received liposuction from a private surgeon in another hospital. After the procedure, the patient gained 25 lb within 3 months, resumed compulsive vomiting, and continued to have suicidal ideation. She stopped treatment at the clinic and was lost to follow-up.

Discussion.—The physician should be alert to a relatively thin young woman asking for lipectomy. Individuals with bulimia are usually within 5 lb of normal weight. The patient should be asked about a history of amenorrhea, binge eating, weight fluctuations, and dieting behavior. The physician should also ask the patient about her expected degree of satisfaction from the surgery, and any expectations that the surgery will change her life. Major discrepancies between the physician's and patient's evaluation of the patient's body or expectations may indicate potential psychological problems.

► I did not realize bulimia was such a well-hidden disease and the minimal bulges we occasionally see may not be recognized as such. This article re-emphasizes the need for contact with all physicians concerned.

P.W. McKinney, M.D.

Circumferential Liposuction of Knees, Calves, and Ankles
Ersek RA, Salisbury AV (Southwest Texas State Univ, Austin)
Plast Reconstr Surg 98:880–883, 1996   4–76

Background.—There is concern about performing liposuction in the ankles and calves because of the prolonged postoperative edema that follows. Good results have been achieved using long, small-tipped Illouz-style catheters for liposuction of the ankles, calves, and knees.

Technique.—Anesthesia is provided with valium followed by IV ketamine. This regimen maintains muscle tone in the calves, reducing the chances of thrombi. Liposuction is done using a super-wet technique, with infiltration of up to 1 L or 0.15% xylocaine with epinephrine in Ringer's lactate. Special blunt-tipped catheters measuring longer than 45 cm are used. Cannulas measuring 4 or 5 mm are used for small- to medium-sized calves, 6 mm for larger calves. To reach the calves, an incision is made in the crease behind the knee and a natural crease just above the Achilles tendon. Both sides must be symmetric, with some subcutaneous fat left behind to provide shape to the calves and ankles. These incisions provide complete circumferential access to the ankle and dorsum of the foot. After the wounds are closed, the entire extremity is tightly wrapped in Ace bandages, tightest at the toes. The bandages are then taped and left in place for 1 week. The patient is to keep the extremities elevated whenever possible. Postoperative massage is done at 1 week, and the patient wears custom-made support hose 24 hr/day for at least 6 weeks.

Results.—Good results were achieved with this technique in more than 100 patients. It is possible to remove liters of subcutaneous fat from the ankles, calves, and knees with reasonably smooth results. The procedure causes agonizing pain when walking for the first few days, and the pain continues for weeks. The patient must understand that the final results will not be visible for 6 weeks or even longer. Thereafter, gratifying results are usually seen. Uneven resection is an occasional problem, but can be corrected by a touch-up procedure within a few months. There have been no problems with infection, persistent edema, or pulmonary embolism.

Conclusions.—This technique of circumferential liposuction of the knees, calves, and ankles can safely recontour the entire leg with few complications. It should not be done in patients with a history of deep phlebitis, hypercoagulopathy, or thrombosis.

▶ Worthwhile results have been achieved with the technique described, but the patient must be prepared for a long healing period with edema and drainage.

P.W. McKinney, M.D.

Postliposuction Histologic Alterations of Adipose Tissue

Carpaneda CA (Brasília, Brazil)
Aesthetic Plast Surg 20:207–211, 1996

4–77

Objective.—Liposuction is a widely accepted technique that produces well-known laboratory and clinical changes. However, the histologic findings underlying these changes remain unclear. Histologic changes in the adipose tissue after suction-assisted lipectomy were studied.

Methods.—The study included 7 patients undergoing suction-assisted lipectomy of the inferior abdominal wall before classic abdominoplasty. The abdominoplasties were planned in 5 patients and performed because of patient dissatisfaction with the results of suction-assisted lipectomy in 2. The surgery permitted histologic examination of the adipose tissue changes after suction-assisted lipectomy. Time from liposuction to abdominoplasty ranged from 5 days to 6 months.

Findings.—On histologic examination, the area treated by liposuction showed large amounts of dead adipocytes and free fat. The pockets created by liposuction were filled with serum hemorrhagic material, which gradually evolved into a healing process; irregular scarring was noted by 30 days. The scars, which matured better when positioned perpendicular or oblique to the surface, provided a new lobular appearance to the adipose tissue and a new supportive framework for the skin. Healing was characterized by increased collagen synthesis at first, followed by a gradual reduction in collagen and a remodeling process.

Discussion.—The histologic changes of adipose tissue after suction-assisted lipectomy are described. Liposuction causes vessel and nerve damage and avulses fragments of adipose tissue, producing hemorrhage and altered sensibility. The free fat that remains and the scarring that follows may take months or even years to resolve completely.

▶ Patients must be aware of the patience required for a final result (from 6 months to a year in the body). They may return in 3 months and complain of being "bloated," which probably reflects the intermittent swelling normally seen in extensive liposuction.

P.W. McKinney, M.D.

Mechanical Properties of Skin and Liposuction
Henry F, Van Look, Goffin V, et al (Univ of Liège, Belgium)
Dermatol Surg 22:566–568, 1996   4–78

Introduction.—The mechanical functions of the skin are partly influenced by the underlying subcutaneous fat. Since liposuction removes some of that fat, setting the skin under tension, it could lead to changes in the overall viscoelastic properties of the skin. Changes in skin extensibility and elasticity after liposuction were investigated.

Methods.—The study included 44 patients, 19 to 59 years of age, who underwent liposuction. The mechanical properties of the skin at the liposuction site were measured 5 to 8 months postoperatively using a noninvasive suction device, the Cutometer SEM 474, with an 8 mm probe. The measured viscoelastic values were compared with the "internal standard" of the skin of the inner forearm.

Results.—The biomechanical properties of the skin at various liposuction sites were not significantly different from those of the forearms. Cutaneous laxity was rarely observed at the liposuction sites.

Conclusions.—Liposuction does not appear to result in increased skin laxity, and thus does not increase clinical signs of skin aging. There is large variation in the extensibility of skin at liposuction sites, while biologic elasticity is almost always greater where liposuction has been performed.

▶ It doesn't loosen the skin; on the contrary it seems that it may shrink it.[1] There are already many examples of skin retraction in the literature. Suction deflates the skin, but it is able to contract to some degree. This difference has to be explained to patients in terms they can understand.

P.W. McKinney, M.D.

Reference

1. Maillard GF, Scheflan M, Bussien R: Ultrasonically assisted lipectomy in aesthetic breast surgery. *Plast Reconstr Surg* 100:238–241, 1997.

Fat Injection: Long-term Follow-up
Chajchir A (Barrancas Med Ctr, Buenos Aires, Argentina)
Aesthetic Plast Surg 20:291–296, 1996   4–79

Objective.—Fat transplants have been used with varying results to correct soft-tissue defects. Aspirating fat carefully and avoiding injury to delicate tissue during injection can prevent scarring. Results of patients treated between 1984 and 1994 were retrospectively reviewed and evaluated.

Methods.—Patients were carefully selected and counseled regarding expectations. A small cannula is used to remove fat globules from the abdomen, trochanter, thigh, knee, or gluteals into a sterile glass receptacle using a pump at 20% to 30% of power with a vacuum not exceeding –10 mm Hg or −30 kPA. The fat globules are placed in a syringe, and parallel cylinders of fat are injected with a trocar at low pressure into a well-irrigated site. After the area is massaged to distribute the fat, the donor area is compressed to prevent edema and bruising.

Results.—Patients were evaluated 3 times a week for 2 weeks and then monthly thereafter (Fig 3 and Fig 4). If reabsorption of material occurs, a second procedure is performed 6–12 months later using another donor site. Skin quality and cellular tissue improved, particularly in women. Complications included edema, hematomas, infection, reabsorption, cysts, and deformities as a result of excess material.

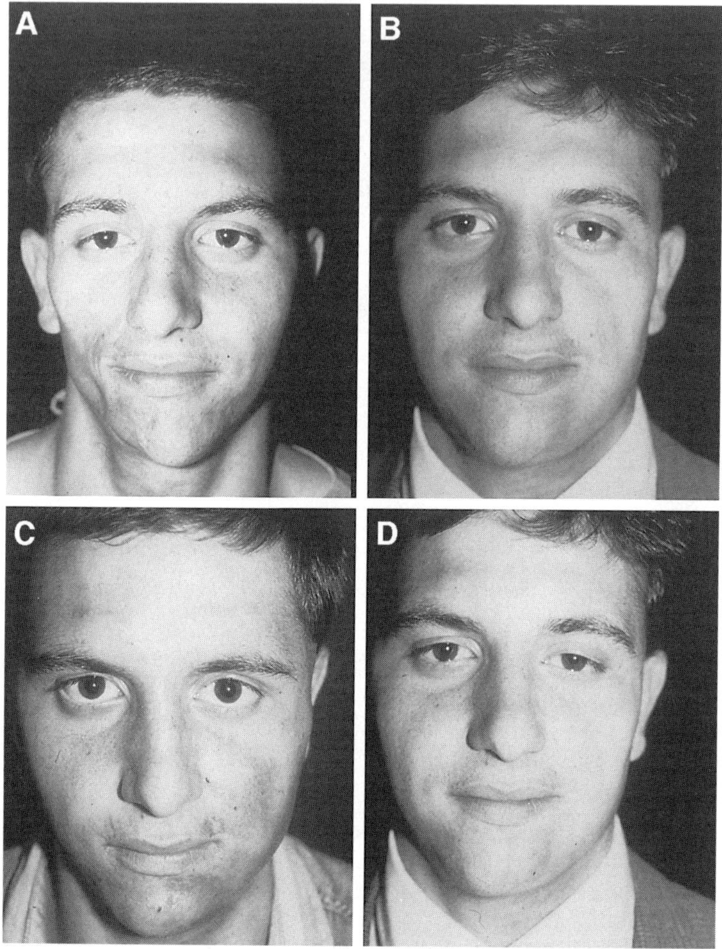

FIGURE 3.—A, patient with scleroderma. **B,** after first fat injection. There was a notable improvement in all the tissues, skin, and cellular and muscle tissue as a result of better irrigation of the area. **C,** same patient 3 years after the first fat injection. **D,** patient 2 years after the second fat injection. With this second injection a noticeable improvement in the volume was obtained. (Courtesy of Chajchir A: Fat injection: Long-term follow-up. *Aesthetic Plast Surg* 10:291–296, 1996. © 1996 Springer-Verlag New York Inc.)

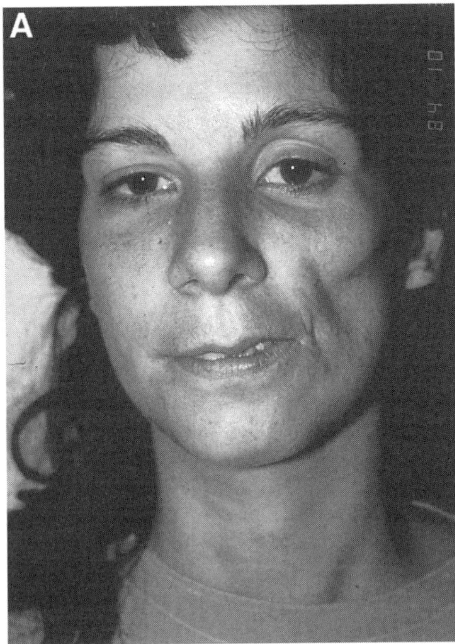
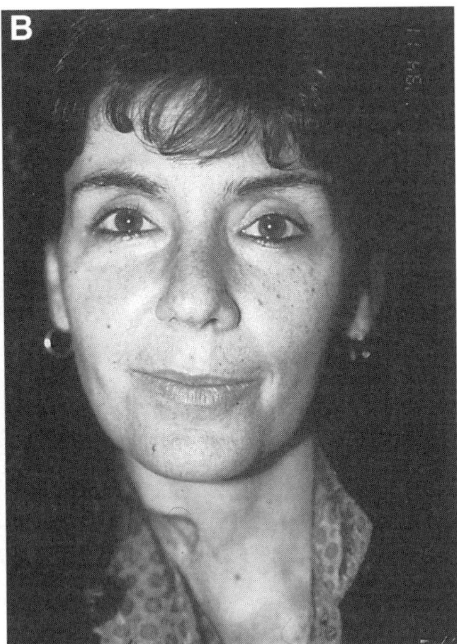

FIGURE 4.—**A,** patient with hemifacial atrophy (Romberg's disease) and **B,** 9 years after 2 fat grafts. The first 1 was in 1984, and the second was in 1987. (Courtesy of Chajchir A: Fat injection: Long-term follow-up. *Aesthetic Plast Surg* 10:291–296, 1996. © 1996 Springer-Verlag New York Inc.)

Conclusion.—Long-term results of fat injection to correct soft-tissue deformities in this study are satisfactory but depend, to a large extent, on harvesting and injecting techniques and the choice of the recipient site.

▶ This is a worthwhile improvement in the treatment of a difficult-to-treat disease. Note that it is applied in areas under less muscle action than one finds in the glabella or the nasal labial fold, where many authors believe it doesn't last. Fat injections are very dependent on technique, and the recipient site.

P.W. McKinney, M.D.

Additional Reading

Ramirez O: Cervicoplasty: Nonexcisional anterior approach. *Plast Reconstr Surg* 99:1576–1585, 1997.

▶ I'm fascinated by the suture suspension technique. I remember Dr. James Smith introducing the umbilical tape technique at the American Society of Plastic and Reconstructive Surgeons meeting in New York in the '80s. The wide undermining in plastysma plasty and suture suspension gives very good results with or without a lower rhytidectomy. Do we need a permanent suture? Do we need it to interlock or will a dissolvable suture do the work and leave, as I feel it would in most situations. Giampapa[1] feels that the permanent suture is necessary to allow the scar to form properly, and the interlocking technique prevents slippage.

Reference

1. Giampapa V: Neck recontouring suture suspension tech, presented at the 26th annual meeting of ASAPS in Boston, 1993.

Morello DC, Colon GA, Fredricks S, et al: Patient safety in accredited office surgical facilities. *Plast Reconstr Surg* 99:1496–1500, 1997.
▶ This is important documentation as office facilities are user-friendly. Hospitals are prone to other agendas which obstruct patient care, not to mention hospital-based "staph." This, of course, leaves a problem for all plastic surgeons in that leaving the hospital setting reduces our exposure. However, except in rare circumstances, there is really very little choice.

Connell BF, Shamoun JM: The significance of digastric muscle contouring for rejuvenation of the submental area of the face. *Plast Reconstr Surg* 99:1586–1590, 1997.
▶ I have never recognized this entity before and now will have to look for it. The question that comes to my mind is why this muscle should be so large, except perhaps in singers, when all other muscles of the body atrophy in the age group we are treating.

Ostad A, Kageyama N, Moy RL: Tumescent anesthesia with a lidocaine dose of 55 mg/kg is safe for liposuction. *Dermatol Surg* 22:921–927, 1996.
▶ In pharmacologic texts, 5–7 mg/kg per hour is the "official" dosage—it is good to have it documented that 55 mg/kg is safe when epinephrine and suction are used.

Ersek RA, Mann GE II, Salisbury S, et al: Noninvasive mechanical body contouring. A preliminary clinical outcome study. *Aesthetic Plast Surg* 21:61–67, 1997.
▶ It seems a mild reduction is possible with this machine, and it may be similar to certain deep massage treatments. It is worth a try in that it is harmless, and many have advocated it for the use of postsuction and for "cellulite."

Har-Shai Y, Lindenbaum E, Ben-Itzhak O, et al: Large liponecrotic pseudocyst formation following cheek augmentation by fat injection. *Aesthetic Plast Surg* 20:417–419, 1996.
▶ We know that some of the injected fat does not survive and some of what is injected is most likely oil, so we should be alert to the fact that these cysts are going to develop. Would small amounts cause less of these cysts?

P.W. McKinney, M.D.

5   Breast

Silicone and Augmentation

Characteristics of Women With and Without Breast Augmentation
Cook LS, Daling JR, Voigt LF, et al (Fred Hutchinson Cancer Research Ctr, Seattle; Univ of Washington, Seattle; Univ of Utah, Salt Lake City; et al)
JAMA 277:1612–1617, 1997   5–1

Objective.—Although silicone breast implants have been associated with myriad illnesses, most epidemiologic studies have failed to establish a connection. Because the characteristics of women with and without implants may be different and therefore may confound epidemiologic studies, interviews were conducted to identify any differences between the 2 groups.

Methods.—The case–control cross-sectional analysis involved personal structured interviews with 80 women who underwent breast augmentation between the ages of 17 and 49 years and 3,490 women who did not; the analysis included records of major life events and photographs of oral contraceptive and hormone preparations used to enhance recall of past exposures.

Results.—Women with implants were better educated, less likely to be overweight, more likely to drink and smoke, younger at first pregnancy, younger at first birth, had a history of pregnancy terminations, more likely to have a first-degree relative with breast cancer, more likely to have used oral contraceptives and more likely to have used them longer, had more lifetime sexual partners, and more likely to use hair dyes than women without implants.

Conclusion.—Limitations of this study include the small number of women with implants and the 70.7% and 76.7% levels of response among the 2 groups of women. These findings show that the characteristics of women with breast implants are possibly very different from those of women without breast implants and illustrate the potential confounding factors in any analysis of the risk of breast augmentation.

▶ This article has sparked a great deal of interest in the popular media—much of it inappropriate. Various individuals have actually tried to use the data to criticize women who have undergone breast augmentation, that is, "they have abortions, they drink, they use oral contraceptives," etc. Plastic surgeons should work to keep their focus on the major contribution of this article: the fact that any studies comparing women with and without breast implants must take into account these, and perhaps many others as yet undescribed, differences between the study groups.

R.L. Ruberg, M.D.

Complications Leading to Surgery After Breast Implantation

Gabriel SE, Woods JE, O'Fallon WM, et al (Mayo Clinic and Found, Rochester, Minn)
N Engl J Med 336:677–682, 1997

5–2

Introduction.—As many as 2 million women in the United States have had breast implantation. A previous study showed no increased risk of connective-tissue or autoimmune disorders among women with breast implants compared with those without. However, there is some concern that local complications may be an important problem, but this is difficult to prove because there has not been a population-based study. The occurrence of surgically treated local complications in the population-based cohort of women living in Olmsted County, Minnesota, was analyzed.

Methods.—Breast implants were placed in 749 women between 1964 and 1991. After the initial procedure and after any subsequent implantation, complications were identified, such as capsular contracture; rupture of the implant; hematoma or bleeding; infection or seroma of the wound; chronic pain; extrusion, leakage, or sweating of the implant; necrosis of the areola, nipple, or flap; wound dehiscence; or malfunction of the filler port of a tissue expander.

Results.—There were 450 additional implant-related surgical procedures for 208 women (27.8%) during a mean follow-up of 7.8 years. There were 359 procedures (79.8%) done for at least 1 clinical indication, thus constituting a complication. The others were anticipated, staged procedures or were done because the woman requested a size change or aesthetic improvement. Of the 749 women involved, 178 had complications (23.8%). Capsular contraction was the most frequent problem (131

TABLE 3.—Estimated Cumulative Incidence of Complications According to the Tme After and Reason for Implantation

REASON	TIME AFTER INITIAL IMPLANTATION					
	60 DAYS		270 DAYS		5 YEARS	
	%	95% CI	%	95% CI	%	95% CI
Cosmetic	3.7	2.5–5.1	5.7	4.0–7.6	12.0	9.1–15.2
Cancer	4.0	2.1–6.6	19.1	13.9–24.0	34.0	27.2–41.3
Prophylactic	3.4	1.1–6.9	16.0	10.4–22.6	30.4	23.1–38.4

Note: Cumulative incidence was estimated by the Kaplan-Meier method.
Abbreviation: CI, confidence interval.
(Reprinted by permission of *The New England Journal of Medicine,* courtesy of Gabriel SE, Woods JE, O'Fallon WM, et al: Complications leading to surgery after breast implantation. *N Engl J Med* 336:677–682, copyright 1997, Massachusetts Medical Society.)

women), followed by implant rupture (5.7%), hematoma, and wound infection. Among women with cosmetic implants, the rate of complications was significantly lower (12% at 5 years) than among those who received implants after mastectomy for breast cancer (34% at 5 years) or prophylactic mastectomy (30.4% at 5 years) (Table 3).

Conclusion.—Local complications are experienced among women who have had breast implantation during the subsequent 5 years. Those who had implants for cosmetic reasons had significantly fewer complications than those who had implants after mastectomy for cancer or for cancer prophylaxis.

▶ This is an important study, not only for its conclusions, which were known intuitively by most plastic surgeons, but because it establishes a database that should be reproducible by other investigators. The major question is whether this retrospective chart review documents those complications that may have led to surgery in the opinion of other surgeons, i.e., the degree of capsular contracture. Another potential concern is whether the techniques and types of implant used during the time period studied varied and would these factors have altered some of the authors' conclusions?

S.H. Miller, M.D.

▶ This is really a valuable article because the information is probably as reliable as can be collected. There should be no bias—no patients lost to follow-up, no bias created by self-reporting, etc.. These are the facts. Tell them to your breast implant patients.

R.L. Ruberg, M.D.

Use of Antipolymer Antibody Assay in Recipients of Silicone Breast Implants
Tenenbaum SA, Rice JC, Espinoza LR, et al (Tulane Univ, New Orleans, La; Louisiana State Univ, New Orleans; Arizona Rheumatology Ctr, Phoenix; et al)
Lancet 349:449–454, 1997   5–3

Introduction.—It is not known whether autoimmune disease is increased in recipients of silicone-containing breast implant (SBI). Serum antibodies to an antigen of apparently high molecular weight have recently been detected in many SBI recipients. The antigen is a complex of synthetic polymers. An antipolymer antibody (APA) assay was developed that is similar to Western immunoblotting. Recipients of SBI and nonexposed controls were evaluated for presence of APA to determine whether there are any between-group differences in proportions of APA; whether the severity of clinical signs and symptoms are associated with APA in SBI recipients, and whether there is a correlation between the presence of APA and ANA.

Methods.—Serum samples were evaluated for APA and ANA in female SBI recipients (with and without symptoms), nonrecipients with autoimmune diseases, and healthy nonrecipient controls. Severity of signs and symptoms were compared with assays for APA and ANA.

Results.—In SBI recipients, positive APA results were observed in: 1 of 34 (3%) with limited symptoms, 2 of 26 (8%) with mild symptoms, 7 of 16 (44%) with moderate symptoms, and 13 of 19 (68%) with advanced symptoms. Only 4 of 23 (17%) healthy non–SBI-exposed controls and 2 of 20 (10%) nonexposed women with classic autoimmune diseases tested positive for APA. The rate of positive ANA results was significantly higher for women with classic autoimmune diseases, compared to SBI subgroups (70% vs. 0% to 33%).

Conclusion.—Findings suggest that the APA assay can objectively distinguish between SBI recipients with limited or mild signs and symptoms, those with severe signs and symptoms, and patients with specific autoimmune diseases. The APA and ANA assays may provide clinically important information when compared in a single patient.

▶ The authors report that they were able to detect antipolymer antibody in 3% of patients with SBIs and limited symptoms of systemic (autoimmune-musculoskeletal) disease, 8% of those with SBI having mild symptoms, and 68% of those with advanced symptoms. They conclude that their test for APA can be used to distinguish between patients with SBI having limited symptoms and those with more severe symptoms.

There are several technical problems with this study. The most telling is that the control group were normal women without SBI and without fibromyalgia. A control group of patients with fibromyalgia having similar degrees of "symptoms and severity" should have been included. Inclusion of such a control group is certainly warranted when one notes that one of the principal authors[1] of this *Lancet* article published an abstract in 1996 entitled "Development of a laboratory marker for fibromyalgia patients who do not have silicone breast implants." This suggests that the authors may have developed an assay for fibromyalgia. However, they have not shown that their assay is sensitive or specific for SBIs.

S.H. Miller, M.D.

Reference

1. Gluck OS, Tesser JRP, Tenenbaum SA, et al: Development of a laboratory marker for fibromyalgia. *Arth Rheum* 39(s):S90, 1996.

Lack of Association Between Augmentation Mammoplasty and Systemic Sclerosis (Scleroderma)

Hochberg MC, Perlmutter DL, Medsger TA Jr, et al (Univ of Maryland, Baltimore; Univ of Pittsburgh, Pa; Univ of California, San Diego; et al)
Arthritis Rheum 39:1125–1131, 1996
5–4

Background.—Reports of connective-tissue disease in women who had undergone augmentation mammaplasty with silicone gel–filled breast implants started to appear in the 1980s. In a review of the English-language literature published from 1979 through June 1993, 38 of 57 patients with definite connective-tissue disease had a diagnosis of systemic sclerosis (SSc). The etiology of this uncommon disease is unknown, but several occupational and environmental factors have been associated with its development. A multicenter case-control study tested the hypothesis that augmentation mammoplasty with silicone gel–filled breast implants is associated with subsequent development of SSc.

Methods.—Cases were 837 women with a clinical diagnosis of SSc who were recruited from 3 scleroderma clinical research centers. Controls were 2,507 women who were race-matched and age-matched to cases in 3 strata: younger than 45 years, 45 to 64 years, and 65 years and older. Cases and controls completed a questionnaire that included sections on sociodemographic variables, gynecologic and obstetric history, and history of breast surgery.

Results.—Cases and controls were similar in mean age at interview, percentages of those currently married, and rate of high school graduation. Neither breast surgery nor augmentation mammaplasty were reported with significantly greater frequency in cases than in controls (Table 2). Among cases, the interval between augmentation mammaplasty and diagnosis of SSc ranged from 4 to 21 years (median, 11 years). Although none reported complications of the implants, 2 underwent removal because of the diagnosis of scleroderma, 1 for hardening, and 1 for hardening and leakage. Controls had undergone implantation a median of 10 years before the interview; 5 reported complications and 1 had the prostheses removed because of breast pain.

TABLE 2.—Frequency of Breast Surgery and Augmentation Mammoplasty in 837 Women with Systemic Sclerosis (Cases) and 2,507 Age-, Race-, and Sex-matched Local Controls

	Cases	Controls
Breast surgery, no. (%)*	117 (17.9)	463 (18.5)
Augmentation mammoplasty, no. (%)	11 (1.31)	31 (1.24)†

*Data available on 653 cases and 2,507 controls.

†Odds ratio (95% confidence interval) estimated from multiple logistic regression model with adjustment for age, race, and site was 1.07 (0.53–2.13), whereas that estimated from conditional logistic regression model with adjustment for age was 1.11 (0.55–2.24).

(Courtesy of Hochberg MC, Perlmutter DL, Medsger TA Jr, et al: Lack of association between augmentation mammoplasty and systemic sclerosis (scleroderma). *Arthritis Rheum* 39:1125–1131, 1996.)

Discussion.—As in other epidemiologic studies, these data from the largest case-control study of the subject to date do not support the hypothesis that silicone gel–filled breast implants are associated with a significantly increased risk of development of SSc. Not addressed here is the possibility of an association between the implants and other connective-tissue diseases.

▶ This article is an important addition to the growing body of scientific knowledge that refutes the various anecdotal and unsubstantiated claims of diseases "caused" by silicone gel–filled breast implants. The work is very carefully done by a respected group of epidemiologic researchers. It is important to note that the study specifically examined the relation of implants and scleroderma and did not address a relation with any other connective-tissue disorders.

R.L. Ruberg, M.D.

Outcome of Mammary Prostheses Explantation: A Patient Perspective
Svahn JK, Vastine VL, Landon BN, et al (Univ of California, San Diego)
Ann Plast Surg 36:594–600, 1996   5–5

Objective.—Although the overall satisfaction rate is high after implantation with silicone gel-filled mammary implants (SGMI), adverse publicity, older age of patients with implants and influence of patient groups have resulted in frequent requests for explantation. Patient satisfaction rates after surgery and determinants for surgery were studied.

Methods.—A postoperative self-assessment questionnaire sent to 100 consecutive white females who underwent removal of SGMIs 6 to 12 months after surgery was completed by 63 patients, aged 24 to 69 years. Patient indications for surgery were suspected connective-tissue disorder as a result of implants (43 patients), painful breast with signs of capsular contraction (37 patients), fear of side effects of silicone (31 patients), fear of implant rupture (25 patients), breast deformity (21 patients), and MRI with evidence of rupture or leak (20 patients). Association between preoperative, operative, and postoperative factors and patient perception of surgical outcome were analyzed statistically.

Results.—Surveys were completed by 45 patients who had original surgery for esthetic reasons and 18 patients who had surgical reconstruction (Table 4). Eight of 11 patients with no medical problems were satisfied. Pain, anxiety, and depression were reduced, whereas confidence in the medical establishment and family and domestic life improved in 49 patients after surgery. However, 14 others with pain before explantation continued to have pain and other symptoms after surgery. Outcome, including appearance, was described as expected by 21 patients, better than expected by 26, worse than expected by 7, and no response by 7. Sixty patients said the informed consent helped them to accept the outcome. If they thought implants were safe, 15 patients would have them again, and 41 would not. Seven patients did not answer the question.

TABLE 4.—Postoperative Characteristics and Outcome of Explantation Surgery

Variable	Satisfied N = 51	Group Dissatisfied/ No Response N = 12	p value
Postexplantation complication			
No	35 (56%)	5 (8%)	0.548
Yes	16 (25%)	7 (11%)	0.405
Scarring	6	4	—
Seroma/infection	3	5	—
New chronic pain	3	2	—
Other (e.g., exacerbation of general problems)	4	2	—
Overall breast and body image change after explantation			
No change	9 (14%)	3 (5%)	0.937
Improvement	39 (62%)	3 (5%)	0.155
Worsening	2 (3%)	2 (3%)	0.400
No response	1 (2%)	4 (6%)	0.011
If convinced that SGMIs are safe, would like them back			
Yes	10 (16%)	5 (8%)	0.392
No	37 (59%)	4 (6%)	0.315
No response	4 (6%)	3 (5%)	0.332

(Courtesy of Svahn JK, Vastine VL, Landon BN, et al: Outcome of mammary prostheses explantation: A patient perspective. Reprinted with permission from *Ann Plast Surg* 36:594–600, 1996.)

Conclusion.—This information should be helpful in counseling patients who are thinking about breast implant removal.

▶ Previous studies of women undergoing SGMI extirpation have shown that patients with *local* symptoms achieve long-term relief, whereas those with systemic symptoms do not. This study did not examine the reasons for extirpation so presumably some patients in the series wanted their implants out because of symptoms (68% had "symptoms" attributed to SGMI), and others had a different motivation (e.g., involvement in SGMI litigation, silicone fears, etc.). In this diverse group the authors found that about 80% of patients noted an improvement in "quality of life"—a complex and largely subjective standard—as a result of implant removal. The information provided in this study should be helpful in counseling patients who are contemplating breast implant extirpation.

R.L. Ruberg, M.D.

Aesthetic Outcome of Breast Implant Removal in 85 Consecutive Patients

Netscher DT, Sharma S, Thornby J, et al (Baylor College of Medicine, Houston)
Plast Reconstr Surg 100:206–219, 1997

5–6

Introduction.—Concerns ranging from possible implant rupture to local breast discomfort secondary to symptomatic capsular contracture to the possible association of implants with systemic illness are causing women to

TABLE 2.—Percentage Change by Category for Each of Removal Only and Removal With Mastopexy

	Removal Only			Removal plus Mastopexy		
	Worse	Same	Improved	Worse	Same	Improved
Ptosis	58.6	27.6	13.8	5.6	5.6	88.8
Profile contour	86.2	6.9	6.9	66.7	22.2	11.1
Aesthetic proportion	72.4	17.2	10.4	44.4	16.7	38.9
Symmetry	44.8	24.1	31.1	22.2	38.9	38.9
Combined score*	82.8	3.4	13.8	33.3	0.00	66.7

*$P = 0.001$.

(Courtesy of Netscher DT, Sharma S, Thornby J, et al: Aesthetic outcome of breast implant removal in 85 consecutive patients. *Plast Reconstr Surg* 100:206–219, 1997.)

visit their plastic surgeons in increasing numbers. The women had implants either for cosmetic reasons or because of mastectomy for breast cancer or bilateral subcutaneous mastectomy. When the women come back to the surgeon asking for breast implant removal, it has been difficult to advise these patients properly because the esthetic outcome of removal has not been predictable. The records and outcomes of women who had implants removed in a 2-year period were reviewed.

Methods.—The review included 85 women who had implant removal, of which 69 originally had cosmetic augmentation and 16 had breast reconstruction with silicone gel implants. Removal of implants alone was conducted on 39 of 69 patients with cosmetic augmentation and 27 had mastopexy accompanying removal. Reaugmentation with saline-filled implants was performed on 3 women and 1 woman had replacement with saline-filled implants Autogenous tissue transfer was performed for 15 of 16 women who had breast reconstruction. Using a 5-point scoring system, preoperative and postoperative photographs of all women were rated. Patients also filled out a questionnaire.

Results.—Adverse esthetic results occur among cosmetic augmentation patients who have implant removal only. When mastopexy is performed in conjunction with implant removal, the postremoval appearance of many patients with cosmetic augmentation actually will be improved over their preoperative appearance (Table 2). A particular outcome can be predicted for women with certain body types. For example, unsatisfactory esthetic outcomes resulted in women with asthenic builds and older women with lax, striated breast skin if they had implant removal only. Favorable results were found with women selected for autogenous breast reconstruction with good outcomes resulting with latissimus dorsi and transverse rectus abdominis myocutaneous flaps.

Conclusion.—A more pleasing esthetic outcome results if patients have mastopexy in conjunction with breast implant removal. This may not apply for women who are full-breast, full-framed, or youthful, and asthenic with elastic skin and modest augmentations.

▶ In this series, most patients showed esthetic improvement when implant removal was combined with mastopexy. This should be useful information to

present to patients requesting implant removal — but it is not an "absolute."
I (and probably the authors as well) would emphasize the need to treat the
whole patient, not just the patient's breasts. Other considerations (additional
costs, additional scars) may lead some patients to choose implant removal
alone, even when advised of the results of this study.

R.L. Ruberg, M.D.

Textured or Smooth Implants for Breast Augmentation: Three Year Follow-up of a Prospective Randomised Controlled Trial

Malata CM, Feldberg L, Coleman DJ, et al (Univ of Bradford, England; Bradford Royal Infirmary, England)
Br J Plast Surg 50:99–105, 1997

5–7

Introduction.—The most frequent complication of augmentation mammaplasty is fibrous capsular contraction around silicone breast implants. Adverse capsular contracture (Baker grades III and IV) has been decreased by implant surface texturing. This has been shown to reduce capsular contracture around static and dynamic implants. An assessment was made as to whether the lower adverse capsular contracture rates seen in the short-term with textured silicone gel-filled breast implants persisted in the medium-term.

Methods.—In a randomized, double-blind study, 53 women had subglandular breast augmentation mammaplasty and were randomized to textured or smooth silicone gel-fillled implants. Results were tabulated 1 and 3 years later, and the degree of capsular contracture was determined by the Baker scale.

Results.—For smooth implants, the incidence of adverse capsular contracture was 59%, whereas for textured implants, the incidence was 11%

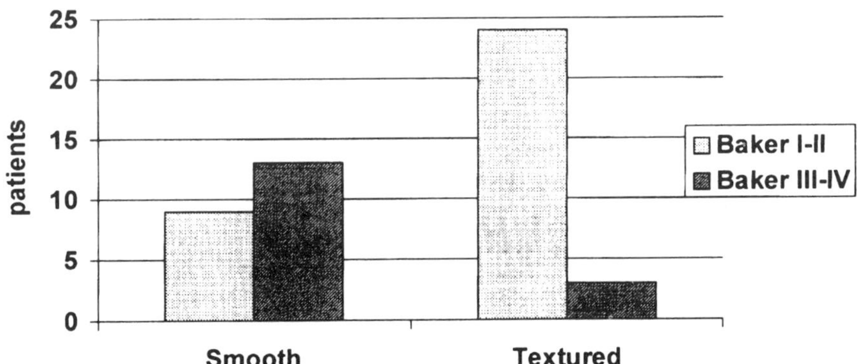

FIGURE 3.—Incidence of capsular contracture at 3 years (including implants exchanged). There was a significant difference between the textured and smooth implants ($P = 0.001$, Yates' correction of the chi-square test). (Courtesy of Malata CM, Feldberg L, Coleman DJ, et al: Textured or smooth implants for breast augmentation: Three-year follow-up of a prospective randomized controlled trial. *Br J Plast Surg* 50:99–105, 1997.)

(Fig 3). Between the 1- and 3-year assessments, 8 women (31%) with smooth prostheses had breast implant exchange. In the textured implant group, 2 women (7.4%) had revisional surgery. In women with textured implants who had revisional surgery, the capsule was lined with a synovial-like fluid with no close adherence of the textured implant envelope to the capsule.

Conclusion.—In augmentation mammaplasty, the effect of textured implants in reducing capsular contracture found at 1 year was maintained at 3 years, as evidenced by the adverse capsular contracture and revisional breast implant surgery rates. These effects of textured implants may be long lasting. Further studies are needed to determine to what degree silicone breast implant surface texturing reduces capsular contracture at 5 and 10 years postoperatively.

▶ Is a 3-year follow-up enough? Probably not. What I really want to see is the 10-year data. But this is a start.

R.L. Ruberg, M.D.

Microbial Growth Inside Saline-filled Breast Implants

Young VL, Hertl MC, Murray PR, et al (Washington Univ, St Louis)
Plast Reconstr Surg 100:182–196, 1997

5–8

Introduction.—Many believed that the silicone envelope of a breast implant was impermeable to large and highly charged molecules that might serve as nutritional substrates for microbial growth, thus the subject of intraluminal contamination of saline-filled breast implants largely has been ignored. Some reports, however, have surfaced of fungal and bacterial species surviving inside saline-filled implants. The issue of microbial growth in the restricted environment of saline-filled implants or tissue expanders has not been widely published. Whether common microorganisms could survive and multiply in saline over a period of time was investigated.

Methods.—The bacteria tested in the in vitro and in vivo experiments were *Staphylococcus aureus, Staphylococcus epidermis, Escherichia coli, Corynebacterium jeikeium, Enterobacter cloacae, Klebsiella pneumoniae,* and *Pseudomonas aeruginosa.* Also included in the test were 3 fungal species: *Aspergillus fumigatus, Paecilomyces variotii,* and *Candida albicans.* The in vitro study involved 9 microorganisms being inoculated into sterile bottles containing 125 mL of 0.9% sterile saline IV fluid, which were incubated for 2 weeks. The in vivo study involved 61 white rabbits with 122 implants who received an experimental implant inoculated with one of the test organisms and a control implant. At 1-, 3- or 6-months, the rabbits were sacrificed, and cultures were taken.

Results.—The in vitro study had 4 organisms surviving in flasks of sterile saline for 2 weeks: *A. fumigatus, C. albicans, K. pneumoniae,* and *P. variotti.* In the in vivo study, none of the control implants had positive cultures. In the experimental implants, however, there were positive cultures for 7 of the 10 inoculated organisms: *S. epidermidis, E. coli, E. cloacae, K. pneumoniae, P. aeruginosa, A. fumigatus,* and *P. variotii.* The capsular cultures showed that 17% (21 of 122) were positive and surrounded inoculated and sterile implants. Capsules that were culture positive, in most instances, contained an organism that was different from the implant that was inoculated in the group.

Conclusion.—In a restricted saline environment for extended periods of time, several types of bacteria, particularly the gram-negative species, and fungi can grow and reproduce. Before it is known how safe saline-implants are more research would be helpful.

▶ In addition to providing new information about microbial growth inside implants, this article has an excellent review of much of the previously published data regarding breast implants and infection.

R.L. Ruberg, M.D.

The Tuberous Breast Deformity: Classification and Treatment
von Heimburg D, Exner K, Kruft S, et al (St Markus Hosp, Frankfurtam Main, Germany; Johann Wolfgang Goethe Univ Teaching Hosp, Frankfurtam Main, Germany)
Br J Plast Surg 49:339–345, 1996   5–9

Introduction.—Several reports have offered descriptive terminology for the so-called tuberous breast deformity, and a number of different operative procedures have been proposed. There is no consensus on nomenclature for tuberous breast deformity. The degrees of tuberous breast deformity and the results of operative correction were evaluated in a retrospective study.

Patients.—Forty patients with 68 tuberous breast deformities were operated on over a 20-year period (Fig 6). Based on the preoperative photographs, the breasts were classified into the following 4 categories: type I, hypoplasia of the lower medial quadrant; type II, hypoplasia of the lower medial and lateral quadrants, with sufficient skin in the subareolar region; type III, hypolasia of the lower medial and lateral quadrants, with deficient skin in the subareolar region; and type IV, severe breast reconstruction with a minimal breast base. In the study sample, 28% of breasts had type I deformities, 26% had type II deformities, 18% had type III deformities, and 28% had type IV deformities. Just 48% of breasts studied had areolar prolapse, which is typically regarded as a major symptom of tuberous breast deformity. At least 2 years' follow-up was available in 51 breasts of 31 patients.

Outcomes.—In type I breasts, reduction mammaplasty of adequately sized breasts or augmentation mammaplasty of the hypoplastic breasts yielded excellent results. The same procedure provided good results in type II deformities, when combined with additional spreading of the breast

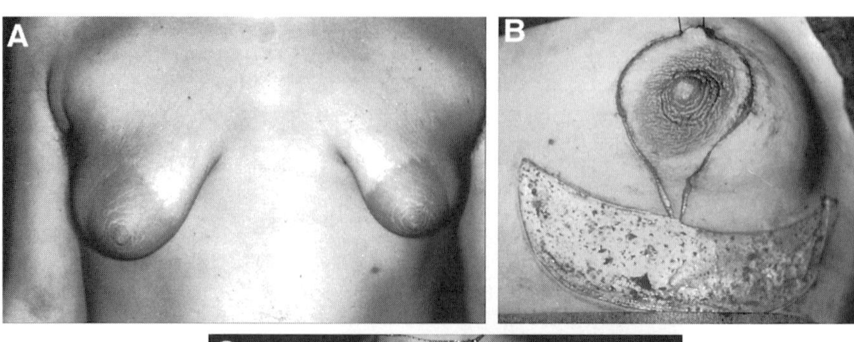

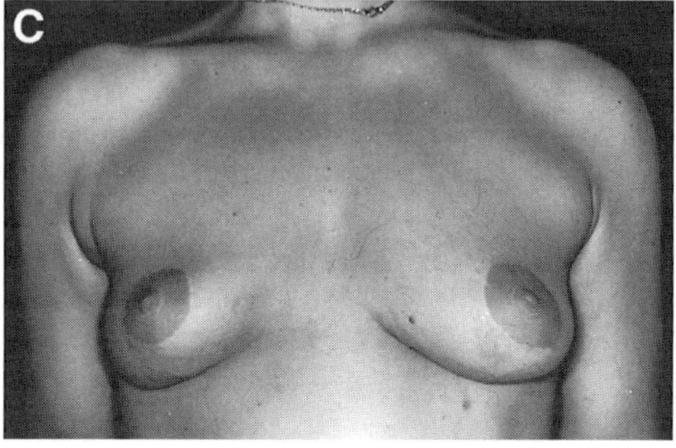

FIGURE 6.—**A**, type III left breast, type II right breast, **B**, correction of the left breast with a de-epithelialized flap. An incision is made along the lower border of the de-epithelialized area. The incision is extended to the upper border medially and laterally to create two tips of the flap, which form the breast cone. In this case, the periareolar area was de-epithelialized and the two inferior triangles of skin were interlocked around the areola, similar to the Maillard technique. **C**, 6 years postoperatively. The right type II breast deformity was corrected with a modified Maillard technique. Note the Z-plasties on both breasts. No implants were used. (Courtesy of von Heimburg D, Exner K, Kruft S, et al: The tuberous breast deformity: Classification and treatment. *Br J Plast Surg* 49:339–345, 1996.)

tissue. However, in types III and IV, these procedures yielded an unsatisfactory breast shape and "second crease" deformity. When these deformities were treated by flaps or tissue expansion, the results were successful in terms of shape, volume, and symmetry.

Conclusions.—The classification and treatment of tuberous breast deformity are evaluated. These deformities fall into significantly different types, and the treatment of choice depends on the type of deformity. The authors' proposed classification will aid in establishing an accepted nomenclature for tuberous breast deformity.

▶ This is a good review article for a difficult problem. The key to success is the surgeon's expertise with a variety of reconstructive options and a realistic patient.

S.H. Miller, M.D.

Personal Approach to Surgical Correction of the Extremely Hypoplastic Tuberous Breast
Muti E (Turin, Italy)
Aesthetic Plast Surg 20:385–390, 1996   5–10

Background.—Correcting small tuberous breasts continues to be difficult. No single technique is effective in the treatment of the many kinds of deformity encountered in these patients. A method for treating extremely hypoplastic tuberous breasts and its outcomes was reported.

Methods and Outcomes.—The underlying goal of the operation is to transform a hypogastric tuberous breast into a simple hypoplasia without discarding gland tissue, which is used to thicken the most deficient region. Differently shaped glandular flaps are turned to correct the deformity. A

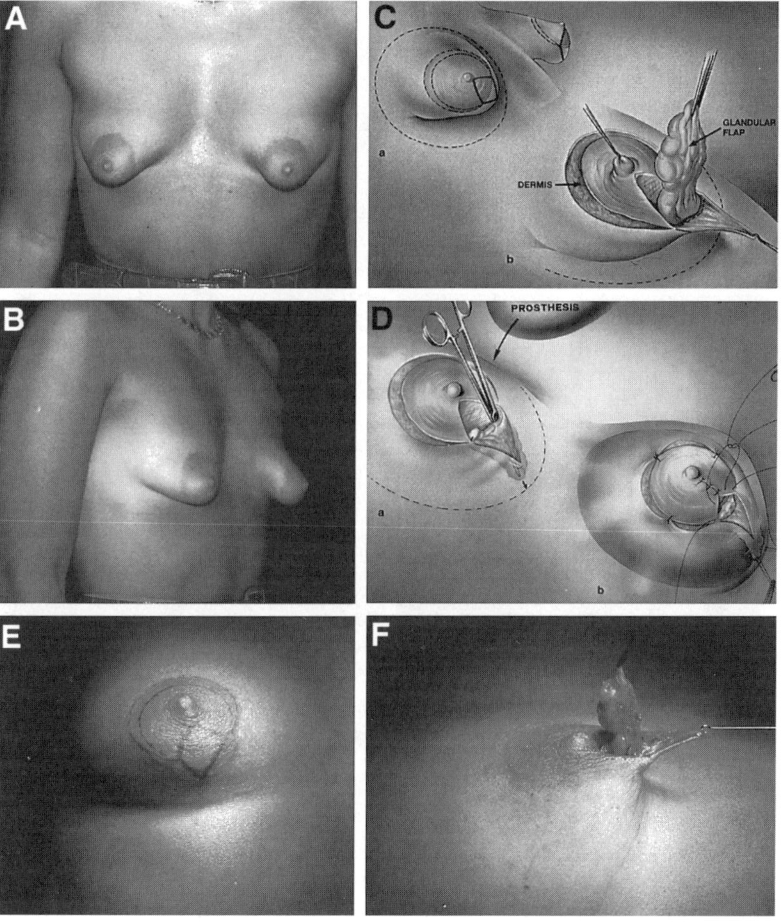

(Continued)

FIGURE 2 (cont.)

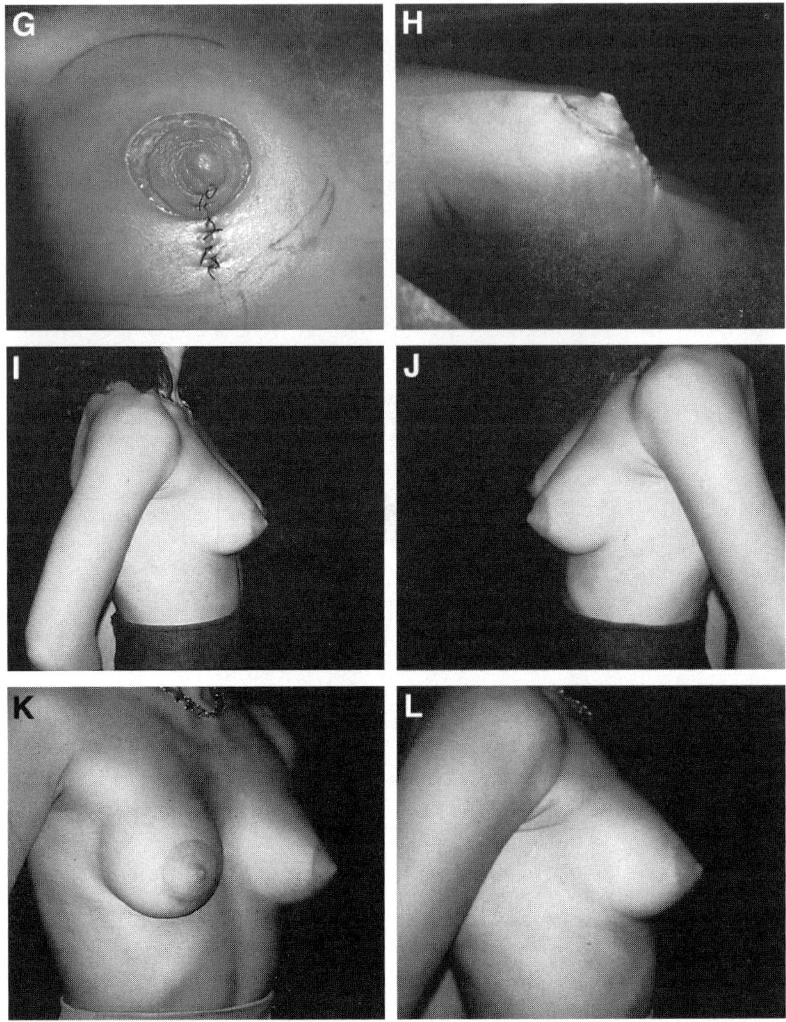

FIGURE 2.—Preoperative front (**A**) and side (**B**) views of hypoplastic tuberous breasts. C, preoperative markings (*a*); the triangular glandular flap shaped and raised (*b*). **D**, the glandular flap folded deeply toward the new lowered sulcus (*a*). The prosthesis has been inserted through the existing surgical breach (*b*). **E**, intraoperative cutaneous mark. **F**, Intraoperative view of the flap being shaped and raised. **G**, Suturing of the lower pole after the skin has been exercised. **H**, the end of the operation. One-year postoperative right (**I**) and left (**J**) side views. Five-year postoperative oblique (**K**) and side (**L**) views. (Courtesy of Muti E: Personal approach to surgical correction of the extremely hypoplastic tuberous breast. *Anesth Plast Surg* 20:385–390, 1996, Figure 2. Copyright 1996 Springer-Verlag.)

prosthesis is then inserted. When necessary, areola size and position are corrected, and the skin of the inferior pole is adjusted. To date, 10 patients have been treated in a one-stage operation (Fig 2). At a minimum follow-up of 5 years, total, recurrence free aesthetic correction of the usual deformities was achieved.

Conclusions.—In this technique, the malpositioned gland tissue is moved to the area of greatest deficiency. The gland flaps will have a shape and amplitude that vary from one patient to another based on the initial anatomical situation. A prosthesis is inserted only when the deformity is corrected. In addition to gland flap mobilization, it is sometimes useful to perform maneuvers used for other methods, such as radial incisions on the deep surface of the gland or the hypodermis to permit better arrangement of tissue covering the prosthesis or telescoping of the areolar-periareolar tissue.

▶ The results shown are quite good. No mention is made of the effects of gland flap mobilization on postoperative nipple sensation.

S.H. Miller, M.D.

Reduction

Blood Loss of Scalpel Versus Cutting Cautery in Bilateral Reduction Mammoplasty Procedures

Hurst LN, Kaila S (London Health Sciences Centre, Ont, Canada)
Can J Plast Surg 4:195–197, 1996   5–11

Objective.—In patients undergoing bilateral breast reduction surgery, the use of cutting electrocautery for subcutaneous dissection has no adverse effects on wound healing. This technique of dissection is assumed to reduce bleeding, but there are no data in the literature to verify the assumption. Blood loss was compared in women undergoing cutting cautery vs. scalpel dissection.

Methods.—A pilot study showed no difference between the 2 techniques in healing or complications. Two groups of randomly selected patients undergoing bilateral reduction mammaplasty were compared: 22 who had scalpel dissection and 39 who had dissection with cutting cautery. The 2 groups were operated on in 1983 and 1993, respectively. Preoperative and 1-day postoperative hemoglobin levels were compared.

Results.—The mean postoperative hemoglobin level was 101 g/L in the scalpel dissection group vs. 107 g/L in the electrocautery dissection group. The difference of 6 g/L was significant at the 95% confidence level.

Conclusions.—In patients undergoing bilateral reduction mammaplasty, the use of cutting electrocautery dissection is associated with a slight but significant reduction in blood loss when compared with scalpel dissection. Especially given the desire to avoid transfusion, reduced blood loss is an advantage of cutting electrocautery dissection.

▶ The difference in postoperative hemoglobin levels between the scalpel and the cutting cautery groups was small but statistically significant. I think the real benefit may be in operative time because of a reduced need for establishing hemostasis during resection with the cautery. I make the skin incision with a knife and do the rest of the procedure with the cutting cautery.

R.L. Ruberg, M.D.

Reduction Mammaplasty: The Results of Avoiding Nipple-Aerolar Amputation in Cases of Extreme Hypertrophy

Chang P, Shaaban AF, Canady JW, et al (Univ of Iowa, Iowa City)
Ann Plast Surg 37:585–591, 1996   5–12

Introduction.—In women with very large breasts undergoing reduction mammaplasty, nipple-areola necrosis may occur. To avoid this complication, amputation and subsequent transplantation of the nipple-areolar complex has been recommended. Rates of nipple necrosis and other complications were compared in women undergoing varying amounts of resection during reduction mammaplasty.

Methods.—The study included 172 consecutive women undergoing bilateral reduction mammaplasty. Their average age was 33 years. All procedures were performed by the inferior breast pedicle technique without amputation of the nipple-areolar complex. The average weight resected from both breasts was 1,946 g, with a range of 548–5,100 g. Mean nipple-areolar transposition was 10 cm. Complications were compared in 4 groups based on weight of resection: less than 1,000 g, 1,000–1,999 g, 2,000–2,999 g, and 3,000 g or greater. The analysis focused on nipple complications, including nipple necrosis and loss of nipple sensibility.

Results.—The overall complication rate was 42%, including a 15% major and 27% minor complication rate. The major complication rate was similar across all 4 groups. There were 2 cases of nipple-areolar complications, for a rate of 1.2%, and 7 cases of loss of nipple-areolar sensibility, for a rate of 4.1%. Neither of these complications was more frequent in patients with larger resection weights (Table 4).

Conclusions.—This study finds no increase in the risk of nipple and other complications among women with extreme breast hypertrophy who are undergoing inferior breast pedicle reduction mammaplasty without nipple amputation. Particularly because most women undergoing breast reduction surgery are young, nipple amputation should be avoided if possible. This decision should not be based solely on the size of the planned breast reduction.

TABLE 4.—Patients With Complications by Group

Complication	Group I	Group II	Group III	Group IV	Total
Major complications	4 (15.4%)	11 (14.9%)	7 (14.6%)	3 (12.5%)	25 (14.5%)*
Minor complications	8 (30.8%)	17 (23.0%)	13 (27.1%)	4 (16.7%)	42 (24.4%)†
All complications*	10 (38.5%)	25 (33.8%)	20 (41.7%)	7 (29.2%)	67 (38.9%)‡
Nipple-areolar necrosis	0 (0%)	0 (0%)	1 (2.1%)	1 (4.2%)	2 (1.2%)
Loss of nipple sensibility	2 (7.7%)	5 (6.8%)	0 (0%)	0 (0%)	7 (4.1%)

*One patient (0.6%) had more than 1 complication.
†Four patients (2.3%) had more than 1 complication.
‡Five patients (2.9%) had more than 1 complication.
(Reprinted with permission from Chang P, Shaaban AF, Canady JW, et al: Reduction mammaplasty: The results of avoiding nipple-areolar amputation in cases of extreme hypertrophy. *Ann Plast Surg* 37:585–591, 1996.)

▶ There are a few advantages to free nipple graft breast reduction as compared with pedicle techniques. One advantage may be reduced time of surgery; a second would be improved survival of the nipple-areola complex. This article certainly seems to negate the latter theoretical advantage, although 2 patients in this series of 172 did have nipple-areola necrosis and both were patients with much larger breasts. In the group with the largest amount of breast tissue removed (greater than 1,500 g per side), the nipple necrosis rate was 4.2%. Is this too high? In general I favor a pedicle technique in younger patients with normal sensation irrespective of the size of the breast. However, in older patients with giant breasts and limited sensation, the free nipple graft technique still makes sense to me.

R. L. Ruberg, M.D.

Nipple Sensitivity and Lactation in Two Methods of Breast Reduction
Kappel RM, Dijkstra R, Storm van Leeuwen JB, et al (Sophia Hosp, Zwolle, The Netherlands)
Eur J Plast Surg 20:60–65, 1997   5–13

Introduction.—Several different breast reduction techniques can give satisfactory results. The authors use 2 main techniques: a modification of the wedge reduction of Skoog, with use of a superior dermal pedicle to carry the nipple-areola complex; and a tangential and circumferential breast reduction technique, a modification of the procedure described by Biessenberger, in which the nipple remains in continuity with the gland. Patients undergoing these 2 techniques were compared for nipple sensitivity and lactation.

Methods.—The analysis included 77 breast reductions in 42 patients operated on between 1981 and 1986. The modified Skoog technique was used in 21 patients, and a modified Biessenberger reduction in 21. Mean reduction weight was 420 and 435 g, respectively. At an average follow-up of nearly 6 years, the patients were asked about breast-feeding and nipple sensitivity. The evaluation included nipple sensitivity testing.

Results.—In each group, 8 patients had 11 babies after breast reduction. Four patients in the modified Biessenberger group were able to breast-feed, compared with none of those in the modified Skoog group. Subjective scores for nipple sensitivity were higher in the modified Biessenberger group, although the objective scores showed no differences. Both groups had nipple erection. Breast ptosis was noted in 45% of breasts after Skoog reduction vs. 23% of breasts after Biessenberger reduction.

Conclusions.—In women undergoing breast reduction, lactation and possibly nipple sensitivity are better preserved with a tangential and circumferential breast reduction technique than with a wedge resection technique. If either type of procedure can be performed in a woman of childbearing age who does not yet have a complete family, the duct-saving procedure should be chosen. The modified Biessenberger technique gives good functional and aesthetic results.

▶ Some of the results of this study are expected; others are confusing. One would expect that a breast reduction technique which leaves the nipple adherent to underlying breast tissue is more likely to permit lactation than a technique in which the nipple is left on a superior dermal pedicle. The study confirms this (although the number of patients is quite small). On the other hand, one would also expect better sensation in the same patients, but that was not objectively proved.

I tell all patients (irrespective of the technique used) that nipple sensation and function after breast reduction may be normal but may also be entirely absent. Very few patients decide to forgo breast reduction even when this information is clearly conveyed to them.

R.L. Ruberg, M.D.

Should Breast Reduction Surgery Be Rationed? A Comparison of the Health Status of Patients Before and After Treatment: Postal Questionnaire Survey
Klassen A, Fitzpatrick R, Jenkinson C, et al (Univ of Oxford, England; Radcliffe Infirmary, Oxford, England)
BMJ 313:454–457, 1996   5–14

Purpose.—Hospitals in the state-funded British National Health Service still offer breast reduction surgery. However, there are questions about whether this procedure is justified in such a system. Such operations are likely to be excluded from future service contracts unless there is evidence to show that they should be included. The benefits of breast reduction surgery were evaluated by before-and-after health status assessments.

Methods.—The study included 166 women referred for breast reduction surgery. A questionnaire was sent to each patient before her operation. The questionnaires included several well-validated health status measurement tools, including the "short form 36" (SF-36) health questionnaire, the general health questionnaire, and Rosenberg's self-esteem scale. Follow-up questionnaires were sent to as many women as possible 6 months after the operation. The SF-36 data were compared with those of a previously studied, random sample of women. The patients' scores before and after surgery were compared with those of the general population of women.

Results.—The patients waited an average of 100 days for an outpatient appointment after the date of referral. Eighty-five patients had breast reduction surgery after spending an average of 146 days on the waiting list. Most of the breast reductions were done for physical indications. Postoperative questionnaires were sent to 74 patients, and 58 (68%) responded. The greatest difference in any score between the patients and the general female population was in the pain dimension of the SF-36. The patients differed from the general population on all 8 dimensions of this study

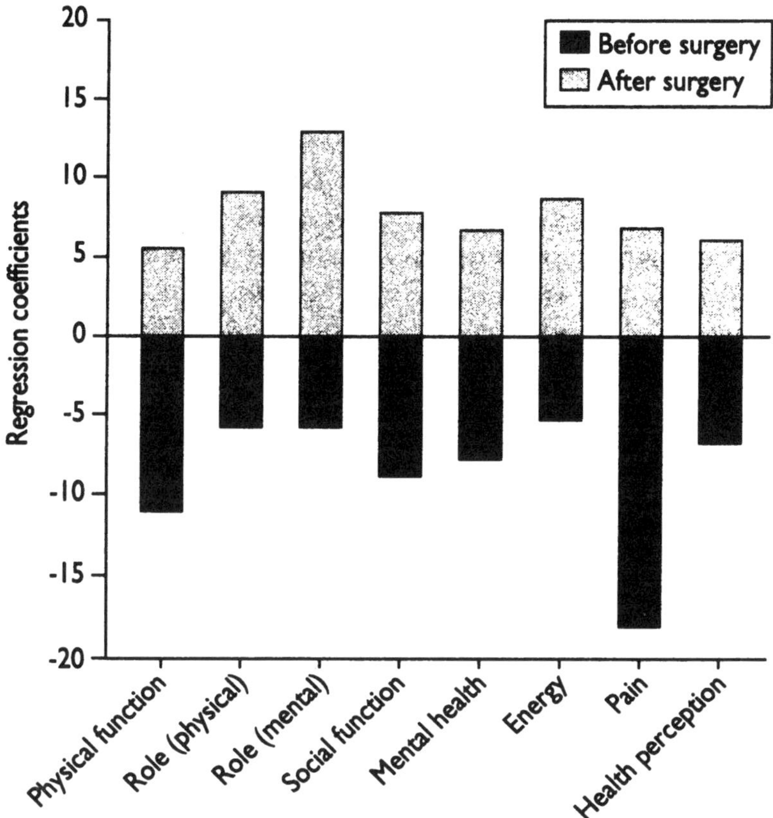

FIGURE 1.—Differences in age-adjusted mean SF-36 scores of patients undergoing breast reduction and women in the general population. (Courtesy of Klassen A, Fitzpatrick R, Jenkinson C, et al: Should breast reduction surgery be rationed? A comparison of the health status of patients before and after treatment: Postal questionnaire survey. *BMJ* 313:454–457, 1996.)

instrument, suggesting that they were in poorer health than the general population (Fig 1). After breast reduction surgery, the patients reported themselves to be in significantly better health than the general population. There was great improvement in Rosenberg's self-esteem scale and moderate improvement in general well-being on the general health questionnaire. The proportion of patients rated as having possible psychiatric disturbance decreased from 41% before to 11% after surgery.

Conclusions.—Women undergoing breast reduction surgery show significant improvement in health status after their operations. The benefits may be compared with those produced by other interventions, such as therapy for peptic ulcer or rheumatoid arthritis. This information should be considered in making resource allocation decisions regarding breast reduction and possibly other cosmetic procedures.

▶ We have ample evidence that breast reduction surgery (using just about *any* acceptable technique) is successful from an anatomical standpoint.

There is a growing body of evidence that confirms the high level of patient satisfaction and relief of symptoms achieved by this procedure. But this study goes 1 step further: using an accepted objective measure of health status (albeit self-reported), the authors conclude that the overall health status of patients requesting breast reduction surgery is worse than that of the normal population, and improves to *better* than that of the normal population if the surgery is done. I would hope that our third-party payors can be swayed by this important study as we try to make the case for the *medical* benefits of breast reduction surgery.

R.L. Ruberg, M.D.

Reduction Mammaplasty: A Safe and Effective Outpatient Procedure

Short KK, Ringler SL, Bengtson BP, et al (Grand Rapids, Mich; The Hunstad Ctr for Cosmetic Plastic Surgery, Charlotte, NC)
Aesthetic Plast Surg 20:513–518, 1996   5–15

Background.—Reduction mammaplasty traditionally has been performed on an inpatient basis, involving a hospital stay of 1–2 days. The safety of outpatient reduction mammaplasty was investigated.

Methods.—The records of 331 patients who had undergone bilateral reduction mammaplasty between 1989 and 1993 were reviewed. One hundred sixty-one were outpatients and 170 were inpatients. Seventy-six percent of the operations were done in the hospital, and 24% were performed at a free-standing surgical facility. The 2 groups were comparable in age, marital status, preoperative health status, surgical technique, and resection weight.

Findings.—Group comparisons showed that the inpatients were significantly heavier, more likely to have a complication, and less likely to receive antibiotics than the outpatients (Table 1). The groups did not differ in incidence of rehospitalization, return to the emergency department, or reoperation. Both groups reported being highly satisfied with their results.

Conclusions.—Reduction mammaplasty can be done safely and effectively on an outpatient basis. The cost savings associated with this approach is significant.

TABLE 1.—Age, Average Actual Body Weight (ABW), and Average Ideal Body Weight (IBW) of Inpatients and Outpatients

	Inpatients	Outpatients
Age	36.2 yr	33.3 yr
ABW	77.5 kg	74.0 kg
ABW – IBW	23.4 kg	18.3 kg

Note: Comparison revealed the inpatient group to be significantly heavier than the outpatient group.
(Courtesy of Short KK, Ringler SL, Bengtson BP, et al: Reduction mammaplasty: A safe and effective outpatient procedure. *Aesth Plast Surg* 20:513–518, copyright 1996, Springer-Verlag.)

▶ I am convinced that outpatient reduction mammaplasty is a safe and effective procedure. I do not believe we can say that this conclusion is unequivocally proved by this article. The study is not prospective and not randomized; the authors acknowledge that there were differences between the inpatient and outpatient groups. Probably the most important difference was that the inpatient group was significantly more overweight than the outpatient group. Thus, it is not really a surprise that the complication rate of the inpatient group was higher than that of the outpatient group.

Despite these criticisms, I still believe that outpatient reduction mammaplasty is appropriate. I currently use a compromise plan in my own practice. Our patients are officially outpatients, but are placed in an observation bed (our "Extended Recovery Unit") overnight. If they have drains, they are removed early in the postoperative morning. Then the patients go home. The costs are significantly reduced, and our patients are happy.

R.L. Ruberg, M.D.

Cancer and Reconstruction

Evaluations of Aesthetic Results in Breast Reconstruction: An Analysis of Reliability
Lowery JC, Wilkins EG, Kuzon WM, et al (Univ of Michigan, Ann Arbor)
Ann Plast Surg 36:601–607, 1996   5–16

Introduction.—Studies of aesthetic results in breast surgery usually rely on an ordinal scale of 4 categories: poor, fair, good, and excellent. These scales are inexpensive and easy to use, but because raters can use their own guidelines, the results can vary considerably from 1 rater to another. Three plastic surgeons were asked to rate the aesthetic results of breast reconstruction using 3 methods: the 4-point ordinal scale, 5 subscales, and a visual analogue scale.

Methods.—Photographs of 50 patients were randomly selected from women who had undergone breast reconstruction at university hospitals between July 1989 and May 1993. Raters were an attending plastic surgeon and 2 senior plastic surgery residents not involved in the patients' care. With the 4-point scale, a rating of poor indicated major aesthetic flaws, fair indicated obvious asymmetry, good reflected only minimal differences between the 2 sides, and excellent was given when the re- constructed breast and the normal breast were comparable. The subscales rated the volume, contour, and placement of the breast mound; the inframammary fold; and breast mound scars; the scale ranged from 0 (poor) to 2 (good). With the visual analogue scale, raters were to indicate the results of reconstruction on a 10-cm line; the left end showed an unreconstructed mastectomy scar and the right had a photograph of a normal pair of breasts.

Results.—The ratings were completed on 2 occasions 4 weeks apart. Intrarater and interrater reliability ranged from poor to good for the 3 methods. The highest reliability was found when plastic surgeons used the subscales, which provided the most detailed analysis of breast appearance. Scales with the least explicit rating criteria also had the lowest reliability.

Discussion.—When instruments used in evaluating the aesthetic results of breast reconstruction lack explicit criteria, the raters must develop and use their own criteria. For results to be comparable across studies, however, more explicit rating criteria are required. And although objective assessments using linear and volumetric measurements may be more reliable, many aesthetic factors are difficult to quantify.

▶ Despite the difficulties inherent in developing criteria by which to judge the results of aesthetic surgery, reliable evaluations by unbiased, trained observers are critical for developing standards to judge outcomes. As the authors have noted, explicit criteria must be developed to limit subjectivity and improve intrarater and interrater reliability. Similar studies for other types of aesthetic procedures are sorely needed.

S.H. Miller, M.D.

Breast Reconstruction With Anatomical Expanders and Implants: Our Early Experience
McGeorge DD, Mahdi S, Tsekouras A (Countess of Chester Hosp, Chester, England)
Br J Plast Surg 49:352–357, 1996   5–17

Introduction.—At the study institution, the method of breast reconstruction after mastectomy is selected according to individual requirements. Anatomically shaped expanders and implants requiring a two-stage reconstruction are preferred to the one-stage technique using the Becker expander/mammary prosthesis in some cases. Results were reviewed for the first 24 breast reconstructions in 19 patients judged suitable for the anatomical expanders and implants.

Methods.—Eighty breast reconstructions were done from August 1994 to April 1995. The most frequently used techniques were the two-stage anatomical expander and implant (30 cases) and the Becker expander/ mammary prosthesis (12 cases). The minimum follow-up for the patients receiving anatomical expanders and implants was 6 months. Data gathered included indications for reconstruction, operative technique, expander size used, on-table inflation volume, number and duration of postoperative inflations, size of the permanent implant, and complications.

> *Technique.*—The expander is inserted through the mastectomy wound for immediate reconstruction. For delayed reconstruction, the mastectomy scar is opened up laterally. The expander is placed in the submuscular pocket and inflated to the maximum volume that will allow tension free closure. Starting 2 weeks postoperatively, patients come once or twice weekly for further inflation of the expander. Two to 3 months after full inflation, the second stage is done through a submammary incision. The expander is then removed and a permanent implant inserted.

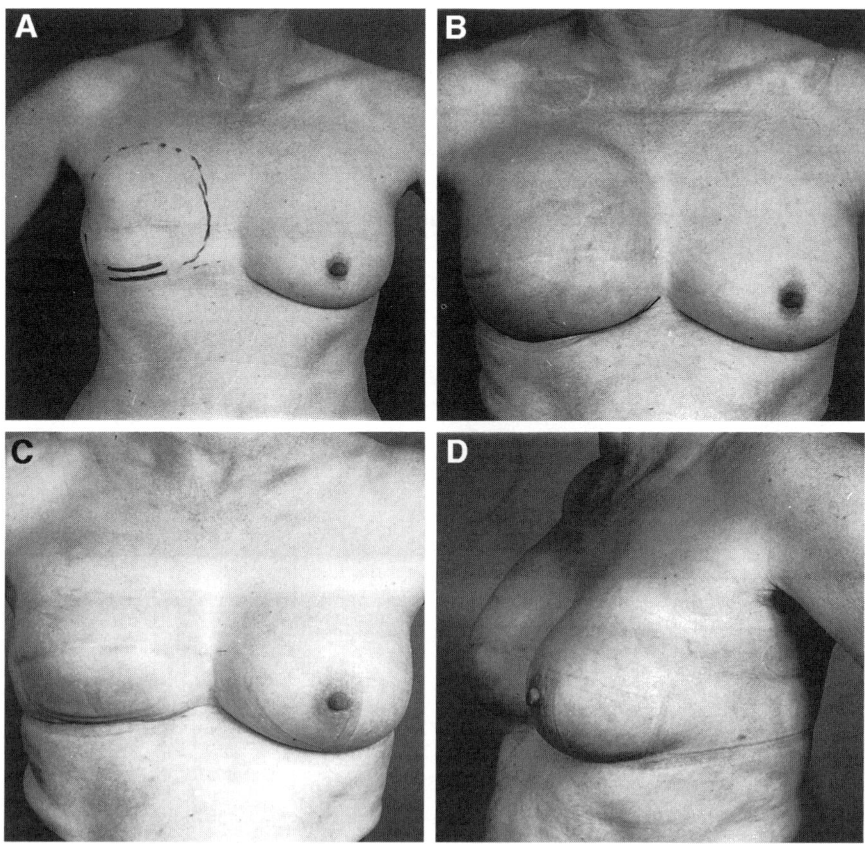

FIGURE 4.—A patient aged 52 years, who underwent delayed right breast reconstruction 2 years after mastectomy. **A,** preoperative view; size of submuscular pocket marked out. **B,** with 500 cc anatomical expander fully inflated. **C, D,** final result, 6 months after replacement of expander with a 450–cc anatomical silicone implant. (Courtesy of McGeorge DD, Mahdi S, Tsekouras A: Breast reconstruction with anatomical expanders and implants: Our early experience. *Br J Plast Surg* 49:352–357, 1996.)

Results.—The most commonly used expander size was 500 cc (range, 400–700 cc); the mean on-table inflation was 215 cc. One to 6 inflations were required. Patients were hospitalized an average of 2.8 days for the first procedure and overnight for the second. One major complication occurred when a woman with bilateral mastectomies and immediate reconstruction with 700–cc expanders experienced overstretching of the skin to the point of incipient ulceration. Salvage reconstruction was done using latissimus dorsi muscle flaps. Overall results were very acceptable, and all patients were pleased with the final outcome (Fig 4).

Conclusions.—Anatomically shaped expanders and implants offer a simple method of breast reconstruction, with aesthetic results superior to those achieved with dome-shaped prostheses. Results are easily reproducible with proper patient selection and good surgical technique.

▶ Although anatomical expanders and implants have been an improvement over round domed implants and expanders, they still produce too much superior fullness in some patients. The resultant asymmetry, especially with the passage of time, may not be overcome by mastopexy alone on the opposite side. Minimizing asymmetry may require the use of an implant on the opposite side or breast reconstruction with autogenous tissue.

S.H. Miller, M.D.

The Vascular Anatomy of the Tendinous Intersections of the Rectus Abdominis Muscle

Whetzel TP, Huang V (Univ of California, Sacramento)
Plast Reconstr Surg 98:83–89, 1996   5–18

Background.—A better understanding of the blood supply in the area of the tendinous intersection may aid in the development of operative methods to improve circulation to transverse rectus abdominis flaps. Therefore, the specific arterial vascular anatomy of the tendinous intersections was delineated through microdissection.

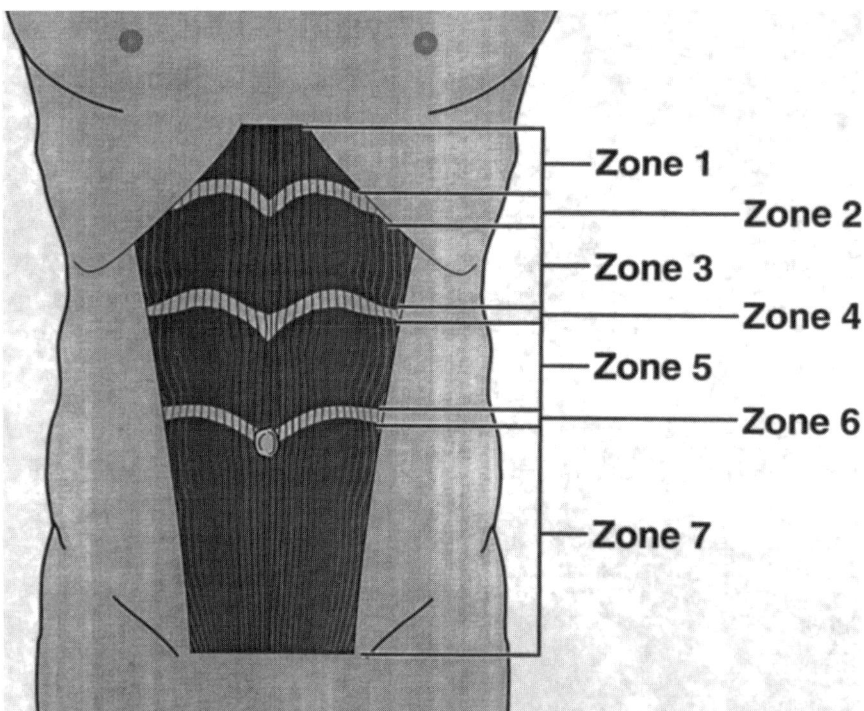

FIGURE 6.—Artist's diagram of anterior abdominal wall with schematic rectus abdominis muscles and their tendinous intersections. Muscle and intersections have been divided into separate numbered zones. *Zones 1, 3, 5,* and *7* represent muscle segments, and *zones 2, 4,* and *6* represent the superior, middle, and inferior tendinous intersections. Perforating vessels were mapped according to the zone at which they pierced the anterior rectus sheath. Umbilicus is usually located centrally in zone 6. (Courtesy of Whetzel TP, Huang V: The vascular anatomy of the tendinous intersections of the rectus abdominis muscle. *Plast Reconstr Surg* 98:83–89, 1996.)

Methods.—Fourteen fresh cadavers were studied. Blue latex was injected into the deep inferior epigastric arteries. Each tendinous intersection was dissected under loupe magnification in 7 specimens. In the other 7, perforator mapping was done at each intersection relative to the rest of the rectus abdominis muscle. Radiographs of barium-latex- injected specimens were obtained in another 2 cadavers.

Findings.—The vascular architecture of the intersections was characterized by transverse arcades arising from either the superior or inferior epigastric arteries. These send branches supplying muscle or the overlying skin. More perforators per square centimeter originated in the intersections than in the rest of the rectus abdominis muscle (Fig 6).

Conclusions.—The vascular architecture of the tendinous intersections consists of a system of transverse arcades that arises from the deep superior epigastric artery or deep inferior epigastric artery to send branches supplying muscle or overlying skin. Thus, for optimal arterial supply, the design of transverse rectus abdominis flaps may be based on intersection location or paraumbilical location.

▶ This study confirms the clinical observations that we and others have made when performing transverse rectus abdominis flap. Special care should be taken during dissection of the tendinous inscriptions and muscle in the periumbilical region.

S.H. Miller, M.D.

Comparison of Resource Costs of Free and Conventional TRAM Flap Breast Reconstruction

Kroll SS, Evans GRD, Reece GP, et al (Univ of Texas, Houston)
Plast Reconstr Surg 98:74–77, 1996   5–19

Background.—Because the free transverse rectus abdominis myocutaneous (TRAM) flap is associated with less donor-site morbidity and a better blood supply with a similar success rate to that achieved with the conventional TRAM flap, it is being used increasingly. However, there have been concerns raised about the cost associated with the free TRAM flap. Therefore, the resource costs of doing breast reconstruction with the free TRAM flap or the conventional TRAM flap were compared. In addition, the costs of doing bilateral mastectomy and reconstruction were compared with those of unilateral mastectomy and reconstruction.

Methods.—The resource costs, defined as the costs required of the hospital, were reviewed for all patients who underwent mastectomy and immediate breast reconstruction between 1986 and 1994. These costs included hourly personnel costs, costs for each day of the hospital stay, laboratory work, and recovery room costs for the initial reconstruction and any subsequent revisions.

Results.—Of the 154 patients with completed breast reconstruction with TRAM flaps, 95 had free TRAM flaps and 59 had conventional

TRAM flaps. There was only a 4.1% difference in the total resource costs for the initial procedure in these 2 groups, with conventional TRAM flaps costing less than free TRAM flaps. However, this was not statistically significant. Revision costs were slightly higher in the conventional TRAM flap group, because of longer hospital stays.

The mean resource cost of unilateral mastectomy with reconstruction was $17,840, compared with $18,729 for bilateral mastectomy with reconstruction, a 5% difference.

Conclusions.—The conventional TRAM flap has a slight cost advantage over the free TRAM flap for the initial procedure. However, the difference is not statistically significant. Similarly, the costs of doing bilateral mastectomy with immediate reconstruction are not significantly higher than the costs of unilateral mastectomy with immediate reconstruction.

▶ Data such as those reported in this study are currently being accumulated by HMOs and other payers, often without appropriate medical input to allow necessary risk adjustment and interpretation of outcomes. We must begin to collect similar data to show cost-effectiveness or cost-benefit, for our reconstructive procedures. These data can then be used to relate patient health status and quality-of-life issues to costs. Studies should be done in academic and community hospital settings alike.

S.H. Miller, M.D.

Bilateral TRAM Flaps for the Reconstruction of the Post Implantectomy/Capsulectomy Breast Deformity
Spiro SA, Marshall D (West Orange, NJ; Miami, Fla)
Aesthetic Plast Surg 20:315–318, 1996   5–20

Introduction.—Women who desire surgical removal of silicone breast implants but decline re-implantation with saline implants are likely to have significant postoperative deformities. In the case presented here, a bilateral transverse rectus abdominis musculocutaneous (TRAM) flap was used in the reconstruction of postimplantectomy breast deformities.

> *Case Report.*—Woman, 53, had nonspecific complaints of fibromyalgia and mastodynia. She had previously undergone subglandular silicone breast implantation but had no evidence of implant rupture or lymphadenopathy. The patient was advised that total capsulectomy would preclude simultaneous mastopexy. Surgery showed near complete disintegration of the implant shells. Six weeks after operation, a substantial deformity was apparent (Fig 2). Because the patient did not want saline augmentation and mastopexy alone would not provide the desired breast volume, she was offered autogenous tissue reconstruction and a bilateral de-epithelialized TRAM flap was used. The same incisions used for capsulectomy/implantectomy were re-entered for flap insetting. At

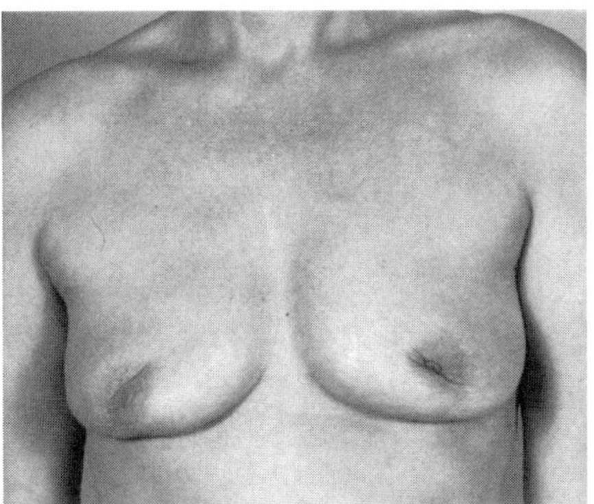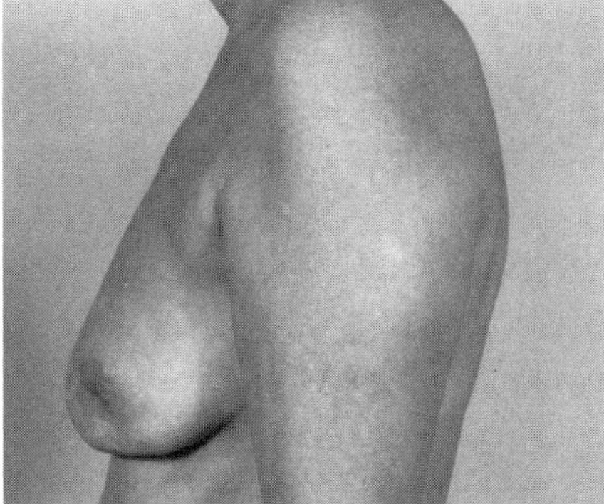

FIGURE 2.—Six weeks after implantectomy and near total capsulectomy. A significant breast deformity remains. There is the expected paucity of tissue in the retroareolar position. (Courtesy of Spiro SA, Marshall D: Bilateral TRAM flaps for the reconstruction of the post implantectomy/capsulectomy breast deformity. *Aesth Plast Surg* 20:315–318, 1996.)

1-year follow-up, the patient's breasts remain soft and symmetric and she is very satisfied with the results (Fig 3).

Discussion.—Although no association between silicone breast implants and connective-tissue diseases has been documented in large outcome

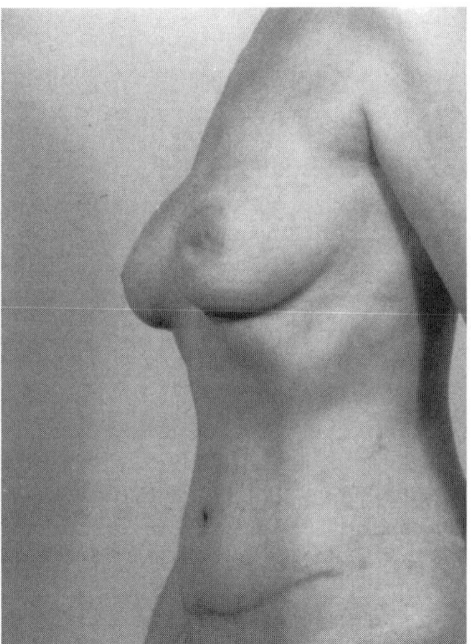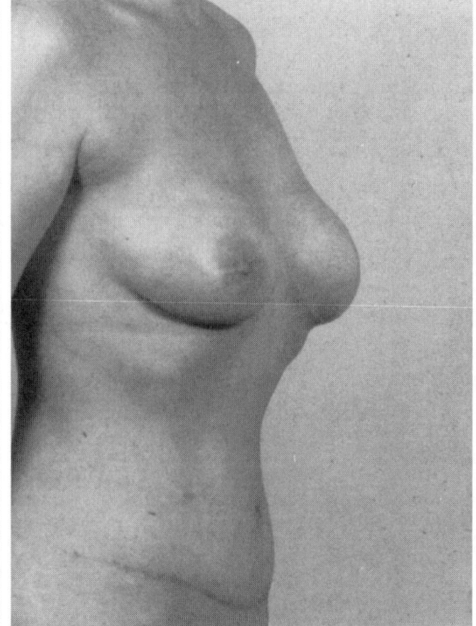

FIGURE 3.—One year after bilateral de-epithelialized transverse rectus abdominis musculocutaneous flaps. Both breasts remain soft. No abdominal bulge or disruption of the inframammary crease is apparent. The patient is also very pleased with the abdominoplasty effect. *Abbreviation: TRAM,* transverse rectus abdominis musculocutaneous. (Courtesy of Spiro SA, Marshall D: Bilateral TRAM flaps for the reconstruction of the post implantectomy/capsulectomy breast deformity. *Aesth Plast Surg* 20:315–318, 1996.)

studies, reports of problems with the implants have caused fear and led some women to have the implants removed. Severe breast deformities may be present after capsulectomy. The procedure described here was not a cosmetic augmentation with autogenous tissue, but a breast reconstruction. A bilateral deepithelialized TRAM flap for reconstruction of postimplantectomy breast deformities can achieve significant esthetic improvement and the secondary benefits of abdominoplasty.

▶ Some might consider this approach a bit of "overkill," but I thought the result presented in this article was impressive. Under the proper circumstances and with appropriate preoperative discussion and counseling, the procedure is probably reasonable.

R.L. Ruberg, M.D.

Abdominal-wall Recovery Following TRAM Flap: A Functional Outcome Study

Kind GM, Rademaker AW, Mustoe TA (Davies Med Ctr, San Francisco; Northwestern Univ, Chicago)
Plast Reconstr Surg 99:417–428, 1997   5–21

Background.—Although the use of the transverse rectus abdominis myocutaneous (TRAM) flap has several advantages that make it popular in breast reconstruction, the effects of the TRAM flap on abdominal wall function have not been assessed prospectively. Abdominal wall function was studied prospectively in a series of patients with breast cancer undergoing reconstruction with free or pedicled TRAM flaps.

Methods.—Twenty-five consecutive patients undergoing breast reconstruction with pedicled or free TRAM flaps were evaluated before and at various intervals after surgery. Abdominal wall function was determined using the B200 Isostation, a triaxial dynamometer. In addition, a physical therapist performed examinations, and the patients completed activity questionnaires.

Findings.—The greatest decrease in performance was noted at the 6–week postoperative test of flexion. The maximum isometric flexion torque of the pedicled TRAM flap group declined to 58% of baseline, a significant difference, and the unilateral free TRAM flap group average was 87% of baseline. By 6 months after surgery, maximum flexion torque had increased to 89% and 93% of baseline in the pedicled and free TRAM flap groups, respectively. The findings of physical therapist assessments and activity questionnaires did not change significantly between groups or over time.

Conclusions.—The harvesting of pedicled TRAM flaps causes greater injury to the abdominal wall than that of free TRAM flaps. Most patients appear to tolerate the ultimate clinical effect well, even when the entire rectus abdominus muscle is lost.

▶ These authors confirm the findings of Suominen, et al. (see following abstract). Their comment on rectus splitting techniques offering no advantage vis-à-vis abdominal wall function is worth noting.

S.H. Miller, M.D.

Sequelae in the Abdominal Wall After Pedicled or Free TRAM Flap Surgery

Suominen S, Asko-Seljavaara S, von Smitten K, et al (Helsinki Univ; ORTON Rehabilitation Centre, Helsinki)
Ann Plast Surg 36:629–636, 1996
5–22

Introduction.—The free microvascular and conventional pedicled transverse rectus abdominis musculocutaneous (TRAM) flaps are widely used for autologous-tissue breast reconstruction. The free TRAM flap provides better blood circulation and a lower rate of edge necrosis than the pedicled TRAM flap. It often is assumed that the free TRAM flap also reduces the rate of abdominal wall complications, but this has never been studied. The abdominal sequelae of free and pedicled TRAM flaps were compared

Methods.—The analysis included 27 patients with free TRAM flap reconstructions and 16 with pedicled TRAM flap reconstructions. They were studied a mean of 23 months after reconstruction. The mean age was 47 years in both groups, and the patients were similar in other demographic characteristics as well. In addition to clinical evaluation, the patients underwent testing of trunk strength using an isokinetic device, a sit-up test, and ultrasonography of the rectus muscles.

Results.—Subjective assessment of the results revealed no differences between groups. Forty-four percent of patients with pedicled TRAM flaps had minor lower abdominal bulges, compared with 4% of those with free TRAM flaps. None of the patients had a hernia. Three patients with free flaps and 1 with a pedicled flap had delayed healing of the abdominal scar. Minor edge necrosis of the breast was present in 44% of the patients with pedicled flaps vs. 8% of those with free flaps. Trunk strength, both in flexion and extension, was similar in the 2 groups. Sit-up performance was also similar and normal for age. The ultrasound studies suggested that the rectus muscle in the free flap group was significantly thinner on the operated side. The patients in the free flap group had a mean muscular defect size of 4.3 × 6.1 cm.

Conclusions.—Patients with pedicled and free TRAM flap breast reconstructions are similar in satisfaction and abdominal muscle strength, although patients with pedicled flaps are more likely to have asymptomatic lower abdominal bulging. The free TRAM flap is preferred when available, but the pedicled TRAM flap gives good results when done by experienced surgeons. Ultrasound studies suggest that harvesting a segment of rectus muscle below the umbilicus may disturb the quality of the entire muscle.

▶ It is of interest that the authors found no difference in sit-up performance nor isokinetic strength testing after free vs. pedicled TRAM flaps. These data would seem to contradict the conclusions of Mizgala et al.[1] and Lejour and Dome[2]. However, in both of the earlier studies, 50% or more of the patients had double pedicled TRAM flap transfers. Although the latter does increase the safety of the transfer, in some patients the price to be paid—increased donor site morbidity—is too high. It would be of interest to re-test these patients longitudinally to determine the long-term subjective and objective effects of rectus muscle loss.

S.H. Miller, M.D.

References

1. Mizgala CL, Hartrampf CR Jr, Bennett GK: Assessment of the abdominal wall after pedicled TRAM flap surgery: The 5- to 7-year follow-up of 150 consecutive patients. *Plast Reconstr Surg* 93:988–1002, 1994.
2. Lejour M, Dome M: Abdominal wall function after rectus abdominalis transfer. *Plast Reconstr Surg* 87:1054–1068, 1991.

Magnetic Resonance Imaging of the TRAM Flap Donor Site
Suominen S, Tervahartiala P, von Smitten K, et al (Helsinki Univ)
Ann Plast Surg 38:23–28, 1997
5–23

Background.—Abdominal wall insufficiency is of concern after surgery with pedicled transverse rectus abdominis musculocutaneous (TRAM) flaps. The use of a free TRAM flap is thought to be less mutilating to the abdominal wall. The quality and size of the rectus abdominis muscles after free and pedicled TRAM flap surgery were investigated using MRI.

Methods.—Twenty-nine women who had had unilateral breast reconstruction with a TRAM flap were included. Nineteen flaps were free, and 10 were pedicled. The free TRAM flap was elevated sparing the lateral third of the rectus muscle; in the pedicled flap procedures, the whole rectus muscle was used. At a mean 22 months postoperatively, T1–weighted, cross-sectional spin-echo images of the abdominal wall were acquired with a surface coil.

Findings.—In the patients undergoing free TRAM flap surgery, the mean area of the rectus muscle in the upper third of the muscle was smaller on the operated side than on the contralateral side. Also, the mean signal intensity of the upper third of the muscle was significantly greater on the operated side. The fat content of the upper third of the muscle was scored higher on the operated than on the nonoperated side. In the patients undergoing pedicled TRAM flap procedures, the remaining rectus comprised a mean 47% of the distance between the lateral muscles, leaving an average 63 mm of the abdominal wall covered by fascia only. There were no hernias in either group.

Conclusions.—Harvesting a free TRAM flap appears to affect the quality of the donor rectus muscle over its entire length. The muscle may have so little contractile power that it is comparable to no muscle. However, it may still contribute to the strength of the abdominal wall and prevent bulging or hernia. The free TRAM flap donor site should be studied prospectively.

▶ This is an interesting evaluation of the effects of harvesting a free TRAM flap on muscle remaining in the donor site. The authors' observation that removal of the insertion of a major portion of the muscle results in atrophy of that muscle is really not a surprise. It is, however, interesting to speculate on why they report so little impairment of the abdominal wall postoperatively. Is it possible that the other abdominal wall musculature hypertrophies in response to the loss of the rectus muscle?

S.H. Miller, M.D.

The Spontaneous Return of Sensibility in Breasts Reconstructed With Autologous Tissues
Shaw WW, Orringer JS, Ko CY, et al (Univ of California Los Angeles School of Medicine; New York Univ)
Plast Reconstr Surg 99:394–399, 1997   5–24

Background.—Alhough some spontaneous return of sensibility is often suspected after autologous tissue breast reconstruction, it has not been well documented. The return of sensibility in a variety of autologous tissue breast reconstructions was investigated.

Methods.—Objective touch-pressure, pain, temperature, and vibratory sensibility were recorded a mean 25.2 months after 33 autologous breast reconstructions. Patients also completed questionnaires.

Findings.—All but 1 patient regained some sensibility. Ninety-seven percent had touch-pressure sensibility; 88%, pain; 64%, heat; 82%, cold; and 100%, high- and low-frequency vibration. Ninety-four percent of the patients said their chest was comfortable to touch after reconstruction, compared to 34% after mastectomy. Mean patient rating of their reconstructions was a 9.3 on a 1–10 scale.

Conclusions.—The spontaneous return of sensibility after autologous tissue breast reconstruction was confirmed in this study. The high degree of patient satisfaction suggests the benefits of sensory return. The mechanism of reinnervation appears to involve both the skin margins and the deep surface of the flap.

▶ One of the more disturbing postoperative events for the patient who has undergone mastectomy is the occurrence of hypoesthesia of the chest and inner surface of the ipsilateral arm. We have noted that patients who undergo either a TRAM flap or a lattissimus dorsi flap reconstruction, with or without an implant, seem to complain less of the "postmastectomy wooden chest syndrome." Although the sensibility has rarely been described in terms of sensuality by my patients, they have clearly described less discomfort. This has been especially true for those who have undergone delayed reconstructions.

S.H. Miller, M.D.

6 Flaps, Microsurgery, and Tissue Expansion

Experimental

Ischemia-Reperfusion Injury in Skeletal Muscle: CD18–Dependent Neutrophil-Endothelial Adhesion and Arteriolar Vasoconstriction

Zamboni WA, Stephenson LL, Routh AC, et al (Univ of Nevada, Las Vegas; Southern Illinois Univ, Springfield)
Plast Reconstr Surg 99:2002–2007, 1997

6–1

Introduction.—Previous studies have suggested that the low-flow state of ischemia-reperfusion injury of skeletal muscle involves neutrophil-endothelial adhesion in venules and progressive vasoconstriction in arterioles. The neutrophil membrane CD18 adhesion ligand may play a role in cell adhesive function during reperfusion, though this has yet to be proved definitively. An in vivo microscopic study was performed to determine whether the neutrophil-endothelial adhesion associated with skeletal muscle ischemia-reperfusion is dependent on CD18 function, and whether this interaction affects the vasoactive response in nearby arterioles.

Methods.—The study used an in vivo microscopy preparation of transilluminated gracilis muscle. Three groups were compared: a sham group undergoing no ischemia and receiving no treatment; a group undergoing 4 hours of global ischemia only; and a group undergoing 4 hours of ischemia plus treatment with monoclonal antibody against CD18. Thirty minutes before reperfusion, the mouse monoclonal antibody that bids the rat leukocyte function antigen 1 CD18 chain was infused into the contralateral femoral vein. Over 15 seconds of observation, the number of leukocytes rolling and adhering to endothelium was counted in 100 µm venular segments. Arteriolar diameters were measured at intervals during the reperfusion period. All values were normalized to the baseline, preischemic readings for that animal.

Results.—Ischemia-reperfusion produced neutrophil-endothelial adherence in venules. This response was blocked by the monoclonal antibody, though rolling behavior was unchanged. The monoclonal antibody also blocked the progressive arteriolar vasoconstriction produced by ischemia-reperfusion.

Conclusions.—The neutrophil-endothelial adherence function observed in ischemia-reperfusion of skeletal muscle appears to be dependent on CD18, though neutrophil rolling does not. For ischemia–reperfusion-induced arteriolar vasoconstriction to occur, neutrophil CD18 function must be present. The CD18-dependent nature of neutrophil-endothelial adhesion and arteriolar vasoconstriction may account for the harmful microcirculatory events occurring with ischemia-reperfusion injury of the skeletal muscle.

E- and L-Selectin Adhesion Molecules in Musculocutaneous Flap Reperfusion Injury

Stotland MA, Kerrigan CL (Royal Victoria Hosp, Montreal)
Plast Reconstr Surg 99:2010–2020, 1997   6–2

Objective.—There is uncertainty regarding the role of various proinflammatory lipid and peptide mediators in reperfusion injury. If the factors influencing leukocyte adhesion to the microvascular endothelium could be defined, it might lead to new forms of treatment for reperfusion injury. A pig latissimus dorsi flap model was used to study expression of the E- and L-selectin adhesion molecules in reperfusion, and to assess the potential benefits of E- and L-selectin blockade.

Methods and Findings.—A series of experiments were performed using pig latissimus dorsi musculocutaneous island flaps that were first subjected to 8 hours of ischemia and then reperfused for a variable period. The microvascular endothelium showed specific immunostaining with the monoclonal antibody EL-246, which cross-reacts with both E- and L-selectin. The intensity of this staining was greater in reperfusion than under baseline conditions or during ischemia. Flow cytometric analysis demonstrated that EL-246 specifically recognized isolated peripheral porcine neutrophils, compared with an isotype-matched control antibody. Percentage staining was greater than 45% compared with less than 3%, respectively.

In situ hybridization using complementary RNA probes for the detection of endothelial E-selectin mRNA showed early up-regulation during the ischemic period. Later, during the reperfusion period, there was downregulation of E-selectin mRNA. Finally, flaps treated with EL-246 showed significantly greater muscle survival than those treated with vehicle, 38% versus 19%. Survival of skin was 49% versus 29%, respectively.

Conclusions.—In this animal model of musculocutaneous flap reperfusion injury, E-selectin expressed along the microvascular surface is up-regulated during ischemia and down-regulated during reperfusion. In pigs, both L-selectin and E-selectin are recognized by the monoclonal antibody EL-246. Experimental results suggest that blocking E- and L-selectin–mediated leukocyte adherence can significantly reduce musculocutaneous flap reperfusion injury.

▶ These papers (Abstracts 6–1 and 6–2) describe two aspects of the same process: Tissue mediated injury or necrosis related to ischemia and reperfusion. They further work begun in the late 1980's by Vedder[1] and Rees,[2] demonstrating that much tissue loss after flap transfer is neutrophil mediated. These papers advance the understanding of the process by describing a role of cell service integrins on both the endophilial cells (selectin) and neutrophils (CD18) in the process. The conclusion from these papers and other similar experiments is that the release of inflammatory cytokines such as TNF from ischemic tissue results in the up regulation and expression of cell service integrins. These make both cells sticky; neutrophils flowing within blood vessels adhere to the cell surface of the endophilial cells in the vessel wall migrate into tissue, where they can induce tissue mediated injury by oxidant release. The appealing prospect is that local application of mediators or blocking agents is possible, and the tissue manipulation to prevent this process is a potentially achievable goal.

W. Garner, M.D.

References

1. Vedder NB, Bucky LP, Richey NL, et al: Improved survival rates of random flaps in rabbits with a monoclonal antibody that blocks leukocyte adherence. *Plast Reconstr Surg* 93:1035–1040, 1994.
2. Rees R, Punch J, Shaheen K, et al: The stress response in skin: The role of neutrophil products in preconditioning. *Plast Reconstr Surg* 92:110–117, 1993.

Durability of Prefabricated Versus Normal Random Flaps Against a Bacterial Challenge
Ko CY, Shaw WW (UCLA School of Medicine, Los Angeles)
Plast Reconstr Surg 99:372–377, 1997   6–3

Objective.—Previous studies have shown good survival with prefabricated flaps. However, there are few data regarding the durability of these flaps as compared with other types of flaps or normal tissue. The response of prefabricated flaps—with and without an angiogenic growth factor—to a bacterial challenge was studied.

Methods.—Prefabricated abdominal cutaneous-panniculus carnosus flaps were made in rats with the use of a groin fasciovascular tissue carrier. Each flap was inoculated with *Staphylococcus aureus*, 1×10^8 organisms per milliliter. One group of these flaps was treated with endothelial cell growth factor between the carrier and flap tissue, and the other was not. Nonprefabricated, random-pattern flaps were studied as controls.

Results.—Dehiscence occurred in 41% of the prefabricated flaps with angiogenic growth factor, 37% of the standard prefabricated flaps, and 4% of the control flaps. Rates of ulceration were 21%, 29%, and 18%, respectively. Erythema or cellulitis occurred in 40% of the prefabricated flaps with angiogenic growth factor, 44% of the standard prefabricated flaps, and 8% of the control flaps. Necrosis occurred in 9%, 29%, and 0%

of the flaps, respectively. All complications except ulceration were significantly less frequent in the control flaps than in the standard prefabricated flaps. Necrosis was less frequent in the prefabricated flaps with angiogenic growth factor than in the standard prefabricated flaps.

Conclusions.—In the face of bacterial challenge, prefabricated flaps are not as durable as random-pattern flaps. One way to make prefabricated flaps more durable may be to use angiogenic growth factor. Further study is needed to clarify the differences in biological behavior between prefabricated flaps and normal tissue.

▶ This paper addresses the biological behavior of a prefabricated vs. a random flap. The particular property studied was response to bacterial challenge. The bacterial challenge was performed quite early (1 week) and therefore in part assessed flap revascularization rather than the intrinsic or final tolerance of such flaps to bacterial infection. In view of this early time point, the results are not surprising. Prefabricated flaps showed a decreased ability to tolerate an infection at 1 week. Flaps treated with angiogenic factors (endothelial growth factor) had increased resistance to infection. Unfortunately, the authors did not directly measure blood flow in the flaps, so it is impossible to correlate these biological responses with changes in blood flow. Numerous alternate possibilities exist, including alteration of immune function and the induction of secondary growth factors or augmentation or impairment of endogenous defense systems. Understanding the biological behavior of prefabricated flaps is essential for us to understand how they should be used in reconstructive surgery. This article addresses but does not answer these critical questions.

W. Garner, M.D.

Impact of Tissue Expansion on Flap Prefabrication: An Experimental Study in Rabbits

Maitz PKM, Pribaz JJ, Hergrueter CA (Brigham/Children's/Harvard, Boston)
Microsurgery 17:35–40, 1996   6–4

Background.—Previous studies have shown that tissue expansion improves vascularity and thus flap survival. The authors have been studying a rabbit ear model of flap prefabrication using an exteriorized vascular pedicle. If pedicle implantation could be combined with tissue expansion, additional tissue would be provided along with a vascular pedicle to supply it. The ability of tissue expansion to improve survival of prefabricated skin flaps was studied.

Methods.—The model used New Zealand white rabbits. The central artery and vein of the left ear were used to construct a vascular pedicle, which was implanted into the neck. The donor site was closed primarily. When the pedicle was implanted, a 5×14-cm subcutaneous pocket was created beneath the implantation site. The rabbits were divided into 4 groups: 3 groups received tissue expanders of varying size and volume, and

1 group received no tissue expander. Expander sizes were 3 × 5 cm, 4 × 8 cm, and 5 × 14 cm, with volumes of 40, 60, and 100 cc, respectively. Three weeks later, the flaps were transposed to the right ear. Flap survival area was assessed 1 week after transfer.

Results.—The mean percentage of survival area was 39% in the non-expanded flaps, 60% with the 40-cc expander, 61% with the 60-cc expander, and 79% with the 100-cc expander. When compared with the control group, which had no tissue expansion, the area of flap survival was significantly increased in the 3 tissue expansion groups. The area of survival was also significantly greater with the 100-cc expander than with the 2 smaller expanders. The flap survival results were consistent with the findings of rubber injection vascularity studies.

Conclusions.—Tissue expansion appears to be a useful addition to flap prefabrication. These 2-stage procedures can be combined to increase the amount of viable tissue as well as the vascularity of the prefabricated flap. The mechanism by which tissue expansion increases vascularity remains to be determined.

▶ Many protocols for free flap fabrication utilize a tissue expander to allow for primary closure of the donor site. This article addresses a related issue— whether the expander increases the rate at which the prefabrication flap becomes vascularized by the transferred pedicle. There was a clear and significant benefit of expanding the tissue before transfer, thus suggesting that tissue expansion has favorable biological effects on revascularization. This study does not address whether this benefit results from the barrier function of the expander or the tissue expansion process. A control group of unexpanded expanders would have been of significant benefit in the experimental groups and should be the focus of additional study.

W. Garner, M.D.

Experimental Study of Allogeneically Vascularized Prefabricated Flaps

Hirai T, Manders EK, Hughes K, et al (Pennsylvania State Univ, Hershey; Nippon Med School, Tokyo)
Ann Plast Surg 37:394–399, 1996   6–5

Objective.—Prefabricated, neovascularized flaps could be useful for reconstruction in areas of inadequate vascularity, for both free and vascularized island flaps. The use of cryopreserved allogeneic vascular bundles as vascular pedicles for neovascularized prefabricated flaps was described.

Methods.—Experiments were performed in rabbits. First, 8-cm auricular vessels were harvested and preserved in liquid nitrogen. After 30 days, the allogeneic vascular bundles were anastomosed orthotopically under the operating microscope into the auricular vein of a recipient animal. Dorsal flaps measuring 6 × 6 cm were then raised on the implanted allovascular bundle. Eight days later, allogeneically vascularized island flaps were elevated and studied by computed microangiography.

Results.—Thirteen of 15 vessels were patent 8 days after implantation. Anastomoses between the vasculature of the implanted vessels and the recipient sites were demonstrated by computed microangiography. One week after elevation, the flaps showed evidence of viability.

Conclusions.—These animal experiments suggest that allovascular bundles can serve as pedicles for vascularized island flaps. This technique could allow vascularized flaps to be created for transfer anywhere on the body, with no need for autologous blood vessels. Allogeneic microvascular grafts could prove very useful in the transfer of autologous composite flaps and as supercharging vessels of large flaps.

▶ This article is not appropriately titled; however, its content and experimental design are quite interesting. The authors harvested small blood vessels from 1 set of animals, cryopreserved them, and then used these as vein grafts to prefabricate flaps. Because inbred rabbit strains were used, there were no allogenetic mismatches; however, freezing the vessels mimics the processing of a variety of bioengineered vessel conduits. Because these conduits might be available in the future, this study assesses the ability of this technique in creating a prefabricated flap. These cryopreserved blood vessels were successful in allowing flap fabrication; therefore the stage is set for creation of prefabricated flaps using a vascular conduit when a vascular pedicle is not immediately available in the reconstructive area. Bioengineered blood vessel substitutes will probably reach clinical practice soon. It is likely that we will be using these types of constructs for various procedures in the reconstruction of difficult or unusual reconstructions or when utilizing an adjacent donor site is of critical importance.

W. Garner, M.D.

Prefabrication of a Free Flap for Tracheal Reconstruction: An Experimental Study. Preliminary Report

Cavadas PC, Bonanad E, Baena-Montilla P, et al (Hosp La Fe, Valencia, Spain)
Plast Reconstr Surg 98:1052–1062, 1996   6–6

Background.—Reconstructing extensive tracheal defects requiring more than direct anastomosis continues to be a problem. In an experimental study, a free flap for tracheal reconstruction was prefabricated in a goat model.

Methods.—Ten animals were used. A composite cutaneous-chondromucosal premolded, prevascularized flap was obtained in a staged procedure using prefabrication techniques. In the first stage of the procedure, the cartilaginous framework and vascular pedicle were constructed. The second stage was done 50 days later. The inner surface of the neotrachea was lined with nasal mucosa. In the third stage, done 10 days after the second procedure, the flap was elevated and free transferred to reconstruct a 15-cm circumferential defect in the cervical trachea.

Findings.—Three animals died early in the postoperative period. Infection developed in another goat, and free flap failure with early tracheal stenosis occurred in another. The 5 long-term survivors had no significant stenosis. The structure of the neotracheal flap was similar to that of the native trachea, with internal respiratory epithelial lining, cartilage rings, and fibrovascular tissue. Fiberoptic bronchoscopy, done on days 10 and 60, showed no significant stenosis in the long-term survivors.

Conclusions.—In this goat model, pregrafting, premolding, and vascular induction methods enabled the creation of a free flap that structurally resembled the native trachea. The behavior of this flap in tracheal reconstruction seems promising.

Prefabricated Jejunal Free-tissue Transfer for Tracheal Reconstruction: An Experimental Study
Banis JC Jr, Churukian K, Kim M, et al (Univ of Louisville, Ky)
Plast Reconstr Surg 98:1046–1051, 1996   6–7

Background.—Long-segment tracheal defects are difficult to reconstruct. The use of prosthetic materials is problematic because of their propensity for infection and extrusion, and the utility of autologous tissue is limited by poor structural features and technical complexity. A simple composite bioprosthesis was proposed that, through prefabrication and subsequent neovascularization, may provide a functional tracheal analogue that is better than currently used forms of reconstruction.

Methods.—In 10 rats, composite flaps were created by combining an isolated, perfused, mucosectomized segment with an outer covering of ring-reinforced woven Dacron vascular graft. This unit was left in the intra-abdominal milieu for 20 days, at which time it was assessed.

Findings.—Seven rats survived the initial phase. In all animals, the jejunal bioprostheses tolerated negative pressures to −200 mm Hg, rotation of 180 degrees, and flexion to 90 degrees without collapse of the graft segments. Neovascularization of the Dacron graft and dense fibrovascular ingrowth into the interstices of the graft were observed on vascular casts and standard histologic study.

Conclusions.—Prefabrication with autologous and prosthetic components to create a single axial flap for transfer may be feasible in long-segment tracheal reconstruction. Neovascularization permeates the full thickness of the prosthetic component. Dense fibrous ingrowth occurs during the delay period. In addition, this neotracheal analogue has structural characteristics similar to those of the native trachea and a durable submucosal layer that supports epithelial ingrowth.

▶ These studies (Abstracts 6–6 and 6–7) are important not only because reconstruction of extensive tracheal defects has not been consistently successful but also because they clearly show the creative ability of plastic surgeons to develop and apply new skills and techniques to a wide variety of unsolved problems. Ultimately, this one will likely be solved by a combination of autogenous tissues and biocompatible prosthetic materials.

S.H. Miller, M.D.

Vascular Delay Improves Latissimus Dorsi Muscle Perfusion and Muscle Function for Use in Cardiomyoplasty
Carroll SM, Heilman SJ, Stremel RW, et al (Cork Regional Hosp, Ireland; Univ of Louisville, Ky)
Plast Reconstr Surg 99:1329–1337, 1997   6–8

Background.—During muscle transfer for cardiomyoplasty, ischemia of the distal portion of the latissimus dorsi muscle may reduce distal muscle contractility and its mechanical efficacy. Muscle function may be improved by a vascular delay procedure that increases distal perfusion of the latissimus dorsi muscle.

Methods and Findings.—Ten adult mongrel dogs were operated on. Their latissimus dorsi muscles were subjected to a vascular delay procedure on 1 side and a sham procedure on the other. After 10 days of vascular delay, muscle perfusion was measured with a laser Doppler perfusion imager before and after the muscles were elevated as flaps, based only on thoracodorsal neurovascular pedicles. To simulate cardiomyoplasty, the muscles were wrapped and sutured around silicone chambers. A stimulating electrode was then placed around each thoracodorsal nerve, and the muscles underwent simulated contraction in rhythmic and tetanic fashion. Measurements of circumferential and longitudinal force generation and fatigue rates were obtained independently. Compared with non-delayed muscle, delayed muscle showed significantly improved circumferential muscle force. Circumferential and longitudinal fatigue rates were also improved. In addition, improvement was noted in distal, middle, and overall perfusion.

Conclusion.—In this dog model, a vascular delay procedure with a 10-day delay adaptation period significantly improved latissimus dorsi muscle flap perfusion and function, especially in the distal and middle part of the muscle. Delay should be considered as a way to improve clinical outcomes in cardiomyoplasty.

▶ Logically, the delay should improve overall muscle function and increase the likelihood that collateral vascularization of the myocardium will occur. The true test of the worth of delay awaits clinical trials to determine whether cardiac hemodynamics can be reliably improved.

S.H. Miller, M.D.

Deletion of Individual Muscles Alters Rat Walking-track Parameters

Reynolds JL, Urbanchek MS, Asato H, et al (Univ of Michigan, Ann Arbor)
J Reconstr Microsurg 12:461–466, 1996   6–9

Background.—Even using advanced microsurgical techniques of reconstructive surgery, it is often not possible to fully restore sensory and motor function after peripheral nerve injury. Rat walking-track analysis is a useful technique for assessing motor recovery after hindlimb nerve injury and repair. However, the relationship between the footprint parameters used with this model and the functional capacity of individual hindlimb muscles has never been assessed. The relationship between individual footprint measurements and the function of specific hindlimb muscles was assessed in an experimental study.

Methods.—Rats were divided into 5 groups for deletion of specific motors: division of the tendon of insertion of the gastrocnemius, soleus, and plantaris muscles; division of the extensor digitorum longus muscle tendons of insertion; division of the extensor hallucis long muscle tendon of insertion; division of the tibialis anterior muscle tendon of insertion; or division of the tibial nerve at the ankle. Before and after these procedures, the animals underwent walking-track analysis. The investigators investigated the effects of muscle deletion on individual walking-track parameters, such as print length, intermediate toe spread, and total toe spread.

Results.—Each of the 5 groups had specific patterns of change in the footprint parameters. Print length was directly related to the function of the triceps surae and tibialis anterior muscles. Total toe spread was linked to function of the extensor hallucis longus. Intermediate toe spread was affected by function of the extensor digitorum longus.

Conclusion.—Experimental deletion of individual rat hindlimb muscles has specific, predictable effects on individual print measurements on walking-track analysis. The findings have important implications for the use of walking-track analysis as an outcome measure in studies of peripheral-nerve repair. The relationship between walking-track measurements and muscle-force output in reinnervated hindlimbs remains to be determined.

▶ In my naiveté, I assumed that if "minor" muscles were deleted, the overall pattern of the imprint would not change and the gait would remain the same. This article nicely demonstrates a direct relationship between individual print measurement and the function of individual rat muscles. This should at least alert us to comparable clinical problems in lower extremity injuries.

D.J. Smith, Jr., M.D.

Clinical

Galeo-Pericranial Flaps in the Forehead: A Study of Blood Supply and Volumes

Potparić Z, Fukuta K, Colen LB, et al (Eastern Virginia Med School, Norfolk)
Br J Plast Surg 49:519–528, 1996   6–10

Objective.—The use of galeo-pericranial flaps has greatly lowered the complication rate after surgical correction of craniofacial deformities. Although a good blood supply is important to prevent bacterial invasion of the dead space in the cranial base, whether the bulk of the galeo-pericranial flaps is always sufficient to provide an adequate amount of vascularized tissue is not known. The blood supply of the different layers of the forehead was explored, the extent of the axial blood supply was deliniated, and volumes of galeo-pericranial flaps derived from the forehead were estimated.

Methods.—The common carotid arteries of 12 fresh cadaver specimens (24 sides) were injected with colored radiopaque contrast medium. Coronal flaps then were dissected and radiographs obtained. Full-thickness scalp specimens were taken from 5 fresh cadavers and analyzed histologically to study tissue layers and differentiation of blood vessels. Twelve halves of coronal flaps from 6 cadavers were cut horizontally and sectioned, stained with hematoxylin and eosin, and examined at 4× magnification. Volume measurements were made of 4 pericranial, 5 galeal-frontalis, and 4 galeal-frontalis-pericranial flaps.

Results.—The supratrochlear and supraorbital vessels provided the entire blood supply to the anteriorly based galeo-pericranial flaps. Axial vessels were 20 to 70 mm long. Whereas layers above the periosteum were well vascularized, anastomoses in deep layers were not well developed. The blood supply distal to the flap had a random pattern. Pericranial flap volume ranged from 3 to 16 mL. Galeal-frontalis myofascial flaps had axial vessels in the proximal portion above the supraorbital rim. Flap volume here ranged from 13 to 20 mL. Axial vessels found here were 70 mm long. The overall blood supply of the galeal-frontalis-pericranial flap was increased, and flap volume ranged from 31 to 48 mL.

Conclusions.—It was difficult to determine the extent of the blood supply because of the variation in length of the axial vessels. Whereas the proximal portions of the flaps were well vascularized, the distal parts were less well supplied. Use of the composite galeal-frontalis-pericranial flap can increase bulk and vascularity.

▶ This manuscript provides a useful description of the blood supply of anteriorly based galeal-frontalis and galeo-pericranial flaps. The authors point out that although the blood supply is abundant at the base of these flaps, the distal blood supply is questionable. They make the clinical recommendation that pericranium be included with galeal-frontalis flaps in cases of large volume needs, noting the increase in vascularity when this is performed.

This work indirectly supports the contention that pericranium-only flaps, which often are used by neurosurgeons to obliterate anterior dead space, will provide little vascularized tissue and are useful only for such purposes as to augment scarring of dermal patches.

S.P. Bartlett, M.D.

Anatomical Basis for a Fasciocutaneous Flap From the Hypothenar Eminence of the Hand
Omokawa S, Ryu J, Tang J-B, et al (West Virginia Univ, Morgantown)
Br J Plast Surg 49:559–563, 1996   6–11

Introduction.—The hypothenar eminence has rarely been considered as a donor site for a vascularized flap to cover soft-tissue defects of the fingers. Most of the literature describing vasculature of the hand provides detailed descriptions for all areas except the hypothenar eminence, for which only gross anatomical observations are reported. The vasculature and neural anatomy of the hypothenar eminence were explored in 32 fresh cadaver hands to determine the possibility and potential benefits of its use as a donor site for free or pedicled island flaps to repair palmar skin defects of the fingers.

Methods.—Specimens were stored frozen and were allowed to thaw for 12 hours before evaluation. Microfil, a silicone rubber compound, was perfused into the brachial artery at the proximal end of the forearm in 27 hands and into the ulnar palmar digital artery of the little finger at artery origin in 5 hands. The area of perfused skin was measured to determine the skin territory nourished by each artery. Dissections and histologic examinations were performed to determine microvascular and neural networks.

Results.—The hypothenar eminence may be divided into 3 territories, as determined by the type of nutrient artery supplying each territory. The distal half of the ulnar aspect of the hypothenar eminence is supplied by multiple fasciocutaneous branches that stem from the ulnar palmar digital artery of the fifth digit. The proximal half of the ulnar aspect is supplied by perforating branches originating from the hypothenar muscles. The radial border of the hypothenar eminence is supplied by small vascular branches that primarily diverge from the superficial palmar arch through the palmar aponeurosis. The dorsal and palmar branch of the ulnar nerve provides sensory innervation.

Conclusion.—The distal half of the ulnar aspect of the hypothenar eminence is a feasible donor site for a skin flap. Inclusion of the dorsal or palmar cutaneous branch of the ulnar nerve will facilitate sensory potential of the flap.

▶ The authors note that "the relatively important sensation of this area for hands function" is the reason why investigators don't consider this area as a donor site. This statement is true, and although their study is nicely presented, this area is an extremely poor choice for a flap. The resultant diminished sensation might be worse than the defect that is being corrected.

R.E. Salisbury, M.D.

Neurocutaneous Island Flaps in Upper Limb Coverage: Experience With 44 Clinical Cases
Bertelli JA (Joana de Gusmão Children's Hosp, Santa Catarina, Brazil; Universite Rene Descartes, Paris)
J Hand Surg [Am] 22A:515–526, 1997   6–12

Background.—The vascularity of the cutaneous nerve of the upper limb and of the skin are closely connected. Perforators of the main arteries vascularize both skin and nerves. Small longitudinal paraneural vessels in close contact with the cutaneous nerves connect these perforating arteries. The clinical experience with 44 neurocutaneous island flaps for upper-limb coverage was reported.

Methods and Findings.—The flaps were supplied by the vessels around and inside cutaneous nerves. These flaps, which were as large as 4×10 cm, provided reliable coverage of skin defects in the upper limb. The proximally based flaps, free flaps, and flaps based distally on the dorsal side of the hand were extremely safe. Necrosis developed in 1 flap based distally on the medial antebrachial cutaneous nerve of the forearm and in 3 flaps used to reconstruct the thumb.

Conclusions.—Neurocutaneous island flaps are reliable, versatile, and easy to dissect. Major vessels, such as the radial, ulnar, and posterior interosseous arteries, are preserved. The donor site may be closed primarily in most patients, with minimal donor site morbidity.

▶ With the increasing understanding of flap anatomy, increasingly sophisticated designs can be fashioned for upper extremity flaps. Interestingly, these neurocutaneous flaps do not include the deep fascia and therefore are not classified as fasciocutaneous flaps. I am not sure that I am totally comfortable with the concept, although I think that under limited circumstances I would be willing to consider this option for soft tissue coverage.

D.J. Smith, M.D.

Tensor Fasciae Lata Myocutaneous Flap Reconstruction Following Ilioinguinal Node Dissection
Savant DN, Dalal AV, Patel SG, et al (Tata Mem Hosp, Bombay, India)
Eur J Plast Surg 19:174–177, 1996   6–13

Background.—Ilioinguinal block dissections are associated with a high incidence of complications, with rates of wound complications ranging from 50% to 70% and lymphedema occurring in most patients. In an effort to decrease morbidity, a variety of incisions and reconstructive techniques have been attempted. Use of the tensor fasciae lata (TFL) myocutaneous flap after ilioinguinal node dissection at 1 institution was described.

Methods and Findings.—Twenty-five patients underwent TFL myocutaneous flap reconstruction as a means of primary reconstruction after a total of 40 groin node dissections. Overlying skin was excised either prophylactically or because of disease involvement. Primary healing occurred in 82.5% of the flaps. Moderate complications developed in 17.5%. Only 12% of the patients had postoperative lymphedema. The mean length of hospitalization was 14.2 days.

Conclusions.—The TFL flap is safe and reliable in patients with unilateral or bilateral groin dissections. The procedure results in minimal postoperative morbidity and a marked reduction in hospitalization.

▶ The real value of this article is not in showing us that the TFL is a good choice for the closure of large defects in the groin (we know that already!), but in recommending that this flap be used *routinely* to close this area after groin dissection with skin resection (instead of "cranking together" the skin and using the flap for secondary closure if the wound breaks down).

R.L. Ruberg, M.D.

Perineal Hernia Repair Using Gracilis Myocutaneous Flap

Hansen MT, Bell JL, Chun JT (Univ of Tennessee, Knoxville)
South Med J 90:75–77, 1997   6–14

Purpose.—Perineal hernia is a potential complication of major pelvic surgery, especially in women. Several different reconstructive techniques have been described. The use of a gracilis myocutaneous flap was analyzed.

> *Case Report.*—Woman, 67, underwent pelvic exenteration, descending colostomy, and ileal conduit surgery for the treatment of stage II colon cancer. Surgery was followed by chemotherapy and pelvic irradiation. After 5 months, the patient noticed a perineal bulge with pain and discomfort that became worse over the course of 3 years. A reproducible hernia was seen through the vaginal remnant. Repair was accomplished by a combined abdominal-perineal approach. The hernia was reduced through the abdominal incision and the hernia sac was excised through the vaginal introitus. The defect in the pelvic floor was then filled with a right gracilis myocutaneous flap, which was passed through a subcutaneous tunnel into the pelvis. The repair was completed by trimming of the skin paddle and anchoring of the distal end of the gracilis tendon to the sacral promontory. Complications consisted of midline fusion of the labia minora, managed surgically, and lymphedema of the right leg, controlled with a pressure stocking. At 11

months' follow-up, the skin paddle was viable and there were no signs of hernia.

Discussion.—A unilateral gracilis myocutaneous flap can be used for repair of a perineal hernia. This flap provides well-vascularized tissue that is useful in many situations requiring pelvic and perineal reconstruction. When this area has been irradiated, the improved vascularity provided by the gracilis flap may permit repair without the need for prosthetic mesh.

▶ This article documents an unusual but creative use of a flap, well known to reconstructive surgeons' after oncologic reconstruction of the vulva or vagina. This technique should be known by surgeons performing intra-abdominal procedures, and reconstruction in these areas is a new possible application for flap use.

W. Garner, M.D.

Sliding Shape-Designed Latissimus Dorsi Flap

Sawaizumi M, Maruyama Y (Toho Univ, Tokyo)
Ann Plast Surg 38:41–45, 1997

6–15

Objective.—When the latissimus dorsi musculocutaneous flap is used in reconstruction and the resulting donor defect is too wide to close primarily, a skin graft of the donor site may be necessary. A new sliding-shape design of the latissimus dorsi flap is useful in avoiding this problem. Two cases were presented.

Methods.—An oval-shaped defect is divided lengthwise, and these semicircular parts are traced on the latissimus dorsi. The 2 paddles thus formed are rotated and slid side-by-side to provide an oval-shaped flap for covering the defect. Defects of greater than 10 cm have been reconstructed in 7 patients with 4 pedicled and 3 free flaps.

> *Case 1.*—Woman, 18, had a synovial cancer removed from the front of the right femur, leaving an 18 × 15-cm defect. The thoracodorsal vessels of the free flap were anastomosed with the descending branches of the lateral circumflex femoral artery. The leg was functioning satisfactorily after 8 months.
>
> Case 2.—Woman, 57, had a 20 × 18-cm defect after resection of recurrent breast cancer with dermatitis and erosion. The defect was covered with the skin island of a sliding-shape latissimus dorsi flap. After 17 months, the limb was functioning with shoulder abduction of 110 degrees.

Conclusion.—The sliding shape–designed latissimus dorsi musculocutaneous flap is useful for covering large donor site defects with minimum morbidity.

► This paper describes a variation of the latissimus muscular cutaneous flap in which the skin paddles are moved to alter the shape of the donor skin defect. The result is a large cutaneous paddle but a donor site which can be closed primarily. It is a clever modification and should be considered for a wound that would be treated by muscular cutaneous flap transfer.

W. Garner, M.D.

Seroma as a Common Donor Site Morbidity After Harvesting the Latissimus Dorsi Flap: Observations on Cause and Prevention

Schwabegger A, Ninković M, Brenner E, et al (Univ Clinic of Plastic and Reconstructive Surgery, Innsbruck, Austria; Univ Inst of Anatomy, Innsbruck, Austria)
Ann Plast Surg 38:594–597, 1997   6–16

Objective.—Although seroma formation after harvesting the latissimus dorsi muscle (LDM) is a relatively common complication, the causes of it have not been well researched. Results of a prospective study investigating the possible causes of seroma formation and the effects of preventive steps are presented.

Methods.—Between January 1993 and November 1996, 58 free or pedicled LDM flaps were harvested by electrocautery in 15 patients (group 1), by scalpel in 21 patients (group 2), and by scalpel with additional skin flap fixation by tacking of an average of 10–20 Vicryl sutures in 22 patients (group 3). In 46 patients, flaps were harvested as musculocutaneous flaps. Each patient had at least 2 drainage tubes inserted. Patients were followed up for a minimum of 2 months, and those with persistent seromas were treated until resolution.

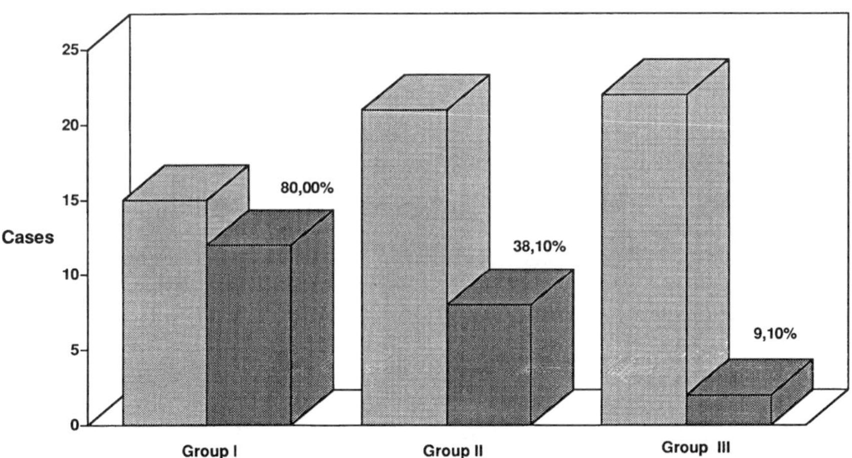

FIGURE 2.—Percentage of seroma formation (*dark gray columns*) compared with total cases (*light gray columns*) within each group. (Reprinted from Schwabegger A, Ninković M, Brenner E, et al: Seroma as a common donor site morbidity after harvesting the latissimus dorsi flap: Observations on cause and prevention. *Annals of Plastic Surgery* 38:594–597, 1997 by permission of Little, Brown and Company, Inc.).

Results.—Seromas developed in 22 patients; group 1 had a significantly higher rate of seroma formation than groups 2 and 3 (Fig 2). Two noncompliant patients required repeated puncture during a 3-week period to promote healing. One group 1 patient required excision of the fibrous capsule to facilitate healing after 10 months.

Conclusion.—The high rate of seroma formation in patients with LDM flaps harvested by electrocautery or scalpel without tacking sutures appears to be caused by friction trauma. Harvesting the flap using a scalpel and tacking sutures significantly decreases the rate of seroma formation.

▶ This technique might be worth a try, although I am not sure I accept the authors' explanation for why it works.

R.L. Ruberg, M.D.

Preventing Seroma in the Latissimus Dorsi Flap Donor Site

Titley OG, Spyrou GE, Fatah MFT (Wordsley Hosp, Stourbridge, England)
Br J Plast Surg 50:106–108, 1997   6–17

Background.—The authors of this article have routinely used the latissimus dorsi flap as a myocutaneous flap in breast reconstruction and as a free muscle flap in lower limb surgery. However, the incidence of donor site seroma after the harvesting of the flaps has been disappointingly high. A quilting technique has been used in an attempt to address this problem.

Methods.—Eleven donor sites treated by the quilting method were studied prospectively and compared with a retrospective group of 16 nonquilted donor sites. Patients in the 2 groups were similar in age range and surgical indications. The quilting procedure involved quilting the donor site skin flaps to the underlying tissues with absorbable sutures.

Outcomes.—After the quilting procedure was introduced, the incidence of donor site seroma declined from 56% to 0%. The quilted donor site group also had a significantly lower mean volume of postoperative drainage—320 mL, compared with 608 mL in the nonquilted group. The drains were removed at a mean of 3.9 days in the quilted group, significantly sooner than the mean of 7.3 days in the nonquilted group. Donor site drainage and time to drain removal did not differ significantly between nonquilted sites at which a seroma developed and those where one did not.

Conclusion.—This procedure is easy to learn, is straightforward in performance, and requires no special instrumentation. Its use is recommended to all surgeons who use latissimus dorsi flaps.

▶ This article describes a simple modification of standard latissimus dorsi muscle harvest. By suturing the overlying skin to the underlying tissue, the authors decreased their seroma formation from 56% to 0%. The amount of drainage was also decreased. The procedure seems straightforward and easy and might significantly reduce the problem of seroma formation.

W. Garner, M.D.

A Theoretical Consideration of Extensions of the Z-plasty Principle
Vegter F, Hage JJ (Academic Hosp of the Free Univ, Amsterdam)
Eur J Plast Surg 20:71–76, 1997   6–18

Introduction.—To deal with congenital or posttraumatic webs and contractures, a variety of local skin flap techniques have been described. With each of the techniques, there is confusion regarding the degree of lengthening that can be obtained and how much lateral slack is needed to allow these flaps to be shifted. The theoretic gains and decreases in width of various procedures are presented.

Z-plasty.—Two triangular skin flaps delineated by a Z-shaped incision make up the Z-plasty. Its 3 incisions are frequently of equal length, and they have 60-degree angles. With a 60-degree Z-plasty, the theoretic gain in length is 74%. The greater the gain in length, the wider the angles. However, disturbing dog-ears may result with angles of more than 100 degrees. Variations include multiple Z-plasties, 4-flap Z-plasty, and 6-flap Z-plasty.

YV-advancement.—When the skin triangle is designed lateral to one side of a scar while a straight incision is made on the other side and perpendicular to it to complete a Y, a YV-advancement has been begun. The new suture line will be V-shaped when the skin triangle is shifted forward along the straight line. To allow the V to be shifted, secondary skin triangles have to be excised bilaterally. The linear scar is lengthened and broken by the advanced tissue triangle. With YV-advancement, the gain in length and lateral narrowing can be about 50%. Variations include multiple YV-advancements, combined double Z-plasty and YV-advancement, and combined rotation and YV-advancement.

Conclusion.—Superior lengthening-to-narrowing ratios can result from the Z-plasty technique and its modifications. Resection of scarred skin can be obtained with combined YV-plasties. In each individual case, the technique to be used depends on position, extent, and orientation of the scar or web.

▶ This interesting, but troublesome article describes several theoretic geometric modifications of Z-plasty and VY-advancement flaps that might be useful in increasing the length of the scar. Unfortunately, the analysis is completely theoretic and there are suggestions for use of these flaps in clinical practice. Of greatest concern to me as a practitioner is that many flaps are quite thin and narrow and would likely not survive in the scarred and injured tissues in which I would like to perform them. On the other hand, thoughtful analysis of a problem can often provide solutions, and this does represent a thoughtful consideration of the Z-plasty. It is to be hoped that the authors will provide us with practical expressions of these thoughts in future articles. Otherwise, their analysis must remain strictly of theoretic interest.

W. Garner, M.D.

Exploring the Use of the Medicinal Leech: A Clinical Risk-Benefit Analysis

de Chalain TMB (Emory Univ, Atlanta, Ga)
J Reconstr Microsurg 12:165–172, 1996

6–19

Purpose.—*Hirudo medicinalis*, the medicinal leech, is increasingly used as an aid to the survival of compromised pedicled flaps and microvascular free-tissue transfers. A growing body of literature describes the safe use of this technique. This review sought to define the clinical risks and benefits of leech use.

Methods.—In a retrospective chart analysis, the investigators identified 18 cases in which medicinal leeches had been used postoperatively. A literature review turned up 36 reports of leech use in 108 cases. Each case was reviewed for data regarding demographics, indications, duration of leech application, antibiotic use, blood transfusions, incidence of infection, and clinical outcomes.

Results.—The flap salvage rate ranged from 70% to 80%. The infection rate was 7% to 20%. In the authors' experiences, there were 2 cases of infection with *Aeromonas hydrophilia*. Once a clinically significant infection occurred, the salvage rate dropped to 30% or lower. Leeches were applied for a mean of 3 days in the authors' experience and 4 days according to the literature. Two thirds of the authors' patients required blood transfusion.

Discussion.—Infection is a significant risk; other risks include blood loss requiring transfusion, loss of leeches into bodily orifices and spaces, allergic reactions, and adverse psychologic reactions. When leeches are used, they are best used early and according to an established protocol. Whenever this decision is made, the potential risks and benefits must be carefully and honestly considered.

▶ As the author notes, leech therapy has been used as a last resort. Increasingly, I have seen leeches used more aggressively and earlier as a therapy for compromised flaps and venous outflow problems. I commend this approach and have adopted it in recent years.

D.J. Smith, Jr., M.D.

Microsurgery

Selection of Appropriate Recipient Vessels in Difficult, Microsurgical Head and Neck Reconstruction

Takamatsu A, Harashina T, Inoue T (Saitama Med School, Japan)
J Reconstr Microsurg 12:499–507, 1996

6–20

Introduction.—It is sometimes difficult to select an appropriate recipient vessel in patients undergoing microsurgical head and neck reconstruction. In the authors' experience with such difficult cases, vessel selection is correlated with the region of reconstruction. They review this experience, including examples of difficult cases in each category.

Experience.—In a 22-year experience, the authors performed 327 microsurgical free flap transfers to the head and neck. In 16 of these cases, scarring and/or radiation made the first choice of recipient vessels unavailable. For patients undergoing scalp and skull reconstruction, this meant that the superficial temporal artery and vein were unavailable. Other small vessels were useful in this situation, such as the posterior auricular artery and vein. Distant neck vessels were sometimes combined with interpositional vein grafts or long pedicled forearm flaps. A distal-tapering anastomotic technique was used to overcome the size difference between these vessels.

For patients undergoing facial reconstruction, the facial and superficial temporal artery and vein are used when available. If these are unavailable, other selections include the tributaries of the external carotid artery and external jugular vein. Failing that, the external carotid artery, internal jugular vein, or flipped-over cephalic vein may be used. There may also be healthy vessels on the other side. Continuous suturing of the posterior wall may be performed if end-to-side anastomosis is done on large, immobile vessels, such as the external carotid artery.

Although bilateral vessels of the neck are generally available for use in reconstruction of the oral cavity, the cephalic vein was flipped over to the upper neck in 1 patient undergoing reconstruction of the oral floor. The contralateral vessels and the tributaries of the subclavian vessel may be used if the ipsilateral vessels of the neck are unavailable for mandibular reconstruction. For neck reconstruction, branches of the subclavian vessels, or the subclavian artery itself, can be used for secondary reconstruction of the cervical esophagus, using free jejunal transfer. Distant recipient vessels can be used in interpositional vein grafting using the saphenous or cephalic vein. The cephalic vein may be used as a free graft, as a pedicle vessel, and for temporary arteriovenous shunt formation.

Conclusion.—Alternative recipient vessels may be used for difficult microsurgical head and neck reconstructions. Adjacent small vessels are usually the first choice in these situations, followed by the major and distant vessels. Healthy vessels must be used for free flap transfers. Special anastomotic techniques and other precautions may be required.

▶ I thought this article was interesting because it concerns a subject to which I have given little consideration. Most of us just assume that there is a plethora of arteries and veins in the head and neck, and if 1 side is not available, the other side will be. The algorithm presented and the analysis are important and emphasize the use of healthy vessels. The section on clever use of the cephalic vein was interesting and intriguing.

D.J. Smith, Jr., M.D.

Endoscopic Sural Nerve Harvest in the Pediatric Patient

Capek L, Clarke HM, Zuker RM (Univ of Toronto)
Plast Reconstr Surg 98:884–888, 1996   6–21

Background.—The sural nerves are the most abundant source of graft material in children who require nerve-grafting procedures. Harvesting of the sural nerve is usually done through a "stocking-seam" posterior leg incision, an approach that provides visualization of the entire sural nerve anatomy. A disadvantage of this approach is the tendency of the donor-site scar to thicken and widen. The technique of endoscopic sural nerve harvest

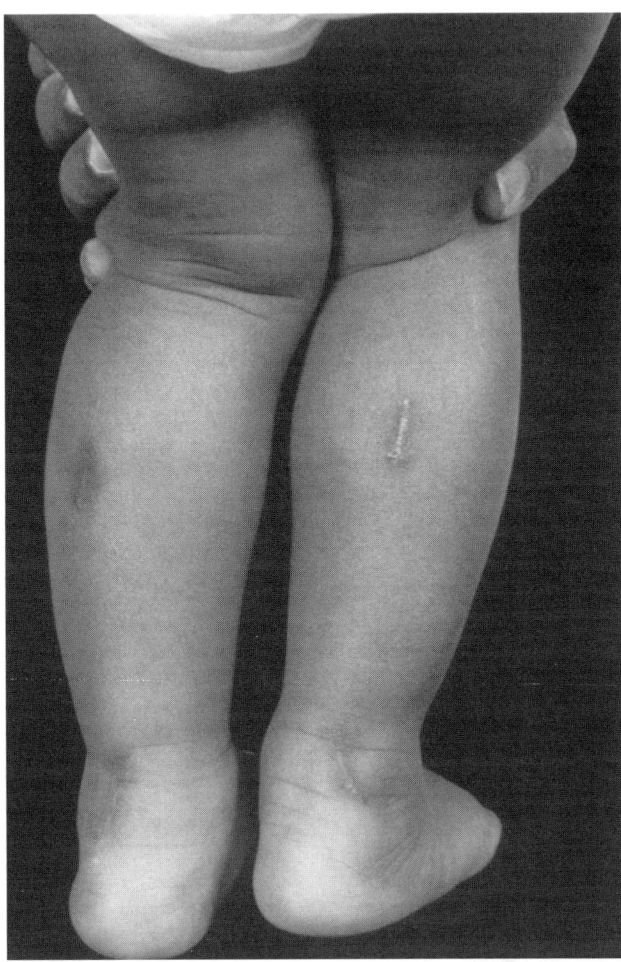

FIGURE 5.—Donor-site scars 6 months postoperatively using endoscopic sural nerve harvest technique. (Courtesy of Capek L, Clarke HM, Zuker RM: Endoscopic sural nerve harvest in the pediatric patient. *Plast Reconstr Surg* 98:884–888, 1996.)

described here minimizes donor-site scarring in children while allowing good visualization and harvest of the maximal length of graft material.

Technique.—Sural nerve harvest is done with the patient under general endotracheal anesthesia. Before harvest, the approximate length of the nerve graft required is determined and the leg is marked as for an open harvest. Two 2-cm incisions are made under tourniquet control for access at the lateral malleolus and the mid-calf. A subcutaneous pocket is dissected around the distal nerve for insertion of the retractor and endoscope apparatus. Tenotomy or Metzenbaum scissors are used to perform blunt dissection of the nerve under endoscopic visualization. The endoscopic view allows the sural nerve to be differentiated from the adjacent lesser saphenous vein. The medial sural nerve is divided in the popliteal fossa proximally, and the lateral sural nerve is identified and harvested when present.

Results.—Eighteen patients ranging in age from 4 months to 16 years (mean, 3.3 years) underwent 27 sural nerve graft harvests using the endoscopic technique. Twenty-five nerves were harvested through 2 small incisions, as described, and 2 legs required extension of the proximal incision for adequate visualization. The mean tourniquet time for a unilateral harvest was 92 minutes. No visible nerve-graft injuries were noted, and no patient had a hematoma, seroma, infection, or wound dehiscence. Postoperative pain and swelling were minimal and scarring was esthetically satisfactory (Fig 5).

Discussion.—Long segments of nerve graft often are required in children undergoing nerve reconstruction. Compared to traditional incisions, the endoscopic technique limits donor-site morbidity while allowing the maximal length of graft to be obtained through 2 short incisions.

▶ We are now firmly in the era of applications of endoscopic techniques to reconstructive surgery in children. The authors were successful in performing endoscopic nerve harvest in infants as young as 4 months of age. The concept and the technique seem appropriate for widespread use.

R.L. Ruberg, M.D.

Ischemia Time and Free Flap Success

Gürlek A, Kroll SS, Schusterman MA (Univ of Texas, Houston)
Ann Plast Surg 38:503–505, 1997   6–22

Introduction.—To surgeons who perform free tissue transfer, flap ischemic time has always been of concern. Irreversible changes, leading to necrosis and failure, occur to the flap after a certain period of ischemia. The likelihood of successful flap transfer may be reduced with increased ischemic time. Flap ischemic times were reviewed to determine whether they affected the success of flap transfer by correlating them with data on flap survival and exploring caused relationships.

Methods.—For 700 free flaps used for breast, head, or neck reconstruction, ischemic time, the time between the interruption and reestablishment of blood supply, was reviewed. A comparison of survival rates was made among patients who had flap ischemic times of 100 minutes or longer and those with flap ischemic times shorter than 100 minutes. A comparison of survival rates was made among patients who had flap ischemic times of 75 minutes or less and those with 120 minutes or more. Those who had flap ischemic times of 180 minutes or more were also studied for success rates.

Results.—Flaps that survived had a mean ischemic time of 91.25 minutes; those that failed had a mean ischemic time of 111.64 minutes. The difference in ischemic time between the failures and successes was not statistically significant. There was no difference found in success rate between the patients who had flap ischemic times of more than 100 minutes and those with less than 100 minutes. There was no difference between the patients who had flap ischemic times of less than 75 minutes and those with more than 120 minutes. Among patients who had flap ischemic times of more than 180 minutes, there was a slight trend toward more flap loss, but the difference was not significant.

Conclusion.—Provided that ischemia is not prolonged past 3 hours, or to the point where the no-reflow phenomenon occurs, ischemic time is irrelevant to flap survival.

▶ This issue is of interest to all who do microsurgical reconstruction: Does the time that a free tissue transfer remains ischemic influence its medium- and long term-success? The simple answer is no. If the flap is revascularized quickly enough to prevent the no-reflow phenomenon, the relative ischemia time has no relationship to flap survival. This fact will likely be useful in the planning of procedures, such as when to begin arterial versus venous anastomoses, when to inset the flap, and other similar planning questions.

W. Garner, M.D.

Free Tissue Transfer in Pediatric Patients
Serletti JM, Schingo VA Jr, Deuber MA, et al (Univ of Rochester, NY)
Ann Plast Surg 36:561–568, 1996   6–23

Objective.—Free tissue transfer in adults for the reconstruction of soft-tissue defects is common. However, few series have been reported in children. An experience with this surgical technique including perioperative anticoagulation and guideline development for tissue selection with pediatric free flaps was presented.

Methods.—Twenty free tissue transfers were performed in 19 pediatric patients, aged 3 to 17 years (6 girls). Eight patients were 6 years of age or younger. The defects were located on the legs or feet in 12 patients, were the result of tumor ablation in 3, and followed infection in 1. Donor tissues included the latissimus dorsi muscle in 7 patients, radial forearm flap in 7, rectus abdominis muscle in 4, and scapular fasciocutaneous flap in 2.

> *Case 1.*—Boy, 3 years, experienced extensive tissue loss to the heel and posterior ankle plus a compound fracture of the calcaneus from a lawn mower injury. After débridement, he received a latissimus dorsi flap graft 4 days later, was discharged 8 days later, and at 36 months' follow-up had no growth impairment and was wearing regular footwear.
>
> Case 2.—Girl, 4 years, had the big toe amputated and metatarsal bone exposed in a lawn mower accident. After débridement, the metatarsal was covered with a free sensate radial forearm flap, followed by an end-to-end anastomosis of the venae comitantes to the saphenous vein. Anastomosis was repeated because of venous thrombosis unresponsive to repeated urokinase treatment and the flap survived. At 13 months recovery was uneventful.
>
> Case 3.—Boy, 14 years, had a synovial cell sarcoma removed from the dorsum of the left foot. After irradiation and chemotherapy, the tibialis anterior, extensor hallucis longus, and extensor digitorum longus tendons were removed and the defect was reconstructed with a composite radial forearm flap, harvested flexor carpi radialis, and palmaris longus. The patient was discharged 7 days after surgery and had normal function and contour.

Results.—After an average follow-up period of 31 months, these free flap transfers are surviving with no significant morbidity other than the venous thrombosis described. There has been no mortality. Hospitalization has averaged 13 days. An equinus deformity 3 years after heel reconstruction developed in 1 patient and a contour deformity developed in another patient with a gunshot wound to the foot. Growth was normal and functional losses at the donor sites were not significant in 16 of 17 patients with leg or foot injuries.

Conclusion.—Free tissue reconstruction is a safe and effective procedure in pediatric patients that yields satisfactory functional results with no abnormal growth problems at donor sites.

▶ This paper is a summary of 20 free tissue transfers in 19 pediatric patients. Clinical information, demographics, and success are well described. The paper provides excellent documentation that these procedures are as safe and effective in children as in adults. The conclusion from this and other clinical series is that the use of free flap transfers should not be withheld from patients based on age if their clinical conditions warrant such procedures.

W. Garner, M.D.

Microvascular Free-tissue Transfers in Elderly Patients: The Leeds Experience

Malata CM, Cooter RD, Batchelor AGG, et al (St James's Univ, Leeds, England)
Plast Reconstr Surg 98:1234–1241, 1996   6–24

Objective.—Many of the problems surrounding free-tissue transfer in the elderly depend upon the definition of the word elderly. Chronological age frequently bears little relationship to the aging process. Results of a study of the efficacy and safety of microvascular head and neck free-tissue transfers in an elderly population were presented.

Methods.—Between 1986 and 1991, 39 microvascular head and neck free-tissue transfers were performed in 33 patients (12 females), aged 70 to 83 years, at St. James's University Hospital, Leeds, England.

Results.—Most defects were the result of resected malignancies or excision of radionecrotic ulcers. Fourteen patients had coexisting medical conditions. Donor sites included the radial forearm in 20 patients, the rectus abdominus in 6, and the jejunum in 5. The average hospital stay was 17 days. There were 17 complications (Table 3). Three of 5 compromised flaps were salvaged for an overall failure rate of 5% and a success rate of 94.9%.

Conclusion.—Free-flap transfers are safe in the elderly. Age alone should not be used to exclude such patients.

▶ This article summarizes a 5-year experience with free flaps in a geriatric population. The majority of them (80%) were done for head and neck cancer reconstruction. In general, the results were similar to those achieved in a younger population, suggesting that, in suitable candidates, free-flap reconstruction should not be denied to the elderly.

W. Garner, M.D.

TABLE 3.—Postoperative Complications

Complication	Frequency
General	
Myocardial infarction	1
Chest infection	1
Pleural effusion	1
Minor bleeding from tracheostomy	1
Donor site	
Lymphangitis of forearm	1
Cellulitis of arm and forearm	1
Fractured radius	1
Recipient site	
Bleeding	5
Compromised flap viability	5

(Courtesy of Malata CM, Cooter RD, Batchelor AGG, et al: Microvascular free-tissue transfers in elderly patients: The Leeds experience. *Plast Reconstr Surg* 98:1234–1241, 1996.)

Free Latissimus Dorsi Muscle Transfer Using an Endoscopic Technique
Cho BC, Lee JH, Ramasastry SS, et al (Kyungpook Natl Univ, Taegu, Korea)
Ann Plast Surg 38:586–593, 1997   6–25

Purpose.—Plastic surgeons have applied endoscopic techniques to many different areas of aesthetic surgery, including face lifting, breast augmentation, abdominoplasty, and tissue expander placement. Endoscopy has also been used to harvest various types of donor tissue for free flap transfer, including omentum, jejunum, latissimus dorsi muscle, and rectus abdominis muscle. A technique of endoscopic-assisted latissimus dorsi free muscle transfer is reported.

Methods.—The endoscopic technique was used to harvest latissimus dorsi muscle in 10 patients with soft tissue defects of the lower extremity. The patients were 9 males and 1 female, age range 8 to 54 years.

Technique.—The procedure began with a 5 to 6 cm incision along the posterior axillary line, which permitted direct identification of the thoracodorsal vascular pedicle. Posterior dissection of the latissimus dorsi muscle was carried as far as possible, then continued under endoscopic visualization. This part of the procedure used both 90- and 30-degree angle, 10 mm diameter endoscopes, along with special endoscopic dissectors and extended electrocautery. Endoretractors with suction permitted simultaneous suction and retraction, providing excellent visualization. Dissection was completed above and below the muscle, and the muscle was divided from its lumbar and iliac attachments. This division was often difficult and time consuming. The muscle insertion was left uncut until the vascular pedicle was completely dissected. Microanastomosis was completed, and a meshed split-thickness skin graft was applied to the transferred muscle. The donor site was closed with fixation sutures and a suction drain.

Results.—The muscle harvested by this endoscopic technique ranged from 6 to 10 cm by 15 to 25 cm. The time needed for muscle harvest varied, with an average of 2 to 3 hours. Including the time needed for donor site closure, there was no difference in time required overall. There were no problems with hematoma or seroma at the donor site. To the patients' satisfaction, the donor site scar was short.

Conclusions.—An endoscopic technique of latissimus dorsi harvest for free flap transfer is reported. The endoscopic approach provides reliable and safe results, with smaller scars and reduced donor site morbidity. The endoscopic harvest technique may be especially useful in women, children, and patients who tend to hypertrophic scarring. Successful performance of this technique relies on surgical dexterity and experience, as well as proper instrumentation.

▶ This paper demonstrates the harvest of latissimus muscles through small incisions for use as a free flap. Overall, the harvest was safe and effective, although somewhat lengthy. This would likely decrease in time with experience. This paper suggests a useful expansion of the list of endoscopic procedures which should be considered.

W. Garner, M.D.

The Fate of Lower Extremities With Failed Free Flaps

Benacquista T, Kasabian AK, Karp NS (New York Univ; Montefiore Med Ctr, New York)
Plast Reconstr Surg 98:834–840, 1996   6–26

Introduction.—High amputation rates have been reported after loss of free-tissue transfers to the lower extremity, but little has been documented regarding the fate of lower extremities with failed free flaps. The immediate and long-term outcomes of patients with failed free flaps to the lower extremities was reviewed.

Methods.—Records of 413 free flaps that were transferred to the lower extremity from 1980 to 1992 were reviewed. Data from successful free flaps to the lower extremities were compared with data from failed free flaps. Long-term follow-up was accomplished through telephone inquiries, questionnaires, and physical examinations.

Results.—Of 413 free flaps transferred to the lower extremities over a period of 13 years, 41 flaps in 36 patients (10%) were considered failures (Table 4). Overall, patients with traumatic injuries had a failure rate of 11%, compared with a rate of 6.7% in patients with nontraumatic defects. The most common causes of flap failure were venous thrombosis (34%), infection (20%), and arterial thrombosis (12%). Previous attempts at wound closure had been made in over half the extremities with failed free flaps.

The amputation rate in patients with failed flaps was 22% (8 of 36 patients) within 2 months of failure, compared with amputation rates of 4.6% at 2 months and 6.9% at 2 years in patients with successful free flaps. The amputation rate after a failed free flap in patients with tibia-

TABLE 4.—Subsequent Salvage Procedures

	All Patients	Tib/Fib Fracture Patients
Amputation	8 (22%)	6 (35%)
Granulation	1	1
STSG	15	5
FTSG	1	0
Local flap	4	3
Distant pedicled flap	2	2
Free flap	7	2
Other	1	0

Abbreviations: Tib/Fib, tibia-fibula; *STSG,* split-thickness skin graft; *FTSG,* full-thickness skin graft.
(Courtesy of Benacquista T, Kasabian AK, Karp NS: The fate of lower extremities with failed free flaps. *Plast Reconstr Surg* 98:834–840, 1996.)

fibula fractures was 35% (6 of 17 patients). The mean number of procedures done to save the extremity in patients with failed flaps was 3.3. Twenty-four of 36 patients (67%) were available for long-term follow-up (mean, 6.2 years). Four of 24 patients underwent amputation after flap failure. Three of the 4 patients with flap failure died (2 patients had AIDS). Before death, all 3 patients were ambulating with a prosthesis. The fourth patient had bilateral amputations, had a psychiatric history, and was wheelchair-bound. All 20 patients with salvaged lower extremities were ambulating and none had undergone amputation at follow-up. Seven patients (35%) reported mild drainage or intermittent breakdown of their wounds. Eleven patients complained of decreased ankle motion.

Conclusion.—The majority of extremities can be salvaged after an initial free-flap loss. At long-term follow-up, most patients had not required subsequent amputation and were ambulating. Although many patients had wound problems, they preferred their salvaged extremities to an amputation.

▶ This paper makes a valuable contribution to our understanding of the role and natural history of lower extremity injury free-flap treatment. The paper describes a 10% failure rate of a large series (413 flaps) over a 13-year period. Both the causes of failure and the secondary reconstructive procedures are discussed. The paper provides well-thought-out rationale for the failure and is extremely useful and quite honest in discussing the clinical response to treatment. The low overall amputation rate supports the protocol for this reconstructive scheme in a majority of patients. The paper should be read by all practitioners who care for patients with lower extremity traumatic injuries and attempt to reconstruct the resulting defects.

W. Garner, M.D.

Single-stage Revascularization and Free Flap Coverage in the Treatment of Ischemic Lower Limb Lesions

Van Landuyt K, Vermassen F, Monstrey S, et al (Univ Hosp, Ghent, Belgium)
Eur J Plast Surg 19:245–252, 1996   6–27

Background.—Several reports have been published on combined revascularization and free tissue transfer in the treatment of ischemic gangrenous lesions of the lower limb. The authors presented their experience with this strategy, emphasizing the value of a 1-stage approach.

Patients and Outcomes.—Fifteen men and 5 women with end-stage peripheral vascular disease and gangrenous defects of the lower limb were treated with a revascularization procedure combined with a free tissue transfer for 3 years. Patient age ranged from 26 to 86 years. Two patients died perioperatively. One free flap was lost, necessitating replacement. Minor complications—such as partial loss of the skin graft, superficial wound dehiscences, and decubitus ulcers—were not uncommon, despite preventive measures. However, all surviving patients began ambulating early after surgery, usually starting at the third postoperative week.

Conclusion.—Gangrenous lesions of the lower limb have traditionally been treated in staged amputations. With a more aggressive strategy combining revascularization and free tissue transfer, the surgeon can limit the level of amputation, and patients can begin ambulation and rehabilitation early, with no need for major orthotic aid. Performing the vascular procedure, débridement, and free tissue transfer in 1 operation markedly decreases the number of procedures without substantially increasing operative time.

▶ This article summarizes an experience with simultaneous limb revascularization and free flap transfer to treat patients with lower extremity tissue loss caused by severe atherosclerotic disease. In 20 consecutive patients, there was only 1 failure. Two patients died perioperatively. The authors described their technique and perioperative management. This article describes the best-case scenario regarding treatment of these patients, and these results can be looked at as the goals for successful treatment of these severe problems. The 95% success rate suggests a high degree of selectivity of patients. In suitable patients, this combined approach is likely to be successful.

W. Garner, M.D.

What You See Is What You Get: Lack of Significant Postoperative Contour Change in Muscle Transplants to the Lower Leg
Isenberg JS (Univ of Oklahoma, Oklahoma City)
Ann Plast Surg 38:46–49, 1997

6–28

Background.—Muscle transplants are generally believed to undergo significant atrophy postoperatively, leading to progressive improvement in the appearance of the reconstruction. The contrasting view that such transplants retain most of their bulk after inset, undergoing minimal atrophy after surgery, was studied prospectively.

Methods.—Twenty patients undergoing muscle transplant reconstruction of Gustillo type IIIB lower limb wounds during a recent 4-month period were studied. They were 17 men and 3 women aged 20–78 years. Reconstruction was done primarily with the rectus abdominis transplant. All patients had bony fixation through an external frame (Table 2).

Findings.—Intraoperative and postoperative limb transplant circumference measurements were surprisingly consistent in all patients. At 6 months after surgery, the maximum transplant projection had decreased minimally.

Conclusions.—This prospective study showed minimal reductions in limb circumference at the 6-month follow-up in patients undergoing muscle transplant reconstruction of Gustillo type IIIB lower limb wounds. In fact, any contour prominence present during surgery persists after surgery.

▶ This article provides a valuable message for the surgeon using free transfer of muscle for reconstructive purposes: to get the contour right in

TABLE 2.—Limb Transplant Maximum Circumference

Patient No.	Intraoperative (cm)	Six Months Postoperative (cm)
1	33.3	32.8
2	41.4	39.9
3	42.2	41.3
4	35.6	33.8
5	28.5	27.4
6	27.2	26.6
7	36.8	35.7
8	43.1	42.3
9	40.3	39.5
10	47.3	45.6
11	23.9	21.9
12	33.6	32.4
13	45.3	43.2
14	37.8	36.5
15	39.8	38.0
16	25.6	24.1
17	44.4	43.2
18	29.1	27.9
19	36.3	35.2
20	32.6	30.8

(Reprinted from Isenberg JS: What you see is what you get: Lack of significant postoperative contour change in muscle transplants to the lower leg. *Ann Plast Surg* 38:46–49, 1997 by permission of Little, Brown and Company, Inc.)

the final result, get it right in the operating room. Of course, in many traumatic situations, the final aesthetic appearance is far from the most important consideration when trying to salvage a badly damaged limb. But the lesson is still useful, and certainly applicable in other more elective reconstructive cases.

R.L. Ruberg, M.D.

Leg Morbidity and Function Following Fibular Free Flap Harvest

Shpitzer T, Neligan P, Boyd B, et al (Toronto Hosp; Univ of Toronto)
Ann Plast Surg 38:460–464, 1997   6–29

Objective.—The vascularized fibula is the preferred donor site for reconstruction of major segmental mandibular defects. Although this method provides many advantages, donor site morbidity can result. Results of a study that examined the early postoperative donor site morbidity associated with removal of the fibular free flap and that determined the presence of any long-term deficits of donor leg function are presented.

Methods.—Fifty consecutive free fibular flap mandibular reconstructions were performed in 47 patients during a 3-year period for a variety of reasons (Table 1). Bone segments removed averaged 8.3 cm. Skin paddles were also removed in 38 patients. In 31 patients, skin graft closure of the donor site was required. All patients were given physical therapy. Patients were followed up for an average of 17 months. Leg function was deter-

TABLE 1.—Causes of Mandibular Reconstruction With Free Fibular Flap

Etiology	No. of Patients
Neoplasia	30
Osteoradionecrosis	8
Fracture of a reconstruction plate	4
Osteomyelitis	2
Self-inflicted gunshot wound	2
Failed plate reconstruction (exposed plate)	1
Total	47

(Reprinted from Shpitzer T, Neligan P, Boyd B, et al: Leg morbidity and function following fibular free flap harvest. *Annals of Plastic Surg* 38:460–464, 1997 by permission of Little, Brown and Company, Inc.)

mined by physical examination and by asking patients to complete a questionnaire.

Results.—Four flaps failed. One of 3 patients who underwent another free vascularized contralateral fibular transfer, experienced flap failure a second time. Infection developed in 1 noncompliant patient shortly after surgery, and the patient required a second skin graft. Patients were able to ambulate and were pain free by week 5. Complications were mild and included weakness of the big toe ($n = 5$), stiffness and instability of the joint ($n = 1$), ankle instability ($n = 2$), donor site pain ($n = 1$), and mild edema ($n = 1$). On examination, 5 patients had restricted range of motion of the ankle joint: 5 had restricted range of plantar flexion of the big toe and, of these, 2 also had dorsiflexion restriction; and 4 had motor weakness of the ankle.

Conclusion.—There is minimal short-term and long-term leg morbidity and loss of function after fibular free flap harvest. Patients' reported symptoms were generally described as mild.

▶ This article provides useful information, documenting the minimal morbidity from fibular harvest. Even if a skin graft is needed to close the donor site, the results are still quite good.

R.L. Ruberg, M.D.

Free Tissue Transfer in Treatment of the Recalcitrant Chronic Venous Ulcer

Weinzweig N, Schuler J (Univ of Illinois, Chicago; Cook County Hosp, Chicago)
Ann Plast Surg 38:611–619, 1997   6–30

Introduction.—Recalcitrant venous stasis ulceration is often refractory to conservative management and skin grafting. It is suggested that long-term cure for these ulcers must involve a dual surgical approach that addresses both the tissue-related and hemodynamic components. Reported are outcomes of 20 consecutive muscle free flaps in 18 patients with 19 recalcitrant chronic venous ulcers.

Methods.—The surgical approach included wide excision of the ulcer and surrounding liposclerotic tissue bed and replacement of a free flap with multiple, competent microvenous valves and normal microcirculation. Patients had nontraumatic, nonosteomyelitic venous ulcers present for an average of 3.5 years and had failed conservative therapy and an average of 2.4 skin grafts.

Results.—Free tissue transfers were successfully performed in 18 of 20 flaps. The 2 failures were secondary to intractable vasospasm. One patient underwent a successful repeat muscle free flap. The mean defect after excision of the ulcer and surrounding lipodermatosclerotic skin was 238 cm². Free flap donor tissues were: 13 rectus abdominis, 5 latissimus dorsi, 1 gracilis, and 1 serratus muscles. Recipient vessels were: 12 posterior tibial, 6 anterior tibial, and 2 peroneal. Only one vein (usually one of the venae comitantes) was anastomosed in end-to-end fashion in all except 1 patient. Important complications were: 3 infection with partial flap and/or skin graft loss, 2 partial skin graft loss, and 1 minor abdominal wound dehiscence. There were no recurrences within flaps, but 1 patient had breakdown at the junction between the flap and the residual adjacent liposclerotic skin. Three patients were lost to follow-up. Follow-up was an average of 32.7 months.

Conclusion.—Patients with recalcitrant chronic venous ulcer can have long-term cure when the diseased tissue bed is replaced with healthy tissue containing competent microvenous valves and a normal microcirculation. This can be performed in 1 reconstructive procedure.

▶ Sporadic reports of free flap coverage of chronic venous ulcers have surfaced. Originally, I was skeptical. Increasingly, we have used free flaps in carefully selected sub-populations with comparable results. Our series is not nearly as large, but this certainly is an option.

D.J. Smith, Jr., M.D.

Vascularized Toe Joint Transfer to the Hand

Chen SH-T, Wei F-C, Chen H-C, et al (Chang Gung Mem Hosp, Taipei, Taiwan; Stanford Univ, Palo Alto, Calif)
Plast Reconstr Surg 98:1275–1284, 1996   6–31

Background.—Treating injured metacarpophalangeal and proximal interphalangeal joints, especially in young persons, has long been difficult. The outcomes of vascularized toe joint transfer to the hand in one large series were reported.

Methods.—Thirty-three patients underwent 36 vascularized toe joint transfers between 1984 and 1993. The current analysis did not include the results of 3 toe joint transfers to elbow and temporomandibular joints or 4 transfers of toe joints to hands in patients lost to follow-up. Twenty-seven patients with 29 vascularized toe joint transfers comprised the final study. The patients were 21 males and 6 females. One procedure was done for congenital deformity and the rest for posttraumatic reconstruction. Mean follow-up was 32.4 months.

Findings.—The average range of motion in toe metatarsophalangeal joint to hand metacarpophalangeal joint transfers was 34 degrees; in toe proximal interphalangeal joint to hand metacarpophalangeal joint transfers, 32 degrees; and in toe proximal interphalangeal joint to hand proximal interphalangeal joint transfers, 24 degrees. Patients had to have well-functioning muscle and associated tendons effecting joint motion to achieve a greater-than-average range of motion. The outcomes of 2 immediate free vascularized toe joint transfers to complex injuries involving loss of the metacarpophalangeal joint were good.

Conclusions.—The use of toe joint transfer is encouraged in the treatment of selected complex hand injuries. However, achieving normal range of motion in the joint of the reconstructed digit is still a major challenge.

▶ I have watched with interest since the initial reports of toe joint transfer. Isolated cases have been reported with variable success. Some authors are encouraging while others are not sure of the benefit. This article presents a large series and outlines a number of the important modifications to allow for successful use of vascular toe joint transfer. I enjoyed reading the modifications that they use and will incorporate them into my own practice.

D.J. Smith, Jr., M.D.

Aesthetic Refinements in Toe-to-Hand Transfer Surgery
Wei F-C, Chen H-C, Chuang DC-C, et al (Chang Gung Med College, Taipei, Taiwan)
Plast Reconstr Surg 98:485–490, 1996   6–32

Objective.—Toe-to-hand transfer has become a widely used technique for reconstruction of the thumb and fingers. Techniques to improve the cosmetic appearance of the thumb are a key part of the success of such procedures; cosmesis of the donor foot is a consideration as well. Techniques for improving the cosmetic results of toe-to-hand transfer surgery were reviewed.

Thumb and Finger Reconstruction.—Cosmetic procedures are needed because the toes do not accurately duplicate the appearance of the thumb or finger. The cosmetic appearance of the reconstructed thumb can be improved by surgical reduction of the soft tissue, bone, interphalangeal joint, and nail and by secondary pulp reduction and contouring procedures. To reduce anteroposterior bulkiness in the reconstructions using the lesser toes, minimal adipofibrous tissue should be included under the plantar skin flap, particularly in the area of the metatarsophalangeal joint. Transferred lesser toes can develop an unsightly claw or drumstick appearance. This can be avoided by performing the repair in tight extension and temporary K-pin fixation of the proximal and distal interphalangeal joint in extension, followed by long-term use of an extension splint at night. Several different measures can help to smooth the transition between the amputated digit and the reconstructed toe, including adequate soft-tissue coverage, cruciate skin incisions, extensive mobilization, and thinning and trimming of the skin flaps of the amputation stump. When the distal digit is being reconstructed, primary closure may be enhanced by skeletonizing the medial and lateral neurovascular bundles of the harvested toe. This prevents problems related to the skin graft on the sides of the new digit.

Donor Foot.—Other procedures are available for improving the appearance of the donor foot. The span of the foot can be preserved by salvaging the last 0.5–1.0 cm of the proximal phalangeal stump of the great toe. In patients undergoing transfer of 1 of the lesser toes or the second and third toes together, an optimal web space should be reconstructed, rather than preserving the proximal phalanx. The donor foot should be closed primarily, without skin grafting.

Discussion.—The most important goal in toe-to-hand transfer surgery is the objective function of the reconstructed digit. However, the better the appearance of the reconstructed hand, the better the patient will accept and use it. The aesthetic refinements discussed in this article lead to high levels of patient satisfaction.

▶ This article is long overdue. A number of authors have talked about individual refinements. This article discusses the overall aesthetic approach to toe-to-hand transfer. Clearly, we have come a long way from the time when successful transfer meant the revascularization of the toe. We now need to concentrate on attaining the highest quality functional and aesthetic result possible.

D.J. Smith, Jr., M.D.

Radial Forearm Flap Donor-site Complications and Morbidity: A Prospective Study

Richardson D, Fisher SE, Vaughan ED, et al (Walton Hosp, Liverpool, England)
Plast Reconstr Surg 99:109–115, 1997   6–33

Introduction.—The radial forearm flap gives good results in the reconstruction of orofacial defects. The few studies of donor-site morbidity associated with this flap have been retrospective in nature. The donor-site complications and morbidity associated with the radial forearm flap were studied prospectively.

Methods.—The study included 100 patients with orofacial defects who were undergoing reconstructive surgery using a radial forearm flap. A standard technique was used in raising the flaps and closing the donor sites. The patients were systematically assessed before, during, and after surgery.

Results.—Follow-up included 86 patients at 3 months and 74 at 1 year; forty-nine of the latter patients had fasciocutaneous flaps and 25 had composite flaps. Sixteen percent of the patients had partial loss of the donor site skin graft, with tendon exposure occurring in 13%. Twenty-two percent had delayed healing of the split-thickness skin graft at the donor site. Seventeen percent of patients with composite flaps had radial fracture. Thirty-two percent of patients had reduced superficial radial nerve sensation, 14% had cold intolerance, and 28% reported poor aesthetic results. Restricted function of the donor arm was noted in 16% of patients with fasciocutaneous flaps and 36% of those with composite flaps, including all of those with radial fracture. The patients with restricted function all had reduced forearm circumference, grip strength, pinch strength, and wrist movement, compared to patients with normal function.

Conclusions.—This prospective study finds a low rate of long-term donor site morbidity in patients undergoing reconstructive surgery with fasciocutaneous radial forearm flaps. The good results and low morbidity achieved with this flap make it the flap of choice for intraoral reconstruction and other indications. Morbidity is higher with composite flaps, particularly if radial fracture occurs.

▶ This paper should be regarded as the "definitive" study of donor-site complications of radial artery forearm flap. Previous studies showed somewhat similar results, but were done retrospectively. This is a prospective study. The findings should be used in preoperative discussions with patients for whom this procedure is being considered, especially if there are other options.

R.L. Ruberg, M.D.

Results of Functioning Free Muscle Transplantation for Elbow Flexion

Chuang DC-C, Carver N, Wei F-C (Chang Gung Med College, Taipei, Taiwan)
J Hand Surg [Am] 21A:1071–1077, 1996   6–34

Introduction.—Functioning free muscle transfer (FFMT) may be used for muscle reconstruction when no musculotendinous donor units are available locally. Patients with brachial plexus injury need reconstruction of elbow flexion. There have been few reports of the use of FFMT for this purpose. A 6-year experience with FFMT for restoration of elbow flexion, using various nerves for reinnervation was evaluated.

Methods.—The experience included 38 patients undergoing FFMT for reconstruction of elbow flexion, most because of brachial plexus injury in motorcycle accidents. Thirty-two patients had been paralyzed for more than 1 year, and 26 had not been operated on previously. The gracilis muscle was transferred in 34 patients and the rectus femoris in 4. Reinnervation was accomplished using the musculocutaneous nerve in 3 patients (who had traumatic biceps loss) (group 1), the intercostal nerves in 31 patients (group 2), and the spinal accessory nerve in 4 patients (group

3). The Medical Research Council grading system was used to evaluate the results. Muscle strength of M4 was considered a successful result.

Results.—All 3 patients in group 1 had successful results within 1 year. In group 2, the success rate was 78% when 3 intercostal nerves were transferred. Complete rehabilitation took an average of 2 years. When 2 intercostal nerves were used, rehabilitation took 3 years, and the final muscle strength and range of motion were not as good. Muscle strength was no better than M2–M3 for the 4 patients in group 3, even after 3 years of rehabilitation.

Conclusion.—For patients with traumatic biceps loss, a nerve-reinnervated FFMT provides better results than regional latissimus dorsi transfer. When the intercostal nerves are used for reconstruction after brachial plexus injury, it is best to use 3 nerves for reinnervation. The results are not as good when the spinal accessory nerve is used, probably because of the need for interposition grafts.

▶ I used to be somewhat skeptical and pessimistic about the return of function of the elbow. My major experience was with latissimus transfer, and I was not overly impressed with the results. Free-flap transfer clearly is superior and is the preferred method of transfer. This article has changed both my approach to restoration of elbow flexion as well as my approach to patients with this problem.

D.J. Smith, Jr, M.D.

The Tensor Fascia Lata Free Flap in Abdominal-wall Reconstruction
Williams JK, Carlson GW, Howell RL, et al (Emory Univ, Atlanta, Ga; Indiana Univ, Indianapolis)
J Reconstr Microsurg 13:83–90, 1997   6–35

Background.—When possible, the pedicled tensor fascial latal (TFL) flap is preferred for use in reconstruction of the abdominal wall. However, the size and location of the abdominal defect sometimes preclude use of the TFL flap. In this situation, microsurgical tissue transfer may provide greater reconstructive freedom. Use of the TFL flap as a free flap for reconstruction of full-thickness defects of the abdominal wall is reported.

Experience.—The retrospective study included 7 patients who had full-thickness abdominal wall defects reconstructed with TFL free flaps (Table 1). The wounds ranged in size from 208 to 375 cm^2; and most were infected or contaminated. Eighty-six percent of the wounds involved the epigastrum. The TFL free flap had several key advantages, starting with elimination of the arc of rotation. This allowed the flap to be horizontally situated with the fascia placed in the position of greatest tensile strength. There was also less need for undermining than with a pedicled flap. The ability to use a single flap precluded the need for multiple donor sites. There was a 30% rate of donor site complications, including dehiscence of the native skin after skin grafting. No cases of total flap loss occurred.

TABLE 1.—Characteristics of the Abdominal Wall Defects

Patient (Age)	Infection/ Contamination	Size (cm^2)	Location (Per Umbilicus)	Underlying Disorder (Initial Operation)
1 (59 yrs)	No	15 × 15	Infra	Leiomyosarcoma of the jejunum
2 (47 yrs)	No	20 × 22	Infra/supra	Adenocarcinoma of the colon
3 (49 yrs)	No	13 × 16	Supra	CABG/sternal dehiscence
4 (27 yrs)	Yes	24 × 12	Infra/supra	Crohn's disease
5 (44 yrs)	Yes	20 × 12	Supra	Gastroesophageal reflux/ Nissen fundoplication
6 (53 yrs)	Yes	?	Infra/supra	Perforated ulcer of duodenum
7 (35 yrs)	Yes	15 × 25	Infra/supra	Multiple abdominal stab wounds

Abbreviation: CABG, coronary artery bypass grafting.
(Reprinted with permission from *Journal of Reconstructive Microsurgery*, Williams JK, Carlson GW, Howell RL, et al: The tensor fascia lata free flap in abdominal-wall reconstruction. *J Reconstr Microsurg* 13:83–90, 1997, Thieme Medical Publishers, Inc.)

Conclusions.—For patients with full-thickness defects of the abdominal wall, the TFL free flap is an attractive reconstructive option. Its use is not hindered by a limited arc of rotation, and it results in increased vascularity of the distal part of the flap. Microsurgical transfer of the TFL free flap is a particularly useful option for large defects or those located over the umbilicus.

▶ Defects of the abdominal wall present a challenging problem in many cases. When the defect is truly full thickness (i.e., none of the components of the abdominal wall can be closed), the TFL can provide durable complete coverage. Because of limitations in the arc of rotation, the TFL as a free flap makes good sense for the middle or upper parts of the abdomen. When the fascia defect is large but the skin can be mobilized for complete closure, I have used a free graft of the fascia lata as an autogenous tissue patch. This is especially useful in cases in which synthetic material has failed or is contraindicated—and of course is much easier to do than the TFL as a free flap.

R.L. Ruberg, M.D.

Cigarette Smoking, Plastic Surgery, and Microsurgery

Chang LD, Buncke G, Slezak S, et al (Johns Hopkins Univ, Baltimore, Md; Univ of Maryland, Baltimore; Univ of California-San Francisco)
J Reconstr Microsurg 12:467–474, 1996   6–36

Objective.—The by-products in cigarette smoke have a thrombogenic effect that inhibits capillary blood flow, increases endothelial permeability, stimulates the action of thromboxane A_2, and inhibits the production and release of prostacyclin. Smoking has a deleterious effect on many plastic surgery procedures.

Facelifts and Cigarette Smoking.—Cigarette smoking is suspected as a cause of retro-auricular flap necrosis by exacerbating tissue ischemia. After facelift surgery, cigarette smokers had a 7.5% chance of a skin slough compared with 2.7% for non-smokers.

The Aging Face and Cigarette Smoking.—Cigarette smokers are 4 times as likely to have premature skin wrinkling, possibly as a result of structural changes in collagen or toxic effects to the skin microvasculature. The risk increases with sun exposure.

Abdominoplasty and Cigarette Smoking.—Reports indicate that the abdominal flap loss in smokers is similar to that of the facelift.

Breast Reconstruction and Cigarette Smoking.—Cigarette smoking significantly increases the risk of epidermolysis in modified radical mastectomy compared with non-smokers (49% versus 14%). During breast reconstruction, the implant loss rate was 33% in cigarette smokers, 14% in non-smokers, and 10% in those who stopped smoking before surgery. Smoking was a cause of non-flap skin loss when autogenous TRAM flap breast reconstruction was used.

Free-Tissue Transfer and Cigarette Smoking.—Whereas cigarette smoking did not appear to affect the success of free-tissue transfers. However, there were significantly more wound problems with skin closures and donor sites in patients who smoked than with donors who did not smoke (17.5% vs. 10%).

Digital Replantation and Cigarette Smoking.—Studies in healthy males have demonstrated a significantly decreased temperature and blood flow to the extremities after cigarette smoking.

Experimental Evidence Linking Cigarette Smoking and Impaired Surgical Healing.—Rats exposed to cigarette smoke had a decreased skin flap survival rate. Cessation of smoke exposure 7 to 14 days before surgery improved the survival of cranially based dorsal flaps in rats. Nicotine injections significantly decreased skin flap survival in animals. Femoral arterial anastomotic patency rates in rats were not affected by cigarette smoke.

Wound Healing and Cigarette Smoking.—Nicotine impairs wound healing in rabbits, increases scar formation in smokers undergoing laparotomies, and increases the incidence of skin necrosis in smokers with cutaneous flaps or full-thickness skin grafts.

Conclusions.—Cigarette smoking is related to decreased survival of cutaneous flaps and digital replantations. Smokers also experience increased wound complications.

▶ This appropriately titled "Clinical Review" summarizes the body of information known about the effects of cigarette smoking on circulatory status in plastic surgery and microsurgery procedures. It is well organized and concise. Appropriate references are provided. It serves as a useful state of the art for practitioners of these procedures. The clinical data from a large series are summarized, and some experimental data are presented when available. Although no new information is presented, this review is an excellent summary of information from a wide variety of sources and will be quite useful to most practitioners.

W. Garner, M.D.

Tissue Expansion

Risk Factors for Complications in Pediatric Tissue Expansion

Friedman RM, Ingram AE Jr, Rohrich RJ, et al (Univ of Texas, Dallas)
Plast Reconstr Surg 98:1242–1246, 1996   6–37

Introduction.—In pediatric plastic surgery, the technique of tissue expansion has found a wide range of applications. At a nominal donor-site cost, tissue expansion provides local tissue of appropriate thickness, texture, color, and sensibility; however, the complication rate can be as high as 40%. To identify risk factors for complications, children who had tissue expansion performed were examined retrospectively.

Methods.—In 82 patients who had a variety of operative indications and anatomical sites, 188 expanders were placed. A review was conducted of their operative reports, medical records, and photographs. The average postoperative follow-up was 15.5 months. The complications were reviewed using the Fisher's exact test.

Results.—In 9% of patients, major and minor complications occurred. Burns and soft-tissue loss, age younger than 7 years, history of 2 or more expansions, and use of internal expander ports were the factors associated with a statistically significant increase in complications. Within the first 90 days, complications were more likely to occur than during any other expansion. Patient gender, wound drainage upon expander insertion or removal, use of customized expanders, operating surgeon, or intra-operative use of antibiotic irrigations were factors that did not influence complication rate.

Conclusion.—If the operative indication does not require prompt surgical attention, delay tissue expansion in children younger than 7 years. Internal expander ports should be avoided in those younger than 7 years. To prevent port displacement, remote expander ports must be positioned and secured carefully. Tissue should be harvested with 1 or 2 expansions. When necessary, expanders can be inflated over an extended period of time. Antibiotic irrigation or wound drainage should not be used routinely.

▶ This article underscores the fact that tissue expansion is not benign and has a significant incidence of complications. The warnings at the end of the article are useful.

R.E. Salisbury, M.D.

Continuous Expansion for the Treatment of Skin Deformities

Nunes PHF, Vargas VEB, Guidi MC, et al (São Paulo, Brazil)
Aesthetic Plast Surg 20:347–349, 1996   6–38

Objective.—Tissue expansion to provide skin for treatment of deformities usually requires insufflation every 3 to 7 days and takes 6 to 12 weeks.

TABLE 1.—Volume Requirements

Patient	Age (years)	Diagnosis	Location	Volume (ml) Expanded	Infused	Expansion time (days)	Reexpansion
1. V.M.	25	Nevus	Right thigh	400 ml	380 ml	10	No
2. E.C.	23	Burn sequela	Scalp	400 ml	350 ml	11	No
3. K.C.	06	Burn sequela	Scalp	400 ml	360 ml	08	Yes
4. E.A.	16	Scar	Neck	400 ml	410 ml	10	Yes
5. R.M.	10	Scar	Right shoulder	400 ml	385 ml	08	No
			Left shoulder	400 ml	360 ml	08	No
6. X.D.	30	Congenital nevus	Back	700 ml	550 ml	09	No
7. R.S.	19	Scar	Chest	600 ml	400 ml	09	No

(Courtesy of Nunes PHF, Vargas VEB, Guidi MC, et al: Continuous expansion for the treatment of skin deformities. *Aesth Plast Surg* 20:347–349, 1996.)

Continuous expansion using an infusion pump, a faster, safer, and more comfortable way of expansion, was reviewed.

Methods.—Between January 1993 and February 1994, expanders were placed in 7 outpatients and after 5 to 7 days, expanded with the aid of an infusion pump set at 1–3 mL/hr of 0.9% saline. Expansion volume varied with the area to be covered (Table 1).

Results.—Expansion time varied between 8 and 11 days, making the entire process 13 to 18 days in duration. There were no complications that caused the process to be discontinued. Pain was treated with analgesics or reduced expansion speed. The thickness of the fibrotic capsule developing around the expander was less than that usually observed with conventional expansion.

Conclusions.—Tissue expansion using an infusion pump is a safe, feasible, and rapid method that is sometimes safer than the conventional expansion method, particularly when the lower limbs are involved. Costs are higher because the process has to be done in a hospital, but outpatient treatment is feasible.

▶ This idea has some merit. I do not think I would use this on a routine basis. Because the patient must remain "hooked up" to an infusion pump throughout the course of expansion, the patient is essentially "disabled" from the start of treatment until completion. When I do conventional tissue expansion, the patients are functional throughout the course of treatment in most cases. I would consider using this approach in a patient who is incapacitated or already hospitalized—for example, because of head injury or respiratory problems after trauma. If I needed tissue for coverage of an open wound, rapid continuous tissue expansion might be included among my surgical options.

R.L. Ruberg, M.D.

External Device for Tissue Expansion: Clinical Evaluation of the Skin Extender
Fan J, Eriksson M, Nordström REA (Univ Hosp, Tromsø, Norway)
Scand J Plast Reconstr Hand Surg 30:215–220, 1996   6–39

Introduction.—Traditional tissue expansion has the disadvantages of: multiple outpatient visits for the filling of the implant, lengthy time to final result, and temporary cosmetic disfigurement. A skin extender device, developed by Blomqvist and Steenfos in Sweden, was evaluated on 10 extremity lesions in 9 adult patients.

Methods.—Defects were: 3 meshed split-thickness skin grafts, 4 scars, 1 nevus, and 2 open wounds. The skin extender is made of 2 silicone or plastic tubes with a bundle of plastic bands placed between them. Using local anesthesia, bands were placed through small incisions on each side of the defect with 2–3 cm intervals between them. The tubes were attached to both ends of each band and tension was applied by the patient by pulling the plastic bands locked by one-way lockers.

Results.—All defects were able to be excised within 3–14 days, except for 1 infected wound in which the plastic bands cut through the skin bridges at the beginning of the extension procedure. Cosmetically disturbing scars resulted from holes in the skin because of the plastic bands.

Conclusion.—The skin extender developed by Blomqvist and Steenfos was able to be applied to open and slightly infected wounds, defects, scars, benign skin tumors, and, in some places where tissue expansion is not possible. This technique is simple, cheap, takes a short time to achieve a result, and has no influence on underlying structures. Disadvantages are the secondary scars caused by the plastic bands and the fact that its use is limited to advancement flaps.

▶ The major concern regarding these devices is whether the width of the final scar and the scarring that occurs secondary to the use of the device will produce a desirable outcome.

S.H. Miller, M.D.

7 General

Wound Healing and Scars

Grafting on Nude Mice of Living Skin Equivalents Produced Using Human Collagens

López Valle CAL, Germain L, Rouabhia M, et al (Saint Sacrement Hosp, Quebec; Laval Univ, Sainte Foy, Quebec)
Transplantation 62:317–323, 1996   7–1

Background.—Although cultured epithelial autografts are available for permanent burn wound coverage, epithelial sheets lack some of the inherent qualities of dermis in vivo. Adding a dermal component would provide some of these properties, thus reducing delays in dermal organization, limiting scar tissue formation steps, and accelerating in situ skin regeneration. It may be possible to produce a clinically useful skin equivalent (SE) by isolating autologous living epidermal cells and dermal fibroblasts from a skin biopsy specimen, amplifying these cells, and seeding them in SE for growth in batches. The results of in vivo transplantation with an SE prepared with human and bovine collagen were evaluated.

Methods and Results.—Transplants were placed in athymic nude mice. Both human and bovine SE showed good adhesion onto the graft bed within the first week after transplantation. By 2 weeks, the graft take rate was 100%, with a well-organized stratum corneum that thickened progressively. The cuboidal morphology of basal cells was maintained in human SE grafts with and without additional dermal matrix components. Indirect immunofluorescence staining confirmed that the grafts were of human origin, and the 2 types of human SE grafts contained equal amounts of human type I collagen. Contraction over time was less with the human SE grafts than with the bovine SE grafts.

Conclusions.—Permanent transplantation of bioengineered SE may soon be an option for burn wound coverage. These experiments suggest that human epidermal cells seeded in SE undergo normal differentiation in situ and then retain their in vivo functional capacities after transplantation. Graft take and histologic evolution is better with anchored SE than with cultured epidermal sheets. A sequential approach to SE transplantation for use in patients with extensive burns is being investigated.

▶ Studies of SEs continue to multiply and the work should be encouraged. The concept has been shown to be sound in the subpopulation of patients with lethal burn injuries, and eventually the techniques that are also cost-effective and affordable will be evident.

R.E. Salisbury, M.D.

From Wound to Scar
Linares HA (Univ of Texas, Galveston)
Burns 22:339–352, 1996

7–2

Introduction.—The complex process of cutaneous wound repair is not fully understood. Various aspects of the biochemical, cellular, and molecular factors involved in the healing of a cutaneous wound are examined, from the immediate first response of the hemostatic process through problems of hypertrophic healing.

The Hemostatic Process.—This process involves blood vessels, platelets, and blood coagulation. The sequence of events in the hemostatic process can be divided into 4 steps: the contact phase, general activation (involving factors IX and X), stabilization, and remodelation. Platelets have a central role in primary hemostasis and trigger the healing process by releasing various local and circulating biological factors. Also involved in the process are polymorphonuclear leukocytes, lymphocytes, mast cells, and macrophages.

The Provisional Matrix/Granulation Tissue/Fibroplasia.—The blood clot is remodeled into a matrix within 48 hours, and this newly constructed matrix within the wound site serves both a structural and a regulatory function for subsequent cell migration. Granulation tissue, the framework for the repair process, provides provisional support for the resurfacing epithelium. Early granulation tissue exhibits collagen fibers that run parallel to the neovessels; with maturity, the newly formed collagen fibers tend to be oriented perpendicular to the vessels. Fibroblast proliferation and extracellular matrix production mark the advance of fibroplasia.

Angiogenesis/The Extracellular Matrix.—Degradation of the basement membrane is the first step toward angiogenesis. The extracellular matrix, which provides tissues with structural support and modulates important processes, has 5 major components: collagen, basement membranes, structural glycoproteins, elastic fibers, and proteoglycans.

Contraction/Re-epithelialization/Beginning of the Permanent Scar.—Within 1 week after injury, the active physiologic process of contraction appears, the forces of which may be produced by fibroblasts and myofibroblasts. Re-epithelialization occurs when epithelial cells initiate a series of mechanisms to cover the new surface. Adequate humidity enhances the advance of epithelial cells. The building up of granulation tissue stops when the migrating epithelia complete the resurfacing of the new connective tissue matrix. The granulation tissue becomes a true scar tissue that matures gradually during a period of at least 6 months.

Potential Solutions for Wound Healing Interferences.—Development of fibrosis may be impeded by blocking the effects of some cytokines. Research has also been conducted on influencing fibroblasts and the extracellular matrix. Growth factors are under investigation as a tool for altering wound healing, and studies of fetal wounds may improve understanding of the normal and abnormal process of adult wound healing.

Conclusions.—The final results of the process of cutaneous wound repair may be normal or abnormal scarring such as hypertrophic, hypotrophic, or atrophic healing. Future studies should investigate why, when, and how an imbalance occurs in the process of healing, which depends upon an adequate balance between the components of a complex biomolecular network.

▶ This is a good comprehensive survey of wound healing with a superb bibliography from someone who has a long and honored interest in human scarring.

R.E. Salisbury, M.D.

Pulsed Electromagnetic Fields in Experimental Cutaneous Wound Healing in Rats

Patiño O, Grana D, Bolgiani A, et al (Universidad del Salvador; Fundación del Quemado, Buenos Aires, Argentina)
J Burn Care Rehabil 17:528–531, 1996   7–3

Introduction.—For the treatment of nonunion bony repair, cutaneous ulcers, musculoskeletal pain, and wound healing, new therapeutic approaches through the application of electrical stimuli are currently being developed. Low-frequency pulsed electromagnetic fields have been used to treat human nonunion fractures. Discrepancies have been shown regarding the effectiveness of electromagnetic fields in skin wound healing. The influence of low-frequency electromagnetic fields on experimental cutaneous wounds in rats was examined.

Methods.—A circular lesion 3 cm in diameter and involving the skin up to the superficial fascia was made in the backs of 22 male Wistar rats. The control group of 8 rats underwent sham treatment; 7 rats were treated with topical nitrofurazone solution, and 7 were treated with pulsed electromagnetic fields of 20 mT. The treatments were 35 minutes twice a day. On days, 0, 7, 14, and 21, planimetry of wounds was performed.

Results.—Significantly lower values were seen in the absolute and relative values of the area and perimeter of the wounds at days 7, 14, and 21 in the pulsed electromagnetic field group than in the control group. Compared with the nitrofurazone solution group, the pulsed electromagnetic field group had significantly lower values only at day 21.

Conclusion.—In rats treated with pulsed electromagnetic fields, a significant beneficial stimulation in the wound healing process was seen. This could lead to the development of a practical tool for clinical and research use. Probably as a result of an increase in the endogenous current induced by the wound, electrical stimulation of the skin accelerates wound healing. To determine the optimal dosage to soft-tissue healing, further studies are required.

▶ This experimentation has been carried out for the past 50 years, and there is increased interest in pulsed electromagnetic fields in orthopedics. It is difficult to understand why their use in soft-tissue wound healing has not been further investigated. One hopes for subsequent studies in which the efficacy of pulsed electromagnetic fields is tested for a longer time (not just 1 hour) and furthermore a directional field issued.

R.E. Salisbury, M.D.

Hyaluronic Acid of Wound Fluid in Adult and Fetal Rabbits

Sawai T, Usui N, Sando K, et al (Osaka Univ, Japan; Aichi Med Univ, Japan)
J Pediatr Surg 32:41–43, 1997   7–4

Objective.—Fetal wounds heal without scar formation and with decreased collagen deposition. Analysis of the fetal extracellular matrix demonstrates a high hyaluronic acid (HA) content. A new biotin HA-link protein assay was used to quantitate the HA content of healing fetal and adult wounds.

Methods.—Wound healing was studied in 118 rabbit fetuses of 24 days' gestation and in 44 nonpregnant adult rabbits. A polyvinyl alcohol sponge implant was placed pervertebrally in subcutaneous tissue of fetuses and paravertebrally in nonpregnant adult rabbits. Implants were removed on days 1, 2, 3, 4, 5, and 7. Wound fluid was extracted, and HA levels were determined using a high-affinity biotin HA-link protein assay. Data were analyzed by analysis of variance.

Results.—The concentration of HA in fetal wound fluid from the 47 fetal implants that survived was significantly increased on day 3 compared with other days, and significantly decreased on day 1 compared with days 3 and 4. On all days, HA deposition was significantly higher in fetal wounds than in adult wounds.

Conclusion.—The fetal wound matrix has a significantly higher HA content than adult wound matrices, demonstrating that the mechanism of wound healing in the fetus is different from the mechanism of wound healing in the adult.

▶ Fetal wounds heal with less scar and fibrosis than adult wounds. Understanding the mechanisms for this difference is of great interest to clinicians who hope to achieve scarless surgery. This paper addresses 1 aspect of that situation in an animal model. The authors find increased amounts of HA, a proteoglycan, in fetal wounds, compared with those of adult rabbits. This finding supports findings of other investigators and provides additional evidence that increased expression of HA may constitute an important part of the difference between fetal scarless healing and adult scar healing.

W. Garner, M.D.

Effects of Electrical Stimulation on Wound Healing in Patients With Diabetic Ulcers
Baker LL, DeMuth SK, Chambers R, et al (Univ of Southern California, Los Angeles; Rancho Los Amigos Med Ctr, Downey, Calif)
Diabetes Care 20:405–412, 1997   7–5

Background.—Understanding which aspects of electric currents are most important to enhance healing effect would enable the development of better guidelines for the treatment of diabetic patients. The efficacy of neurally regulated regional effects of electric stimulation for enhanced wound healing, while minimizing the possible polar characteristics of the stimulation, was investigated.

Methods.—Eighty diabetic patients with open ulcers were enrolled in the prospective study. Stimulation was delivered with an asymmetric biphasic (A) or symmetric biphasic (B) square-wave pulse. The amplitudes used were designed to activate intact peripheral nerves in the skin. Another 2 groups of patients were given very low levels of stimulation current or no electric stimulation (combined and considered the control group). Daily treatments were delivered until the wound healed, the patient withdrew from the study, or the physician changed the overall management plan.

Outcomes.—Stimulation with the A protocol significantly increased the rate of healing compared to the control group. Healing was enhanced by almost 60% in the A group. Stimulation with the B protocol did not significantly increase the rate of healing compared to that in the control group.

Conclusions.—Electric stimulation with an asymmetric biphasic square waveform enhanced the healing rates in these diabetic patients with open ulcers. Further research is needed to determine the optimal choices for stimulus pulse duration and electrode placements in diabetic patients.

▶ The effects of electricity and electric stimulation on wound healing are not well characterized and are poorly understood. A variety of investigators have applied electric stimulation to wounds with positive results, and this is one of such studies. In contrast to other anecdotal studies, this is a comparative trial between 3 different types of electric stimulation. One hundred fourteen wounds were studied in 80 patients. The study concludes a significant improvement in wound closure rates. Unfortunately, this conclusion must be tempered by the fact that there is a significant difference within the patient populations. The successful treatment group was equally divided between Hispanic and non-Hispanic white patients. In contrast, the control groups had a preponderance of Hispanic patients. The effect of this difference is unknown. In addition, vital capacity was much greater in the successfully stimulated group compared to the other treatment groups. Therefore, these results (while intriguing) are not convincing that this specific type of electric current will successfully heal diabetic foot ulcers. This reviewer believes that a larger trial that is more carefully controlled could be performed, and that this may document the effects seen in this preliminary study.

W. Garner, M.D.

Particle-mediated Gene Transfer With Transforming Growth Factor-β1 cDNAs Enhances Wound Repair in Rat Skin

Benn SI, Whitsitt JS, Broadley KN, et al (Vanderbilt Univ, Nashville, Tenn; Dept of Veterans Affairs Med Ctr, Nashville, Tenn; Shriners Burns Inst, Boston; et al)
J Clin Invest 98:2894–2902, 1996   7–6

Objective.—Direct TGF-β1 injection facilitates healing of incisional wounds. Because production and purification of growth factors is expensive, it would be desirable to deliver gene therapy to the wound site and provide for in situ expression of growth factors. Using in vivo gene transfer by particle-mediated DNA delivery to rat skin, the effect of overexpression of TGF-β1 on wound healing was studied.

Methods.—Luciferase reporter gene expression construct with several viral promoters or control DNA was used to enhance particle-mediated

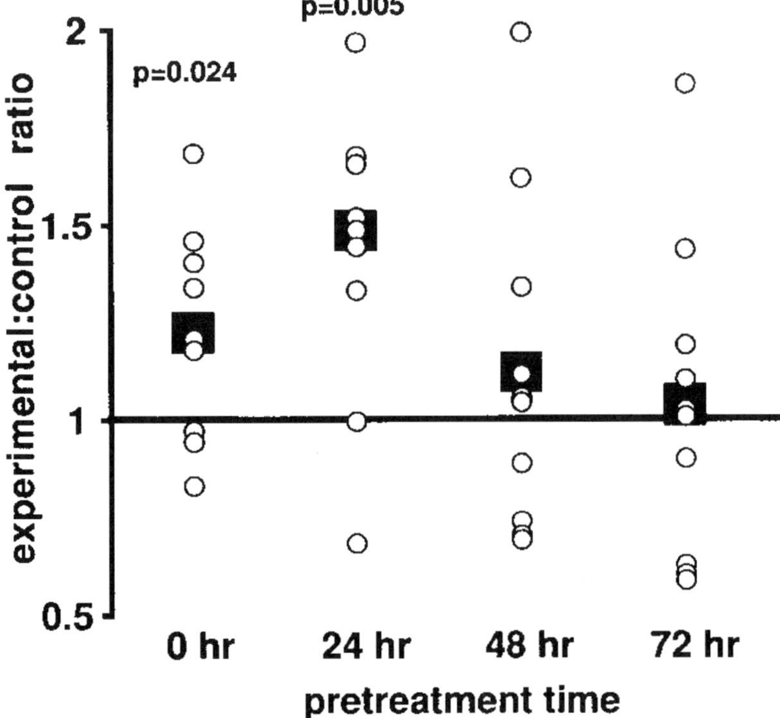

FIGURE 10.—The effect of TGFβ1 gene transfection timing on wound healing. Surgical sites were transfected by particle-mediated gene transfer at 0, 24, 48, and 72 hours before surgery. Incisional strength was measured on tissue harvested 14 days after surgery. Data are expressed as the experimental:control ratio of each of 9 paired wound sites on 5 different animals. Means are shown by *filled squares*. Significance was determined by student's *t* test. P values of 0.05 or less are illustrated. (Courtesy of Benn SI, Whitsitt JS, Broadley KN, et al: Particle-mediated gene transfer with transforming growth factor–β1 cDNAs enhances wound repair in rat skin. *J Clin Invest* 98:2894–2902, 1996. Reproduced by copyright permission of the The American Society for Clinical Investigation.)

gene delivery to cutaneous transfections in healthy and diabetic male Sprague-Dawley rats. The construct was delivered by helium powered gene gun at various pressures at the wound site. Tensile strength of skin incisions were determined. Animals were killed on days 0 to 7, and luciferase activity determined. In vitro expression of TGF-β1 activity was determined. Total RNA was isolated and sequenced using PCR amplification. Tissues were biopsied, and histological and immunocytochemistry studies were performed.

Results.—The force at which the construct was driven into the skin, the promoter and the site (ventral versus dorsal) affected the expression of luciferase. Luciferase activity continued for at least 5 days. Transfected cells consisted mainly of keratinocytes. The cytomegalovirus promoter provoked the highest level of luciferase activity. The transgene was found in RNA isolated from tissue transfected with the cytomegalovirus construct. Biological activity of constructs were verified by determining in vitro activities. Granulation tissue was verified by in vivo activity measurement of TGF-β1 constructs as the site for in vivo transfection. In rats treated with the CMV construct there was a significant increase in the tensile strength of healed incisions at 14 and 20 days after transfection. Optimal timing for transfection was determined to be 24 hours before surgery (Fig 10).

Conclusion.—Wound healing as measured by tensile strength of skin is significantly improved by transfection with TGF-β1 expression constructs.

▶ This paper describes state-of-the-art gene therapy techniques to improve wound healing in an animal model. Studies by Erickson and colleagues have shown the ability of exogenously administered growth factors to improve a variety of wound healing parameters. This well-researched and well-written paper merges these 2 lines of investigation by documenting successful gene transfer and increased levels of cytokines within the wound, simultaneous to an increase in tissue tensile strength of full-thickness incision sites. At present, this technology and technique is costly and not suitable for human use. However, it is likely that in the near future, these techniques will be used to manipulate directly wounds and wound healing.

W. Garner, M.D.

Effect of Macrophage Stimulation on Collagen Biosynthesis in the Healing Wound

Portera CA, Love EJ, Memore L, et al (East Tennessee State Univ, Johnson City; Veterans Affairs Med Ctr, Mountain Home, Tenn)
Am Surg 63:125–130, 1997   7–7

Background.—Previous work has demonstrated that (1–3)-β-D-glucans facilitate healing in experimental wounds. Specifically, glucan phosphate has been shown to enhance early healing of experimental skin wounds in rodents. A separate study showed that this effect of glucan was mediated,

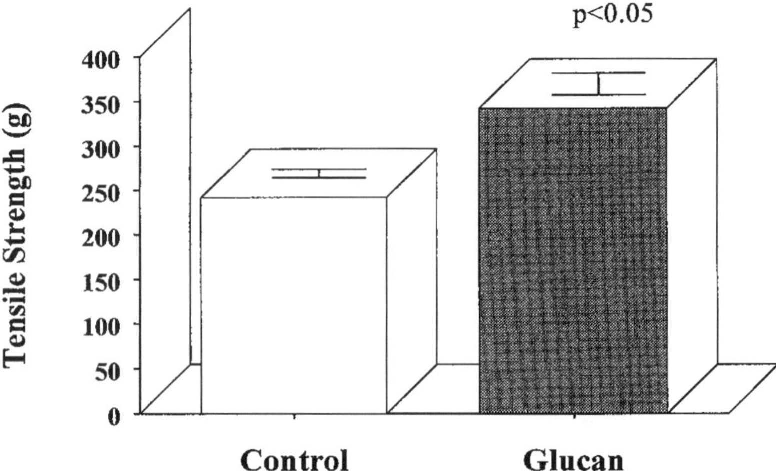

FIGURE 1.—Enhanced tensile strength of day 3 rat, dorsal, full-thickness skin wounds after glucan phosphate administration. Glucan phosphate was administered IV (250 mg/kg) 24 hours before and immediately after surgery. Dextrose served as the control. Skin samples were harvested on postoperative day 3 and analyzed by constant velocity tensiometry. N = 12 per group. (Courtesy of Portera CA, Love EJ, Memore L, et al: Effect of macrophage stimulation on collagen biosynthesis in the healing wound. *Am Surg* 63:125–130, 1997.)

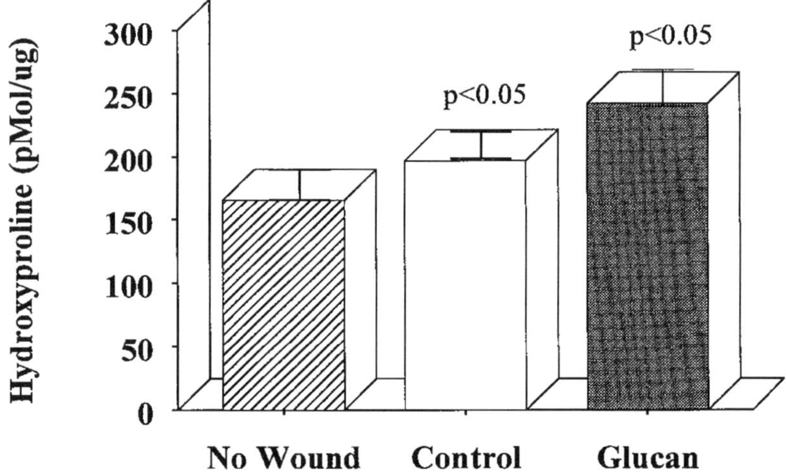

FIGURE 2.—Increased hydroxyproline levels in day 3 rat, full-thickness skin wounds after glucan phosphate administration. Glucan phosphate was administered IV (250 mg/kg) 24 hours before and immediately after surgery. Dextrose served as the control. As an additional control, normal, nonwounded skin was also assayed for hydroxyproline levels. Hydroxyproline levels were established by N-(9-fluorenyl)-methoxycarbon/p-phaladehyde high-performance liquid chromatography. N = 17–27 per group. (Courtesy of Portera CA, Love EJ, Memore L, et al: Effect of macrophage stimulation on collagen biosynthesis in the healing wound. *Am Surg* 63:125–130, 1997.)

in part, by macrophage release of soluble growth factors. The effect of glucan phosphate on wound tensile strength and collagen biosynthesis was studied as a way to investigate the exact mechanism by which $(1-3)$-β-D-glucans accelerate wound repair.

Methods.—Two groups of animals were studied: rats with skin wounds and mice with colon wounds. An injection of glucan phosphate was given 24 hours before the wounds were surgically induced, then again immediately after surgery. The animals were euthanized on postoperative day 3, and the wounds were evaluated for hydroxyproline content (a measure of collagen synthesis) and tensile strength. In both groups, nonwounded samples were also evaluated.

Results.—In the rat skin wounds, tensile strength was 42% higher and hydroxyproline content was 47% higher, in wounds that had received glucan phosphate injections than in nonwounded skin (Fig 1 and Fig 2). Both differences were statistically significant. In the mouse colon wounds, the tensile strength of wounds that had received glucan phosphate was 34% higher than in control tissue, a significant difference. The increase in hydroxyproline content was not significant.

Conclusions.—In these animals, macrophage modulation with glucan phosphate increased the tensile strength of experimental wounds. There was also a positive correlation between glucan phosphate treatment, wound tensile strength, and collagen biosynthesis. Taken together, these data suggest that increased collagen biosynthesis is partly responsible for the early wound repair induced by glucan phosphate.

▶ This study addresses the role of macrophages in stimulating collagen synthesis and tensile strength in an animal model. The results demonstrate substantial increases in tensile strength in both the skin and the colon. These results provide continued support for the idea that wound healing is orchestrated by macrophages. They provide additional evidence that stimulation of these macrophages by a simple chemical compound such as glucans can significantly increase wound healing rates. Clinical applicability of this information is as yet uncertain.

W. Garner, M.D.

Double-blind Randomized Placebo-controlled Trial of the Use of Granulocyte-Macrophage Colony-stimulating Factor in Chronic Leg Ulcers
da Costa RM, Jesus FM, Aniceto C, et al (Hosp Distrital de Leiria, Portugal)
Am J Surg 173:165–168, 1997   7–8

Objective.—As the population ages, chronic wound care becomes an increasingly important health issue. Granulocyte-macrophage colony-stimulating factor (GM-CSF) is an important growth factor involved in wound repair, leading to studies of exogenous GM-CSF to improve impaired wound healing. Animal experiments and preliminary studies in humans have given promising results. A double-blind, randomized, controlled trial of perilesional GM-CSF for the treatment of chronic leg ulcers was done.

Methods.—The study sample comprised 40 patients with chronic leg ulcers of varicose or ischemic causes. They were assigned to receive a single perilesional injection of recombinant human GM-CSF, 400 µg, or placebo. The average wound size was about 10 cm² in both groups. The injections were made in 4 equal doses in the 4 quadrants of the wound. The wounds were assessed at 8, 15, and 29 days, then weekly for 3 months. Healing was compared in the 2 groups.

Results.—The results were so much better in the GM-CSF group that the study was ended early—16 patients were treated in the GM-CSF group and 9 in the placebo group. By day 8, ulcer size had decreased to 7 cm$_2$ in the GM-CSF group, compared with a slight increase in the placebo group. In the GM-CSF group, ulcer healing occurred by 1 week in 19% of patients and by 8 weeks in 50%. In contrast, just 1 of 9 patients in the control group had ulcer healing at 1 week. That was the only ulcer that healed in the control group. Treatment with GM-CSF had no significant side effects and caused no alterations in hematologic or biochemical parameters.

Conclusions.—Recombinant human GM-CSF is an effective treatment for chronic leg ulcers. Good results are achieved in both venous and ischemic wounds with a single perilesional treatment. More research is needed to optimize the indications for treatment, the drug dose, and the dosing regimen. The histologic changes in the ulcer and the perilesional skin must be described as well.

► This article is part of an increasing body of literature showing that the healing of chronic wounds can be accelerated or achieved through the use of exogenous growth factors or other stimulants. In this case, GM-CSF was used in a comparative trial of patients with chronic wounds. The authors describe such positive effects from their treatment that the randomized portion of the study was terminated after partial enrollment into the study.

The article lacks the degree of information one would optimally want to plot wound closure during this treatment; however, the end results of wound closure and decrease in wound size appear to be clearly enhanced by GM-CSF treatment. Follow-up with additional studies to validate this first observation will be necessary before this treatment should be brought into general practice.

W. Garner, M.D.

Tumor Necrosis Factor-α Inhibits Collagen α1 (I) Gene Expression and Wound Healing in a Murine Model of Cachexia
Buck M, Houglum K, Chojkier M (Univ of California, San Diego)
Am J Pathol 149:195–204, 1996   7–9

Objective.—Decrease in collagen synthesis plays an important role in poor wound healing in cachectic patients undergoing surgery. Tumor necrosis factor (TNF)-α has been implicated in the pathogenesis of cachexia. Although it is known that TNF-α inhibits collagen gene expression in vitro, its in vivo effect is not known. The effect of chronically elevated serum TNF-α on collagen metabolism in nude mice inoculated with Chinese hamster ovary (CHO) cells secreting TNF-α is presented.

Methods.—CHO cells (10^7) with or without TNF-α transfection were injected into 4-week-old male athymic nude mice. The mice were killed 14 to 21 days and 28 to 35 days. The mice received incisional skin wounds at 11 days after inoculation to study wound healing. Desmin and TGF-β were assayed immunohistochemically. Collagen α1(l)mRNA was determined by an RNAse protection assay. The *cis*-regulatory region of chimeric collagen α1(l)hGH reporter gene was characterized.

Results.—Two to 3 weeks after injection, TNF-α animals but not control animals began to lose weight and muscle and had serum TNF-α concentrations of 275 pg/ml. Skin collagen production was inhibited by approximately 40% in the TNF-α treated mice. Inhibition of collagen gene expression was confirmed in these mice by demonstrating a substantially decreased level of collagen α1(l) mRNA. TNF-α-treated mice had impaired wound healing with a significant increase in desmin-positive cells in the dermis, a decreased extracellular matrix deposition, increased cellularity in the wounds, and dramatically decreased expression of TGF-β in the skin. Mice expressing hGH, the reporter gene included -2.3 kb of the 5' flanking regulatory region. When the 5' region with only -0.44 kb did not affect transgene expression.

Conclusion.—TNF-α may be a mediator of wound healing in cachectic patients by inhibiting skin collagen α1(l) gene expression and skin TNF-β expression. The *cis* regulatory region of the collagen α1(l) gene is inhibited by TNF-α.

▶ Tumor necrosis factor is an inflammatory cytokine and appears to be very important in the early response to trauma, sepsis, and infection. This study used recombinant molecular biology techniques to create cell strains that produced marked increases of TNF-α. In an experimental model, cells with and without this cytokine were injected into nude mice and the increased amount of TNF-α validated. Standard wound healing parameters were impaired in these TNF-α animals including collagen production, wound contraction and TGF-β synthesis.

Two conclusions can be drawn from this paper:

1. TNF-α induces a cachexic-like state, therefore it is not surprising that overexpression would impair wound healing. This is similar to the condition of patients with end stage malignancy who do not heal as expected.

2. Because TNF-α is an inflammatory cytokine, wounds that are infected or that display excess inflammation from other reasons may, similarly, not heal. Whether removal of the cytokine from nonhealing wounds will change wound-healing activities is as yet an untested possibility.

W. Garner, M.D.

Type I (RI) and Type II (RII) Receptors for Transforming Growth Factor-β Isoforms Are Expressed Subsequent to Transforming Growth Factor-β Ligands During Excisional Wound Repair
Gold LI, Sung JJ, Siebert JW, et al (New York Univ)
Am J Pathol 150:209–222, 1997   7–10

Purpose.—The β_1, β_2, and β_3 isoforms of transforming growth factor β (TGF-β) are involved in regulating cell growth and differentiation and play a critical role in regulating tissue repair and remodeling. The heteromeric receptor complex that transmits signal transduction for TGF-β function is made up of 2 serine/threonine kinase transmembrane proteins, RI and RII. In the process of wound repair, the expression of each TGF-β isoform shows a distinct spatial and temporal pattern. This immunohistochemical study localized RI and RII during the process of repair of full-thickness excisional wounds in sheep.

Methods and Results.—Studies were performed up to 21 days after wounding. Colocalized expression of RI was noted in wounded and unwounded skin and in the same cell types of TGF-β ligands. Throughout the repair process, immunoreactivity for TGF-β receptors lagged 1–5 days behind TGF-β isoform immunostaining. This delay suggested that TGF-β ligands upregulate TGF-β receptors for function or that local processing of TGF-β causes a time lag. As in unwounded skin, all 4 layers of epidermis expressed both RI and RII. There was slight to moderate immunostaining in a wavy pattern and moderate immunoreactivity of hair follicles, sweat glands, and sebaceous glands. No immunoreactivity was noted in the extracellular matrix, fibroblasts, or dermal blood vessels.

Injury was followed by increased expression of RI and RII in the adjacent epidermis. It took 7 days for complete re-epithelialization, and not until that time did the migratory epithelium become completely devoid of TGF-β receptor immunoreactivity. Up until day 5 after wounding, the dermis showed only slight immunoreactivity for RI and RII. At that time, immunostaining for fibroblasts, connective tissue cells, and new blood vessels began to increase and continued to be intense until day 14. Throughout the 21-day study period, fibroblasts active in the production of extracellular matrix components showed slight immunoreactivity for RI and RII. Immunostaining for the ALK-1 (TSR-1) type I receptor—which binds activin and TGF-β—was only slight through the first 7 days after wounding. From days 10–21, this staining became increasingly intense, and suggested a possible switch to a different receptor.

Conclusions.—This study of wound healing demonstrates concomitant expression of TGF-β isoforms and their signal-transducing receptors, thus indicating possible spatial and temporal activity of TGF-β. The findings suggest that although TGF-β ligand is present in wounds, it plays no role in the repair process until RI and RII appear. This could prove useful in the development of receptor antagonists to treat scarring and fibrosis. It is important to study protein expression in vivo to understand the mechanisms observed in vitro.

▶ This article continues the authors' exploration of the role of a particular cytokine (TGF-β) in wound healing. In this case, the activity of this growth factor is documented, as well as the activity of its receptors. The authors document activity of TGF-β the day after injury. The activity of the receptors for the cytokine are delayed until several days later. Both receptors I and II were activated in a similar time course and tissue distribution. This decreases the likelihood that the activity of this cytokine is regulated by differential receptor activity. This is a well-performed and well-written basic paper that further documents what is likely to be an important role of TGF-β in healing of wounds.

W. Garner, M.D.

A Comparative Study of Three Occlusive Dressings in the Treatment of Full-Thickness Wounds in Pigs

Ågren MS, Mertz PM, Franzén L (Univ of Miami, Florida; Faculty of Health Sciences, Linköping, Sweden)
J Am Acad Dermatol 36:53–58, 1997   7–11

Objective.—Whereas occlusion encourages healing of surgically excised partial-thickness wounds, not much information is available on the healing effect of occlusive dressings on full-thickness wounds. Results of a study of tissue response to and effects of hydrocolloid dressing A (Comfeel Ulcer Dressing, Coloplast A/S, Espergaerder, Denmark), hydrocolloid dressing B (DuDERM Convalec, Princeton NJ), and film dressing (OpSite, Smith & Nephew, Hull, UK) on the quality and rate of closure of full-thickness wounds in domestic pigs were reported.

Methods.—Punch wounds (20 mm) were made in the muscular layer of 3 white, female domestic pigs and dressed with 8 × 8-cm hydrocolloid dressing A, hydrocolloid dressing B, and film dressing. After 4 days, the wounds were cleaned and redressed, and after 10 days, wound contracture was determined using the equation $(A_{\text{Day 0}} - A_{\text{Day X}})/A_{\text{Day 0}} \times 100$ where $X =$ 4 or 10 in day X. Wound sections were evaluated by light spectroscopy and planimetry.

Results.—Wound exudate leaked from the 2 hydrocolloid dressings. Hydrocolloid dressing A and film dressing were easy to remove but hydrocolloid dressing B stuck to the skin and the wound. Significantly more foam cells were found in wounds covered with the hydrocolloid dressings than in film dressing. Significantly more extracellular vacuoles, often surrounded by granulomas, were present in wounds covered by hydrocolloid dressing B but not in the other 2 dressings. In the deeper layer of wound tissue, wounds covered by hydrocolloid dressing B had a stronger inflammatory reaction than wounds covered by the other dressings, although in the superficial granulation tissue, the inflammatory response was less severe with hydrocolloid dressing A than the other 2 dressings. Percentage wound contracture and epithelialization were similar for all dressings (Fig 4). The average wound surface covered (57%) was similar for all dressings.

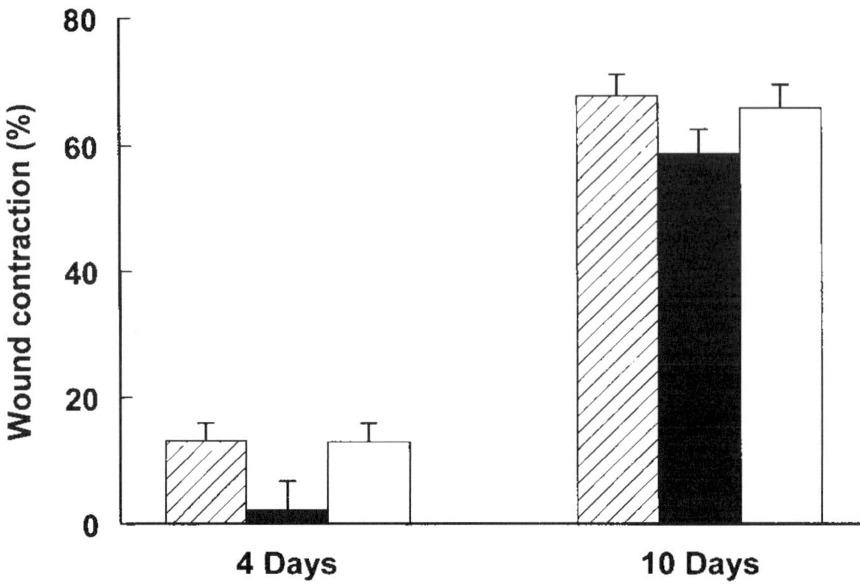

FIGURE 4.—No significant effect of treatment on wound contraction on postoperative days 4 or 10 was found (mean ± standard error of the mean). *Hatched bars*, indicate hydrocolloid dressing A; *solid bars*, hydrocolloid dressing B; *open bars*, film dressing. (Courtesy of Ågren MS, Mertz PM, Franzén L: A comparative study of three occlusive dressings in the treatment of full-thickness wounds in pigs. *J Am Acad Dermatol* 36:53–58, 1997).

Conclusion.—There was no difference in wound contracture or epithelialization of full-thickness wounds in pigs treated with 3 different occlusive dressings.

▶ Numerous studies have demonstrated the increased rate of epithelialization beneath occlusive dressings. The question for the clinician is *Which* occlusive dressing? This paper tests 3 such dressings (2 hydrocolloids and 1 polyurethane film). The results show essentially no difference in the healing responses among the 3. Both wound contraction and epithelialization were unchanged (see Fig 4). This paper suggests that the practitioner should choose an occlusive dressing based on practical considerations of ease of use, patient tolerance, and cost.

W. Garner, M.D.

A Study of the Effects of Epinephrine Infiltration on Delayed Bleeding in a Rat Flap Model
Rey RM Jr, Smoot EC III, Nguyen D, et al (Univ of Tennessee, Memphis; Harbor–Univ of California Los Angeles Med Ctr, Torrance)
Ann Plast Surg 37:406–410, 1996   7–12

Objective.—Whereas epinephrine is known to reduce blood loss, there is little information regarding its effect on homeostasis. One concern is that after the vasoconstrictive effect of epinephrine wears off, smaller vessels might dilate, then bleed, creating a hematoma. The effect of local infiltration of lidocaine and lidocaine/epinephrine on postoperative bleeding was evaluated in the rat model using the McFarlane dorsal skin flap and the ventral pedicled flap.

Methods.—A dorsal McFarlane flap and a ventral pedicled flap were raised on each of 50 Sprague-Dawley female rats. Ventral flaps were infiltrated with 1.5 mL and dorsal flaps were infiltrated with 1.0 mL of either 1% lidocaine hydrochloric acid (HCl), 2% lidocaine HCl, 1% lidocaine HCl and epinephrine (1:100,000), or 0.5% lidocaine HCl and epinephrine (1:200,000). A control group received no infiltrate. Rats were killed 24 hours later. At 26 hours, flaps were opened and the coaguli removed and weighed. Weights were compared statistically.

Results.—There were no significant differences in weights of coaguli among treatment and control groups.

Conclusion.—In this study, there was no difference in delayed bleeding between infiltrated and noninfiltrated flaps treated with lidocaine and lidocaine-epinephrine combinations.

▶ Does infiltration of the skin with lidocaine or lidocaine-containing epinephrine increase or decrease the bleeding in the tissues after wound closure? This paper suggests that there is no difference between no infiltration or infiltration with 2 doses of lidocaine and 2 doses of epinephrine. Unfortunately, the study does not fully answer these important questions. The number of animals in each subgroup is quite small (1–7) and, therefore, differences of as much as tenfold are not considered significant. Whether this is because of small sample size is, in part, addressed by a power analysis done by the authors.

They should be congratulated for this attempt to answer the important question of no difference vs. inadequate sample size. Unfortunately, their power analysis shows a power of less than 80% in at least 3 of 6 comparisons. The authors should have increased the number of samples and sample size to provide more definitive information because the questions they are asking are important ones.

W. Garner, M.D.

Biochemical Analysis of Wound Fluid From Nonhealing and Healing Chronic Leg Ulcers

Trengove NJ, Langton SR, Stacey MC (Univ of Western Australia, Australia; Fremantle Hosp, Australia)
Wound Rep Reg 4:234–239, 1996   7–13

Objective.—The underlying causes of delayed healing in chronic leg ulcers is poorly understood. Analysis of fluid from leg ulcers may provide information about the growth condition of cells within the wound. The biochemical composition of wound fluid collected from chronic leg ulcers at healing and nonhealing phases was compared to determine whether the fluid really is extracellular.

Methods.—Wound fluid and blood samples were collected within 24 hours of admission (nonhealing) and after 2 weeks of dressing and bed rest (healing) from 8 patients (2 females), aged 69 to 89 years, with chronic lower leg ulcers, including those with venous disease treated with compression therapy. Surface area and appearance of the ulcers were recorded, wound fluid and blood samples were analyzed, and bacteriologic characteristics were determined. Comparisons were analyzed statistically.

Results.—Relative to serum levels, wound lactate levels were significantly elevated (10.9 vs. 2.7 mmol/L) and glucose levels (1.8 vs. 6.4 mmol/L) and bicarbonate levels (19 vs. 26 mmol/L) were significantly lower, which indicated an acidotic and anaerobic environment. When compared with the nonhealing phase, the healing phase showed significantly increased levels of bicarbonate, glucose, albumin, total protein, gamma-globulin, and cholesterol and significantly decreased levels of C-reactive protein. Bacteria were cultured from leg ulcers in both phases.

Conclusions.—Protein results of wound fluid analysis indicate that the fluid is an exudate, and the increase in protein and albumin during healing may indicate improved nutritional status. Bicarbonate and glucose results reflect reduced wound hypoxia during healing, whereas decreased levels of C-reactive protein may indicate a lessening in the inflammatory process.

▶ Although measurement of the exudate from venous leg ulcers indirectly suggested a reduction in wound hypoxia and inflammation, it is difficult to determine whether these data significantly increase our knowledge of wound healing. Current trends in wound healing research that focus on cellular molecular biology seem more promising avenues to explore.

R. Rudolph, M.D., F.A.C.S.

Long-term Appearance of Lacerations Repaired Using a Tissue Adhesive

Simon HK, McLario DJ, Bruns TB, et al (Emory Univ, Atlanta, Ga; Univ of Tennessee, Chattanooga)
Pediatrics 99:193–195, 1997   7–14

Background.—Histoacryl Blue (HAB) is a tissue adhesive that reduces laceration repair time, results in less pain, and eliminates the need for suture removal. The short-term cosmetic outcomes have been found to be comparable with those achieved with conventional suturing. The long-term cosmetic outcomes of HAB were compared with those of conventional suturing for laceration repair in children.

Methods and Findings.—Sixty-one children brought to an urban pediatric emergency department for laceration repair between October 1994 and February 1995 were enrolled in the prospective, randomized clinical study. Inclusion criteria were patient age between 1 and 18 years, lacerations of less than 5 cm in length, and no areas of high tension or mobility. Thirty children were treated with HAB and 31 with conventional suturing. Thirty children in the HAB group and 25 in the conventional suturing group were available for follow-up at 2 months, and 17 and 15, respectively, were available at 1 year. These children were comparable to those not followed up in treatment group, demographics, wound characteristics, and initial parental satisfaction. Two plastic surgeons graded the cosmetic appearances of the wounds in the 2 treatment groups. Repairs made with HAB were comparable to those made by conventional suturing at 2 months and 1 year.

Conclusions.—The use of HAB is an excellent alternative to conventional suturing in children requiring cutaneous closure of low-tension lacerations. The long-term cosmetic outcomes of HAB treatment are comparable to those achieved with conventional suturing.

▶ This paper describes the appearance of lacerations closed with a tissue adhesive rather than sutures. It represents the late results of patients randomly allocated to repair using either tissue adhesive or 5–0 or 6–0 Prolene sutures. The results showed no difference in appearance between the 2 techniques in low-tension, low-risk facial wounds. The conclusion from this study can likely be expanded to other forms of wound closure such as steri-strips or the equivalent taping techniques. If the wound edges can be kept in position for an appropriate period of time, the wound will heal with an excellent result. This conclusion will likely save significant anguish from parents wishing the placement of sutures by a board-certified plastic surgeon to obtain the best resulting scar for their injured child.

W. Garner, M.D.

Effectiveness of Silicone Sheets in the Prevention of Hypertrophic Breast Scars
Cruz-Korchin NI (Univ of Puerto Rico, San Juan)
Ann Plast Surg 37:345–348, 1996   7–15

Background.—Silicone gel and elastomer sheets have been widely used to treat hypertrophic scars for many years. Recently, their use to prevent such scars has been investigated. The efficacy of silicone sheets in preventing hypertrophic scars in women undergoing reduction mammaplasties was studied.

Methods.—Twenty women scheduled for bilateral McKissock reduction mammaplasties were included. Beginning at the time of suture removal, the women used a precut silicone elastomer sheet over the scars of 1 breast only; the other served as a control. The silicone sheets were used for 12 hours a day for 2 months.

Findings.—At 2 months, 60% of the untreated scars were hypertrophic, compared with only 25% of the treated scars. This difference was statistically significant. The beneficial effects of the silicone sheets continued to

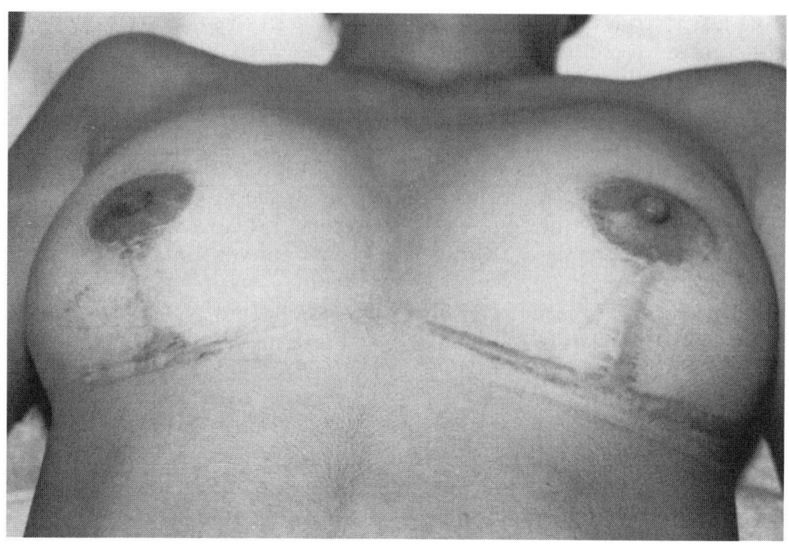

FIGURE 4.—In this patient, the treated right side shows a more dramatic result when compared to the hypertrophic left side. (Courtesy of Cruz-Korchin NI: Effectiveness of silicone sheets in the prevention of hypertrophic breast scars. *Ann Plast Surg* 37:345–348, 1996. Reprinted from *Annals of Plastic Surgery* by permission of Little, Brown and Company, Inc.)

be apparent at 6 months, 4 months after sheet use was discontinued (Fig 4).

Conclusions.—Although the mechanism of action remains unclear, silicone sheets appear to be effective in the treatment and prevention of hypertrophic scars. The adverse effects associated with their use seem to be minor and transient.

▶ This well-designed study provides good evidence for the benefits to be achieved in scar modification by the application of silicone gel sheeting. I think this is really worth using—and I plan to do so, especially in patients whom I consider to be at high risk for hypertrophic scars after breast reduction.

R.L. Ruberg, M.D.

Comparison of Polydioxanone and Polyglactin 910 in Intradermal Repair

Guyuron B, Vaughan C (Case Western Reserve Univ, Cleveland, Ohio)
Plast Reconstr Surg 98:817–820, 1996   7–16

Introduction.—The suture material polyglactin 910 reportedly has longer retention of tensile strength and less traumatic monofilament design than other sutures. The results of intradermal layer closure with 6–0 polyglactin 910 and with polydioxanone were compared.

Methods.—The study included 80 suture sites on 20 consecutive patients undergoing facial rhytidectomy. One side of the rhytidectomy incision was repaired with 6–0 clear polydioxanone and the other with 6–0 polyglactin 910. Superficial closure was always done with 6–0 plain catgut. Because of differences in closure tension and healing potential, the temple and occipital regions of the 2 sides were evaluated separately. The double-blind evaluation included erythema, induration, infection, scar spreading, and hypertrophic scarring. Evaluations were performed at 5 months and 1 year postoperatively.

Results.—Scar spread of more than 1 mm occurred in 16% of incisions repaired with polyglactin 910 and 8% of those repaired with polydioxanone. The rate of hypertrophic scarring, defined as any raised scar, was 8% in both groups. Most of the hypertrophic scars were in the occipital region. Overall, 76% of the sites healed with no visible scarring.

Conclusions.—This study finds no significant difference in the healing of rhytidectomy scars when polyglactin 910 or polydioxanone is used as the suture material. Given their equal results, the author has gone back to using polyglactin 910 because of subjective problems with polydioxanone, namely, extrusion and awkward intraoperative handling.

▶ The suture materials are similar, but there are less bristles to project with polydioxanone (Vicryl and PDS).

P.W. McKinney, M.D.

The Use of Negative Pressure to Promote the Healing of Tissue Defects: A Clinical Trial Using the Vacuum Sealing Technique
Müllner T, Mrkonjic L, Kwasny O, et al (Univ of Vienna)
Br J Plast Surg 50:194–199, 1997   7–17

Objective.—When negative pressure is applied to soft-tissue defects, production of granulation tissue increases significantly. The negative pressure increases skin perfusion while removing debris from the wound bed. The findings to date suggest the need for further study of the use of negative pressure in complicated acute and chronic soft-tissue defects. A trial of a vacuum sealing technique for complicated sacral pressure ulcers, acute traumatic soft-tissue defects, and infected soft-tissue defects was reported.

> *Technique.*—The negative pressure system used polyvinyl foam placed into the defect and covered with a transparent polyurethane dressing. Drainage tubes were connected to vacuum bottles or pump-suction. When the vacuum was switched on, it created negative pressure in the polyvinyl foam, producing a high contact zone in the interface between the wound and the foam. The foam was left in place for about 1 week, as long as the vacuum remained intact. The dressing was changed at 4 to 7 days, at which time granulation tissue was evaluated. Once the granulation bed was

adequate, definitive wound closure could be achieved by 1 of several different approaches.

Methods.—A prospective study was performed in 45 patients with wounds developing after rigid stabilization of lower leg fractures. All of the wounds were complicated by exposed bone and/or implants. Seventeen patients had sacral pressure ulcers, 12 had acute soft-tissue defects, and 16 had infected soft-tissue defects. All patients were treated by the vacuum sealing technique, beginning after irrigation and debridement. Vacuum treatment was deemed successful if the wound was reduced in size by 80% or if the wound bed was covered by granulation tissue.

Results.—The vacuum sealing technique was successful in 84% of patients, including 71% of patients with sacral pressure ulcers, 100% of those with acute soft-tissue defects, and 86% of those with infected soft-tissue defects. The vacuum sealing technique shortened healing time while eliminating any pre-existing infection. In 35 of the 45 wounds, wound closure was achieved by granulation, secondary closure, or split-thickness skin grafting.

Conclusion.—The vacuum sealing technique appears to be a useful alternative for the management of complicated soft-tissue defects. As described in this study, the system enhances production of granulation tissue while keeping the wound bed relatively clean. It is an inexpensive technique and should be helpful adjuvant therapy for the management of infected wounds.

Vacuum-assisted Closure: A New Method For Wound Control and Treatment: Animal Studies and Basic Foundation
Morykwas MJ, Argenta LC, Shelton-Brown EI, et al (Bowman Gray School of Medicine, Winston-Salem, NC)
Ann Plast Surg 38:553–562, 1997   7–18

Purpose.—Vacuum-assisted closure (VAC) is a new technique designed to enhance wound healing by secondary intention, particularly in compromised and debilitated patients. It consists of a system that applies controlled subatmospheric pressure to the wound. A swine model of acute wounds was used to evaluate the effects of VAC on wound healing.

Methods.—Wounds measuring 2.5 cm in diameter were created on the backs of pigs. The wounds were treated by VAC, in which an open-cell foam is placed in the wound, the area is sealed with adhesive tape, and subatmospheric pressure (125 mm Hg below ambient pressure) is applied. The animals were divided into groups for studies of blood flow in the wound and adjacent tissue, as measured by laser Doppler ultrasonography; granulation tissue formation under conditions of continuous and intermittent subatmospheric pressure; bacterial clearance from infected wounds; and nutrient flow, as measured by random-pattern flap survival.

Results.—At the level of subatmospheric pressure applied, there was a fourfold increase in blood flow. Blood flow studies revealed that the effect was optimal with a 5 minutes on/2 minutes off cycle, which was subsequently used for studies of intermittent subatmospheric pressure. Formation of granulation tissue increased by 63% with continuous subatmospheric pressure and by 103% with intermittent pressure. Four days of VAC treatment produced a significant reduction in tissue bacterial counts. Compared with non–VAC-treated controls, the application of subatmospheric pressure significantly increased the survival of random-pattern flaps.

Conclusion.—The subatmospheric pressures applied in the VAC technique provide an environment conducive to wound healing. In this swine model, VAC increased local blood perfusion, hastened granulation tissue formation, and increased nutrient blood flow. The mechanisms of these effects may include removal of excess interstitial fluid, reduced tissue bacterial levels, increased protein and matrix molecule synthesis, and increased cell proliferation.

Vacuum-assisted Closure: A New Method for Wound Control and Treatment: Clinical Experience
Argenta LC, Morykwas MJ (Bowman Gray School of Medicine, Winston-Salem, NC)
Ann Plast Surg 38:563–577, 1997   7–19

Background.—Chronic, nonhealing wounds and wound complications pose difficult problems for patients and physicians alike. Even with various advances, these wounds continue to present treatment challenges. A new approach to wound treatment—vacuum-assisted closure (VAC)—was tested in patients with chronic, subacute, and acute wounds.

Methods.—In VAC, an open-cell foam is placed in the wound, the area is sealed with adhesive tape, and subatmospheric pressure (125 mm Hg below ambient pressure) is applied. This technique was used in a series of 300 patients with wounds: 175 chronic wounds, such as pressure ulcers and stasis ulcers, that had not progressed toward healing for more than 1 week; 94 subacute wounds, such as infected and dehisced wounds and open amputations; and 31 acute wounds, such as acute avulsions, evacuated hematomas, and gunshot wounds. The initial patients were treated in the hospital by the senior author; later patients were managed as outpatients under the care of other practitioners. The VAC system was applied after thorough debridement and meticulous hemostasis. The results of patient follow-up and definitive treatment were reported.

Results.—Ninety-nine percent of the wounds showed increased granulation tissue formation in response to VAC. Subatmospheric pressure treatment continued until the wounds closed completely, split-thickness skin grafting was performed, or a flap was rotated into the granulating wound bed. In chronic wounds, the length of treatment ranged from less than 2 weeks to more than 16 weeks, depending on the size of the wound. There have been no pressure ulcer recurrences at the treated wound site. The subacute wounds showed a more rapid and uniform response than the chronic wounds. Successes in this category included many patients with exposed fixation hardware or bone. Healing was quicker still for patients with acute wounds. Except for 1 patient who died, all wounds were successfully closed. The few complications of VAC were mainly technical in nature.

Conclusion.—The VAC technique produces good results in patients with chronic or otherwise difficult wounds. The application of subatmospheric pressure eliminates chronic edema, thus increasing localized blood flow. The forces applied to the wound lead to enhanced granulation tissue formation. The article includes a discussion of the practical considerations involved in VAC. Further study of this new treatment modality is needed. A large, randomized trial is underway.

▶ This is an intriguing modality (Abstracts 7–17 to 7–19) for dealing with large and infected wounds that heretofore required significant medical resources to achieve wound closure. It would have been of interest had the authors looked more closely and in greater depth at the failures to better define the type of patients in whom this technique is most likely to be effective. Randomized, controlled studies are necessary to determine whether this adjunctive modality is helpful in wound healing. The definition of a chronic wound in the clinical study by Argenta and Morykwas is quite liberal; 1-week-old wounds are not usually classified as chronic.

S.H. Miller, M.D.

Miscellaneous

Reflex Bradycardia in Out-patient Surgery Done Under Local Anesthesia
Hurwitz PJ, Ogilvie M (Surgical Day Care Ctr, Aarau, Switzerland)
Eur J Plast Surg 18:76–78, 1995   7–20

Objective.—Reflex bradycardia occurs as a result of a sustained drop in pulse rate. Reflex bradycardia is synonymously referred to as vasovagal reflex, oculocardiac reflex, and trigeminocardiac reflex because of the variety of clinical signs that accompany it. Experience with reflex bradycardia in patients undergoing plastic surgery who were given local anesthesia was reviewed.

Methods.—Twelve (6 female) of 432 patients undergoing plastic surgery experienced reflex bradycardia. The patients aged 19–62 years, had 5 facial operations, 1 otoplasty, 5 hand operations, and 1 scar correction on the knee.

Results.—Bradycardia ranged from 35 to 56 beats min, and the average pulse drop was 30%, resulting in an irregular heart beat in 4 patients. Atropine (0.5–1.0 mg) restored rhythm.

Conclusion.—Plastic surgeons need to be familiar with forms of brady-cardia that can be manifested by patients under local anesthesia. Use of a pulse oximeter and an IV line are recommended.

▶ A reminder!

P.W. McKinney, M.D.

Treatment of Thromboembolic Complications of Fulminant Meningococcal Septic Shock

Mele JA, Linder S, Capozzi A (Bothin Burn Ctr, San Francisco)
Ann Plast Surg 38:283–290, 1997   7–21

Introduction.—Several causative organisms have been implicated in thromboembolic complication with septic shock, including *Neisseria meningitidis, Hemophilus influenzae,* and β-hemolytic *Streptococcus.* A previously healthy young man had meningococcal meningitis. He had flulike symptoms before admission, with high fever, blurry vision, severe headache, anorexia, photophobia, and an erythematous rash that progressed to a purpura.

Hospital course.—After admission to the hospital, the patient became hypotensive, needed intravenous fluid resuscitation, and continued to have a high fever. His white blood cell count elevated to 31,000 cells/mm^3 and his thrombocytopenia elevated to 50,000 cells/mm^3. His rash progressed to full-thickness skin loss, including subcutaneous fat in many regions and involving the head, neck, and trunk. The lower extremities had the most severe complications, with toes turning black and hard and loss of much skin of the right calf and thigh.

Treatment.—He underwent surgery to débride down to viable tissue; this was followed by wound care. He received wet-to-dry dressings in the areas smaller than 2 cm in diameter. In the larger wounds, delayed primary closure was used to minimize the risk of infection. Several wounds were closed with split-thickness skin grafts. The dorsal foot and heel were treated with local skin flaps. The left foot then received microvascular transplantation. The right foot had the most severe injuries, and the toes were amputated at initial débridement. To obtain a healed wound, below-the-knee amputation was necessary.

Conclusion.—The patient had Waterhouse-Friderichsen syndrome, a fulminating meningococcal septicemia characterized by vomiting, diarrhea, purpura, cyanosis, tonoclonic convulsions, circulatory collapse, and hemorrhage into the adrenal glands. This patient survived after the insult had stabilized. To heal the thromboembolic complications, extensive reconstruction was necessary.

▶ Early treatment of this condition by vigorous intensive care methods reduces mortality. What is most significant is that early diagnosis and treatment have not seemed to alter the morbidity, and massive tissue loss seems to be determined early despite intervention. So far the etiology of this phenomenon and the ability to reverse it are not apparent.

R.E. Salisbury, M.D.

Necrotizing Soft-tissue Infections
Bosshardt TL, Henderson VJ, Organ CH Jr (Univ of California, Davis-East Bay, Oakland)
Arch Surg 131:846–854, 1996   7–22

Objective.—Necrotizing soft-tissue infections (NSTIs) carry a high mortality rate. Diabetes mellitus, IV drug abuse, obesity, malnutrition, older age, peripheral vascular disease, and other systemic diseases contribute to increased NSTI mortality. The causes of NSTIs, the outcomes of patients with NSTIs at a single urban community hospital, and the effect of parenteral drug abuse as a causative factor for NSTIs were evaluated.

Methods.—Between December 11, 1990 and December 28, 1995, the records of 45 consecutive patients (18 women), aged 23 to 84, with NSTIs were reviewed for predisposing factors, interventions, and outcomes.

Results.—Necrotizing fasciitis was diagnosed in 38 patients and necrosis involving the subcutaneous tissue and skin in 7. Risk factors included parenteral drug abuse in 30 patients, diabetes mellitus in 20, obesity in 15, alcohol abuse in 14, and malnutrition in 14. Diabetes, drug abuse, or both was found in 40 patients. The average duration of drug abuse in 19 of 30 patients was 18.84 years, and the drug of choice was heroin in 27 of 30 patients. The proximate cause of infection were determined to be heroin injection in 25 patients, cutaneous infections or ulcers in 5, postoperative infections in 4, perirectal abscesses in 4, and soft-tissue traumas in 3. Necrotizing soft-tissue infections occurred on the extremities in 24 patients, the perineum or buttocks in 9, the trunk in 8, and the head and neck in 4. The patients were treated with fluid resuscitation, surgical débridement, parenteral antibiotics, and supportive therapy. Bacteriology studies showed that 78% of the infections were polymicrobial. Twelve patients (27%) died. Survivors has significantly higher systolic blood pressures than non-survivors on hospital admission and significantly smaller-sized infections. The extent of infection, initial blood pressure, and initial temperature were independent predictors of survival.

Conclusions.—The incidence of NSTIs is increasing in urban areas. Most are polymicrobial. Parenteral drug abuse is a significant cause of NSTIs. The extent of infection is related to risk of mortality. Early, aggressive treatment is critical.

▶ This paper summarizes the clinical outcomes of soft-tissue infections cared for in an urban hospital in the Bay area. The paper's strongest attribute is that it provides a useful summary of epidemiologic information and desribes clinical information, management, survival, and treatment success. Although there is an extensive discussion about various alternative treatments, there is no attempt made to describe how the treatment of this disease has evolved with experience. A review of such a large series of patients is best when the authors summarize how their experience has improved outcome.

W. Garner, M.D.

An Evaluation of the Impact of Social Interaction Skills Training for Facially Disfigured People
Robinson E, Rumsey N, Partridge J (Univ of the West of England, Bristol; Changing Faces, London)
Br J Plast Surg 49:281–289, 1996   7–23

Background.—Individuals with facial disfiguration can have significant psychological problems, largely from difficulties interacting with others. The effects of social interaction skills workshops on the psychological well-being of such patients were described.

Methods.—Sixty-four facially disfigured patients participated in the workshops. Types of disfiguration ranged widely, including scars from burns, cleft lip and palate, birthmarks, facial palsies, cancer-related deformities, and dermatologic problems. Before attending the workshop and 6 weeks and 6 months afterward, the patients filled out the Hospital Anxiety and Depression Scale, the Social Avoidance and Distress Scale, and an open-ended questionnaire. The workshops emphasized social interaction skills to help the patients deal more effectively with others' reactions. Participants shared their experiences and problems in a safe atmosphere. Instruction, modeling, role-playing, feedback, and open discussion were part of the workshop.

Findings.—The high levels of anxiety recorded before the workshop declined significantly 6 weeks after the workshop and remained significantly reduced at the 6-month assessment. Scores on the Social Avoidance and Distress Scale also were significantly lower at follow-up. The patients reported feeling more confident when with others and when meeting new individuals at the 6-week and 6-month assessments. Sixty-one percent of those who had had problems before the workshop reported a positive change afterward.

Conclusions.—The psychological problems of individuals with facial disfiguration need to be addressed. Social interaction skills training appears to effectively relieve many of these problems.

▶ Most plastic surgeons have long, albeit often unknowingly, accepted the unity of the mind-body concept. All too often, our reconstructions fail to return patients to normal, yet we can offer little in the way of further improvement through surgical intervention. The use of directed adjunctive psychological support to teach and inculcate social interaction skills could improve the quality of these patient's lives. Unfortunately, mental health has become an abandoned orphan as health care resources are reapportioned, it is unlikely that these services will be widely in the United States.

S.H. Miller, M.D.

A Late Follow-up of Several Severely Wounded Veterans of World War II

Cannon B (Lincoln, Mass)
Plast Reconstr Surg 98:171–177, 1996

7–24

Introduction.—At the end of World War II, the author and a team of other plastic surgeons were working at Valley Forge General Hospital in Pennsylvania, providing definitive care for the war wounded. After the War, a group of surgeons volunteered for extended service to continue caring for the many patients who were still hospitalized. The author recalls his experience, including long-term follow-up with many of the wounded soldiers.

Organization.—The hospital had a careful triage system, placing the more severely injured men in the "front" wards and those with less severe injuries in the "back" wards, to be followed up later. Operating in the preantibiotic era, the surgeons had 2 operating rooms for "clean" cases and 1 for "septic" cases. The 2 clean operating rooms were organized for maximum efficiency such that 2 operations could be performed simultaneously. From a surgical standpoint, the experience included dealing with very destructive high-velocity missile injuries, massive facial rebuilding with remote flaps and bone grafts, and arduous primary and reconstructive care for the ubiquitous burn and freeze injuries.

Follow-up.—Over the years, the author has interviewed many of the men treated during this experience. The current report summarizes 6 such interviews, including cases of deep freeze injury, shell fragment trauma, high-explosive shell trauma, phosphorus burns, and flame burns in air combat, and flame burns in a ground take-off accident. The definitive treatment of each patient is described. Some of the men have done exceptionally well since their traumatic experience, others less so. A few have kept in close contact and become close friends of the author and his wife.

Discussion.—An experience in a stateside hospital providing definitive plastic surgical care for severely wounded World War II veterans is reviewed. The author emphasizes the satisfaction obtained from that experience, including the expressions of gratitude from the patients he has helped.

▶ A historic treasure.

S.H. Miller, M.D.

The New Medical Marketplace: I. Managed Care

Krieger LM (UCLA Med Ctr, Los Angeles)
Plast Reconstr Surg 98:1095–1101, 1996

7–25

Background.—To best function in the new environment of managed care, plastic surgeons must understand the business principles that underlie managed care. These principles and the specific ways in which managed care companies put these theories into practice were summarized.

Managed Care.—Managed care is a mechanism to decrease health care expenditures by controlling health care utilization. Managed care plans seek to maximize savings and profits by controlling the supply of patients, physicians, and hospitals. All managed care organizational structures integrate financing and delivery of health care. Health maintenance organizations are the most integrated, placing providers at direct or indirect financial risk for providing services. There are 5 types of HMOs: staff model, group model, network model, independent practice association model, and mixed model. Preferred provider organizations act as intermediaries between insurance companies and other health care buyers and providers. Physician-hospital organizations or provider-sponsored organizations are the newest models and range from loosely affiliated independent practice associations and preferred provider organizations to full-service HMOs. Over the years, market evolution has passed through 4 phases.

The mechanisms by which managed care controls the delivery of health care to its members and provider behavior vary by degree of market penetration. In earlier generations, the gatekeeper system was integral to limiting access and cost. Negative and positive incentives are offered to the primary care physician for preventing patients from gaining access. Capitation is a powerful mechanism for increasing profits by minimizing expenditures. In this system, all treatments or referrals provided by the gatekeeper are deducted from his or her monthly stipend, an amount determined by the number of enrollees. In the final generation of market penetration, specialists also are compensated under capitation.

Future Directions.—In the future, managed care will probably become more aggressive in its attempts to expand. Although physicians must face the great challenge of fighting over which treatments will be covered, tools exist to negotiate successfully for the welfare of the patients. The most powerful tool is the cost and outcome study.

▶ This is a good short review, especially the author's description of the well-recognized stages in the evolution of health care delivery systems. It is important for us to understand managed care because it affects our individual practices. It is equally important that we become knowledgeable about its role and potential for dramatically and forever altering health care delivery systems in this country.[1,2]

References

1. Shortell SM, Gillies RR, Anderson DA: The new world of managed care: Creating organized delivery systems. *Health Aff* 13:46–64, 1994.
2. Begun JW, Lippincott RC: *Strategic Adaptation in the Health Profession: Meeting the Challenges of Change.* San Francisco, Jossey-Bass, 1993.

Subject Index

A

Abdomen
  lipoplasty, suction
    intestinal perforation after, 190
    intestinal perforation and peritonitis
      after, 191
  wall
    reconstruction, tensor fascia lata free
      flap in, 265
    recovery after TRAM flap, 226
    sequelae after TRAM flap, 227
Abdominoplasty
  smoking and, 267
  with two fusiform plications, 183
Abrasion
  corneal, in carbon dioxide laser lower
    lid blepharoplasty, 155
Abuse
  drug, parenteral, causing necrotizing
    soft tissue infections, 294
Acne
  scars
    effects of dermabrasion on, 109
    facial, full-face resurfacing with
      Ultrapulse carbon dioxide laser
      with CPG scanner for, 108
Actinic
  keratoses, widespread facial, chemical
    peel *vs.* fluorouracil for, long-term
    efficacy and safety of, 45
Acyclovir
  in prevention of facial herpetic
    infections after chemical peel and
    dermabrasion, 111
Adhesion
  molecules, E- and L-selectin, in
    musculocutaneous flap reperfusion
    injury (in pig), 232
  neutrophil-endothelial,
    CD18-dependent, in
    ischemia-reperfusion injury in
    skeletal muscle, 231
Adhesive
  tissue, long-term appearance of
    lacerations repaired with, 286
Adipose
  tissue, postliposuction histologic
    alterations of, 194
Adolescent
  cleft lip deformities in, secondary,
    correction using dermofat grafts,
    32

cleft lip repair in, effect on maxillary
  morphology in patients with
  unilateral complete cleft lip and
  palate, 27
Aeromonas hydrophilia
  infection after medicinal leech use, 248
Aesthetic
  analysis of eyebrows, 148
  considerations in composite
    rhytidectomy, 139
  outcome of breast implant removal, 205
  refinements in toe-to-hand transfer
    surgery, 262
  results in breast reconstruction,
    reliability of evaluations of, 219
  surgery, 97
    brow, 125
    extremities, 182
    eyelid, 154
    face, 125
    neck, 125
    nose, 167
    quality of life before and after,
      health-related, 97
    skeletal, 116
    skin, 100
    teaching at resident level, 98
    trunk, 182
Agee carpal tunnel release
  system, 70
Aging
  face and smoking, 267
  photoaging, facial
    histologic effects of high-energy
      pulsed carbon dioxide laser for,
      102
    resurfacing for, full-face, with
      Ultrapulse carbon dioxide laser
      with CPG scanner, 108
  treatment of, isolated cervicofacial
    liposuction applied to, 127
Airway
  obstruction in rhinoplasty, septal and
    nasal valvular surgery in correction
    of, 178
  pressure, continuous positive, nasal, for
    obstructive sleep apnea in children
    with craniofacial dysostosis, 16
Ala
  nasal (*see* Nasal, ala)
Allogeneically
  vascularized prefabricated flaps (in
    rabbit), 235

Allograft
cranial bone, cryopreserved onlay,
viability of (in sheep), 2
epidermal, cultured, for deep
partial-thickness burns, 91
vein wrapping,
glutaraldehyde-preserved, of
peripheral nerves, histologic effect
of (in rat), 72
Aluminum
burn injury and, 94
Alveolar
cleft, grafting in
bone, secondary alveolar, 29
morbidity of iliac crest harvest for, 30
Amputation
of lower extremities with failed free
flaps, 256
nipple-aerolar, avoidance in reduction
mammaplasty in cases of extreme
hypertrophy, 214
Anatomical
basis for fasciocutaneous flap from
hypothenar eminence of hand, 241
expanders and implants in breast
reconstruction, 220
Anatomy
surgical, of fat in upper eyelid medial
compartment, 154
vascular, of tendinous intersections of
rectus abdominis muscle, 222
Anchoring
device, new, for tendon reinsertion in
medial canthopexy, 158
Anesthesia
local, outpatient surgery done under,
reflex bradycardia in, 292
tumescent, with lidocaine dose of
55mg/kg for liposuction, 198
Angiogenesis
in wound healing, 272
Angiogenic
growth factor and durability of
prefabricated flaps against bacterial
challenge (in rat), 233
Angiography
in combination with MRI, diagnostic
value in vascular malformations, 34
Animation
surgery, facial, implication of MRI
dynamic analysis of changes in
nasolabial fold in, 132
Ankle
instability after fibular free flap harvest,
260
liposuction of, circumferential, 193

Antibiotics
parenteral, for necrotizing soft tissue
infections, 294
Antibody
antipolymer antibody assay use in
recipients of silicone breast
implants, 201
Antipolymer
antibody assay use in recipients of
silicone breast implants, 201
Apert's syndrome
fronto-orbital advancement in,
extradural deadspace after, in
infant, 14
mental function in, prognosis for, 13
Apnea
sleep, obstructive
craniofacial dysostosis and, nasal
CPAP for, 16
septoplasty for, after cleft lip repair in
infant, 31
Aponeurotic
system, submucosal (*see* SMAS)
Areolar
-nipple amputation avoidance in
reduction mammaplasty in cases of
extreme hypertrophy, 214
Arhinia
total external and internal construction
in, 18
Arm
(*See also* Extremity, upper)
flap, lateral, in reconstruction in
massive upper extremity burns, 93
Arterial
thrombosis causing free flap failure in
lower extremities, 256
Arteriolar
vasoconstriction, CD18-dependent, in
ischemia-reperfusion injury in
skeletal muscle, 231
Ascorbic acid
therapy, delayed, reduced resuscitation
fluid volume for second-degree
burns with (in guinea pig), 77
Aspergillus fumigatus
growth inside saline-filled implants, 208
Atropine
for reflex bradycardia in outpatient
surgery done under local
anesthesia, 292
Augmentation
breast (*see* Mammaplasty,
augmentation)
cheek, by fat injection, large
liponecrotic pseudocyst after, 198

chin, Silastic, progressive bone
  resorption in, labial incompetence
  as marker for, 121
face, lower, with expanded
  polytetrafluoroethylene, 147
lip (*see* Lip, augmentation)
mammaplasty (*see* Mammaplasty,
  augmentation)
penile, guidelines for, 182
pharyngeal wall, autogenous, for
  velopharyngeal dysfunction, 33
Auricular
  graft, composite, correction of
    hypoplastic nasal ala with, 167
Avulsive
  facial injuries, high-energy, 64

B

Bacterial
  challenge, durability of prefabricated
    flaps against (in rat), 233
Ballistic
  facial injuries, high-energy, 64
Bands
  platysma, management of, 130
Bell palsy
  time course of, 56
Biessenberger breast reduction technique
  modified, nipple sensitivity and lactation
    in, 215
Biochemical
  analysis of wound fluid from chronic
    leg ulcers, 285
  changes in muscles affected by
    distraction osteogenesis of
    mandible (in dog), 25
Biodegradable
  positive fixation for endoscopic
    browlift, 149
Biosynthetic
  temporary skin replacement for burns,
    92
Blacks
  photoaged facial skin in, histologic
    effects of high-energy pulsed
    carbon dioxide laser on, 102
Bleeding
  delayed, after flap closure, effects of
    epinephrine infiltration on (in rat),
    284
Blepharoplasty
  lower
    eyelid retraction after, hard palate
      grafts and lateral tarsal strip for,
      161
    transconjunctival, carbon dioxide
      laser, complications of, 155
  new concept in, 165
  transblepharoplasty forehead lift and
    upper face rejuvenation, 152
  transconjunctival, with
    chemoexfoliation, 158
  upper, combined with open coronal
    browlift, safety and efficacy of, 157
Blood
  loss of scalpel *vs.* cutting cautery in
    bilateral reduction mammaplasty,
    213
  supply, and galeo-pericranial flaps in
    forehead, 240
Body
  contour surgery, standardization in
    photography for, 187
  contouring, noninvasive mechanical,
    outcome, 198
  sculpture, 188
Bone
  allografts, cranial, cryopreserved onlay,
    viability of (in sheep), 2
  graft
    alveolar, secondary, for cleft, 29
    cranial, in mandibular condyle
      reconstruction (in monkey), 1
  resorption, progressive, in Silastic chin
    augmentation, labial incompetence
    as marker for, 121
Bony
  deviation of nose, external, unilateral
    osteotomies for, 180
Brachial
  plexopathies, electrodiagnostic testing
    in, 68
Bradycardia
  reflex, in outpatient surgery done under
    local anesthesia, 292
Breast, 199
  augmentation (*see* Mammaplasty,
    augmentation)
  cancer, 219
  deformity
    post implantectomy/capsulectomy,
      bilateral TRAM flap reconstruction
      for, 224
    tuberous, classification and treatment,
      209
  implant
    anatomical, in breast reconstruction,
      220
    complications leading to surgery after,
      200
    deformity after, bilateral TRAM flap
      reconstruction for, 224
    removal, outcome of, 204
    removal, outcome of, aesthetic, 205

saline-filled, microbial growth inside, 208
silicone, 199
silicone, antipolymer antibody assay after, 201
silicone, textured or smooth, for augmentation, follow-up, 207
reconstruction, 219
aesthetic results in, reliability of evaluations of, 219
with anatomical expanders and implants, 220
autologous tissue, spontaneous return of sensibility in breasts after, 229
flap for, TRAM (*see* TRAM flap, breast reconstruction)
smoking and, 267
reduction (*see* Mammaplasty, reduction)
scars, hypertrophic, prevention with silicone sheets, 287
sensibility in, spontaneous return after autologous tissue breast reconstruction, 229
tuberous, extremely hypoplastic, surgical correction of, 211
Brow
surgery, aesthetic, 125
Browlift
endoscopic
fixation for, biodegradable positive, 149
preventing hairline elevation in, 151
open coronal, combined with upper blepharoplasty, safety and efficacy of, 157
Bulimic patient
lipoplasty in, 192
Burn(s), 77
deep
Index of Deep Burn Injury, in children, 84
partial-thickness, cultured epidermal allografts for, 91
edema in skin after, effect of recombinant neutral endopeptidase on (in guinea pig), 94
emotional and psychosocial factors in hospitalized patients after, 85
energy and protein provisions after, in children, 80
hyperbaric oxygen therapy for, 83
massive upper extremity, free flap reconstruction in, 93
microminerals and, essential, 94
ornithine α-ketoglutarate metabolism after enteral administration in, 82
pain
procedural, intensity under conditions of varying physical control by patient, 89
wound debridement, topical 2% lidocaine gel in, 89
prognostic indicators in elderly with, 79
rehabilitation after, critical pathways to enhance, 86
resuscitation (in sheep), 78
second-degree, reduced resuscitation fluid volume with delayed initiation of ascorbic acid therapy for (in guinea pig), 77
skin expansion after, problems, rules, and indications, 83
survivors, pediatric
applying what they have to say to future therapeutic interventions, 88
competence and physical impairment after burns of more than 80% total body surface area, 87
wounds, excised, Dermagraft-transitional covering of, 92
Burning
eyelid, in carbon dioxide laser lower lid blepharoplasty, 155

C

Cachexia
tumor necrosis factor-α inhibits collagen α1 gene expression and wound healing in (in mice), 280
Calves
liposuction of, circumferential, 193
Camera
ultraviolet, use to enhance appearance of photodamage and other skin conditions, 114
Cancer
breast, 219
skin, 45
tongue, neurovascular infrahyoid muscle flap for tongue reconstruction in, 54
Candela SPTL-1 lasers
comparison to other pulsed dye lasers, 100
Canthopexy
medial, tendon reinsertion in, new anchoring device for, 158
Capsulectomy
breast deformity after, bilateral TRAM flap reconstruction for, 224
Carbon dioxide
laser (*see* Laser, carbon dioxide)

Cardiomyoplasty
vascular delay improves latissimus dorsi muscle perfusion and function for use in (in dog), 238
Care
managed, 296
Carpal
tunnel
MRI detection of median nerve compression in, 69
operated, bilateral fast MRI of, 68
release, endoscopic, single-portal, 70
syndrome, electrodiagnostic testing in, 67
Cartilage
concavities, nasal tip, suture correction of, 168
tragal cartilage-temoroparietal and deep temporal fascia sandwich graft technique, modified, for repair of nasal septal perforations, 181
Cast
immobilization in scapholunate dissociation associated with distal radius fractures, 76
Cautery
scalpel *vs.* cutting, blood loss of, in bilateral reduction mammaplasty, 213
CD18
-dependent neutrophil–endothelial adhesion and arteriolar vasoconstriction in ischemia-reperfusion injury in skeletal muscle, 231
Cell
viability of cultured epithelium after freezing storage, 90
Ceramic
containing crosslinked collagen as new cranial onlay and inlay material (in rabbit), 2
Cervicofacial
contours, value of liposuction in improvement of, 125
liposuction, isolated, applied to treatment of aging, 127
Cervicoplasty
nonexcisional anterior approach, 197
Cheek
augmentation by fat injection, large liponecrotic pseudocyst after, 198
Chemical
peel (*see* Peel, chemical)
Chemoexfoliation (*see* Peel, chemical)
Children
burns in
deep, Index of Deep Burn Injury, 84

energy and protein provisions after, 80
of more than 80% of total body surface area, competence and physical impairment after, 87
survivors of, applying what they have to say to future therapeutic interventions, 88
craniofacial dysostosis in, obstructive sleep apnea in, nasal CPAP for, 16
infant (*see* Infant)
lacerations repaired with tissue adhesive in, long-term appearance of, 286
myelomeningocele repair in, tissue expansion in, 39
otoplasty in, endoscopic, 43
plastic surgery in, endoscopic, 42
sural nerve harvest in, endoscopic, 250
tissue expansion in, risk factors for complications in, 268
tissue transfer in, free, 252
Chin
augmentation, Silastic, progressive bone resorption in, labial incompetence as marker for, 121
Chisels
Delta-shaped, in treatment of over-wide nasofrontal angle, 175
Chondrocutaneous
ear helical free flap for reconstruction of defects of nasal tip, columella and/or ala, 55
Chromium
burn injury and, 94
Cigarette
smoking, effect on plastic surgery and microsurgery, 266
Cleft
alveolar, grafting in
bone, secondary alveolar, 29
morbidity of iliac crest harvest for, 30
lip
deformities, secondary, correction using dermofat grafts, 32
repair, effect on maxillary morphology in patients with unilateral complete cleft lip and palate, 27
repair, septoplasty for obstructive sleep apnea in infant after, 31
unilateral complete cleft lip and palate, effect of cleft lip repair on maxillary morphology, 27
palate
hearing histories and, 29
timing of hard palatal closure, 27

unilateral complete cleft lip and
palate, effect of cleft lip repair on
maxillary morphology, 27
Closure
vacuum-assisted (*see* Vacuum, -assisted
closure)
CO$_2$
laser (*see* Laser, carbon dioxide)
Cold
intolerance after peripheral nerve injury,
natural history and severity of
symptoms, 75
sensitivity after nerve injury, long-term
follow-up, 74
Collagen
α1 gene expression in cachexia inhibited
by tumor necrosis factor-α, and
wound healing (in mice), 280
biosynthesis in healing wound, effect of
macrophage stimulation on (in
rodent), 277
crosslinked, ceramic containing, as new
cranial onlay and inlay material (in
rabbit), 2
skin equivalents produced with, living,
grafting of (in mice), 271
Colloid
vs. crystalloid resuscitation after burns
(in sheep), 78
Colony-stimulating factor
granulocyte-macrophage, in chronic leg
ulcers, 279
Columella
reconstruction, chondrocutaneous ear
helical free flap for, 55
Comfeel Ulcer Dressing
for full-thickness wounds, comparative
study (in pig), 283
Competence
of pediatric survivors of burns of more
than 80% total body surface area,
87
Compression
median nerve
detected by MRI of carpal tunnel, 69
recurrent, vein graft wrapping for, 71
Concavities
cartilage, nasal tip, suture correction of,
168
Conchal
bowl skin grafting in nasal tip
reconstruction, 51
Conjunctiva
blepharoplasty through
with chemoexfoliation, 158
lower lid, carbon dioxide laser,
complications of, 155

Conjunctivitis
after blepharoplasty, carbon dioxide
laser lower lid, 155
Construction
nasal, total external and internal, in
arhinia, 18
Contour
body, surgery, standardization in
photography for, 187
cervicofacial, value of liposuction in
improvement of, 125
change in muscle transplants to lower
leg, significant postoperative, lack
of, 258
facial
in craniofacial malformations,
congenital, microsurgical correction
of, 19
new use for temporalis superficialis
fascia in, 141
Contouring
body, noninvasive mechanical, outcome,
198
digastric muscle, for rejuvenation of
submental area of face, 198
Contraction
in wound healing, 272
Copper
burn injury and, 94
Cornea
abrasion in carbon dioxide laser lower
lid blepharoplasty, 155
Corset
for platysma bands, 130
Cosmetic
surgery, nasal tip, and thick skin, 169
Costs
resource, of free *vs.* conventional
TRAM flap breast reconstruction,
223
CPAP
nasal, for obstructive sleep apnea in
children with craniofacial
dysostosis, 16
CPG scanner
Ultrapulse carbon dioxide laser with,
for full-face resurfacing for rhytids,
photoaging, and acne scars, 108
Cranial
bone
allografts, cryopreserved onlay,
viability of (in sheep), 2
graft mandibular condyle
reconstruction (in monkey), 1
onlay and inlay material, new, ceramic
containing crosslinked collagen as
(in rabbit), 2

Craniofacial
  asymmetry and lambdoid stenosis,
    long-term outcomes, 7
  dysostosis, obstructive sleep apnea in
    children with, nasal CPAP for, 16
  malformations, congenital,
    microsurgical correction of facial
    contour in, 19
Cranioplasty
  complex, *vs.* synostectomy for sagittal
    synostosis, 9
Craniosynostosis
  classification of previously unclassified
    cases of, 11
  skull surgery in, posterior, 15
Critical pathways
  to enhance rehabilitation of burn
    patients, 86
Cryopreserved
  allografts, onlay cranial bone, viability
    of (in sheep), 2
  skin, cadaver, for temporary coverage of
    excised burn wounds, 92
Cryospraying
  tumescent dermasanding with, 110
Cryotherapy
  combined with superpulsed carbon
    dioxide laser for facial rhytids, 105
Crystalloid
  vs. colloid resuscitation after burns (in
    sheep), 78
Cultured
  epidermal allografts for deep
    partial-thickness burns, 91
  epithelium, structural changes and cell
    viability after freezing storage, 90
Cutaneous (*see* Skin)
Cynosure Photogenica V lasers
  comparison to other pulsed dye lasers,
    100
Cyst
  after fat injection, 196

D

Deadspace
  extradural, after infant fronto-orbital
    advancement in Apert syndrome,
    14
Debridement
  pain, burn wound, topical 2% lidocaine
    gel for, 89
  surgical, in necrotizing soft tissue
    infections, 294
Deepithelialized
  flaps, buried local, in upper and lower
    lip augmentation, 143

Deformity(ies)
  (*See also* Malformations)
  breast
    post implantectomy/capsulectomy,
     bilateral TRAM flap reconstruction
     for, 224
    tuberous, classification and treatment,
     209
  cleft lip, secondary, correction using
    dermofat grafts, 32
  after fat injection, 196
  skin, continuous expansion for, 268
Degenerative
  conditions, 56
Delta-shaped chisels
  in treatment of over-wide nasofrontal
    angle, 175
Dermabrasion
  effects on acne scarring, 109
  prevention of facial herpetic infections
    after, 111
Dermagraft
  -transitional covering of excised burn
    wounds, 92
Dermasanding
  tumescent, with cryospraying, 110
Dermatofibrosarcoma
  protuberans
    excision for, wide and deep block,
     including underlying muscle, 50
    growth characteristics based on
     tumor modeling and review of
     cases treated with Mohs surgery, 49
    Mohs micrographic surgery *vs.* wide
     surgical excision for, 47
Dermofat
  grafts for correction of secondary cleft
    lip deformities, 32
Dermoids
  facial, endoscopic plastic surgery for, in
    children, 42
Dermolipopexy
  nasolabial, 133
Diabetes mellitus
  insulin-induced lipohypertrophy in,
    liposuction for, 185
  ulcers in, effects of electrical stimulation
    on wound healing in patients with,
    275
Digastric
  muscle
    contouring for rejuvenation of
     submental area of face, 198
    histopathologic and biochemical
     changes after distraction
     osteogenesis of mandible (in dog),
     25

Digital
    replantation and smoking, 267
Disfiguration
    facial, impact of social interaction skills
        training for patients with, 295
Distraction
    osteogenesis of mandible,
        histopathologic and biochemical
        changes in muscles affected by (in
        dog), 25
DNA
    cDNAs, transforming growth factor-β1,
        particle-mediated gene transfer
        with, effect on wound repair (in
        rat), 276
Drainage
    suction, for parotid leakage after
        rhytidectomy, 140
Dressings
    occlusive, for full-thickness wounds,
        comparison of three (in pig), 283
Drug
    abuse, parenteral, causing necrotizing
        soft tissue infections, 294
DuDERM
    for full-thickness wounds, comparative
        study (in pig), 283
Dye
    laser
        flashlamp-pumped, for port-wine
            stains, 5-year assessment of, 36
        pulsed, 585 nm, are they all
            equivalent? 100
Dysostosis
    craniofacial, obstructive sleep apnea in
        children with, nasal CPAP for, 16

E

Ear
    helical free flap, chondrocutaneous, for
        reconstruction of defects of nasal
        tip, columella and/or ala, 55
    prominent, endoscopic-assisted
        correction of, 42
    replantation without microsurgery, 61
    Stahl's, operation for, 36
Edema
    after fat injection, 196
    leg, after fibular free flap harvest, 260
    pulmonary, complicating tumescent
        liposuction, 189
    skin, after burns, effect of recombinant
        neutral endopeptidase on (in guinea
        pig), 94
Elbow
    flexion, results of functioning free
        muscle transplantation for, 264

Elderly
    burns in, prognostic indicators, 79
    rhytidectomy in, management of parotid
        leakage after, 140
    tissue transfers in, microvascular free,
        254
Electrical
    stimulation, effects on wound healing in
        patients with diabetic ulcers, 275
Electrocautery
    latissimus dorsi flap harvested by, and
        seroma formation, 245
Electrodiagnostic
    testing in hand surgery, 67
Electromagnetic
    fields, pulsed, in cutaneous wound
        healing (in rat), 273
Emotional
    factors in burn patients during
        hospitalization, 85
Endopeptidase
    recombinant neutral, decreases edema in
        skin after burns (in guinea pig), 94
Endoscopic
    -assisted intraoral approach for
        masseteric hypertrophy, 43
    -assisted lift, combined with
        conventional, for facial
        rejuvenation, 134
    browlift
        fixation for, biodegradable positive,
            149
        preventing hairline elevation in, 151
    carpal tunnel release, single-portal, 70
    forehead lift, technique, 150
    forehead-scalp flap fixation with K-wire,
        152
    otoplasty, 42
    plastic surgery, pediatric, 42
    rhytidectomy, laser, subperiosteal
        minimally invasive, 137
    sural nerve harvest in children, 250
    technique of free latissimus dorsi muscle
        transfer, 255
Endothelial
    -neutrophil adhesion, CD18-dependent,
        in ischemia-reperfusion injury in
        skeletal muscle, 231
Energy
    provisions for thermally injured
        children, 80
Enteral
    administration in burn patients,
        ornithine α-ketoglutarate
        metabolism after, 82
Enterobacter cloacae
    growth inside saline-filled implants, 208

Epidermal
  allografts, cultured, for deep
      partial-thickness burns, 91
Epinephrine
  infiltration, effects on delayed bleeding
      after flap closure (in rat), 284
Epithelium
  cultured, structural changes and cell
      viability after freezing storage, 90
Escherichia coli
  growth inside saline-filled implants, 208
E-selectin
  adhesion molecules in
      musculocutaneous flap reperfusion
      injury (in pig), 232
Excision
  wide and deep block, including
      underlying muscle for
      dermatofibrosarcoma protuberans,
      50
  wide surgical, *vs.* Mohs micrographic
      surgery for dermatofibrosarcoma
      protuberans, 47
Excisional
  wound repair, type I and type II
      receptors for transforming growth
      factor-β isoforms are expressed
      subsequent to TGF-β ligands
      during (in sheep), 282
Expanders
  anatomical, in breast reconstruction,
      220
Expansion
  skin, in burn patients, problems, rules,
      and indications, 83
  tissue (*see* Tissue, expansion)
Extender
  skin, clinical evaluation of, 270
Extracellular
  matrix in wound healing, 272
Extradural
  deadspace after infant fronto-orbital
      advancement in Apert syndrome,
      14
Extraocular
  muscles, combined paresis and
      restriction after orbital fracture, 66
Extrasynovial
  tendon gliding resistance through A2
      pulley, 77
Extremity
  lower
      (*See also* Leg)
      fate with failed free flaps, 256
      ischemic lesions, single-stage
          revascularization and free flap
          coverage for, 257
  surgery, aesthetic, 182

upper
  burns, massive, free flap
      reconstruction in, 93
  coverage, neurocutaneous island flaps
      in, 242
  lymphedema, postmastectomy,
      microwave heating in, 56
  trauma, 67
Eyebrow
  aesthetic analysis of, 148
Eyelid
  burning in carbon dioxide laser lower
      lid blepharoplasty, 155
  lower
      medial tarsal suspension of, for
          paralytic lagophthalmos, 159
      perforation in carbon dioxide laser
          blepharoplasty, 155
      retraction after blepharoplasty, hard
          palate grafts and lateral tarsal strip
          for, 161
  surgery, aesthetic, 154
  upper, surgical anatomy of fat in medial
      compartment, 154

F

Face
  (*See also* Facial)
  acne scars, Ultrapulse carbon dioxide
      laser with CPG scanner for full-face
      resurfacing for, 108
  aging, and smoking, 267
  animation surgery, implication of MRI
      dynamic analysis of changes in
      nasolabial fold in, 132
  herpetic infections after chemical peel
      and dermabrasion, prevention of,
      111
  injuries, high-energy ballistic and
      avulsive, 64
  lift (*see* Facelift)
  lower
      augmentation of, expanded
          polytetrafluoroethylene, 147
      width, angle-splitting ostectomy for
          reducing, 116
  peel (*see* Peel)
  photoaged, Ultrapulse carbon dioxide
      laser with CPG scanner for full-face
      resurfacing for, 108
  reconstruction, primary, for high-energy
      ballistic and avulsive injuries, 64
  rejuvenation (*see* Rejuvenation, facial)
  resurfacing, full-face, with Ultrapulse
      carbon dioxide laser with CPG
      scanner, for rhytids, photoaging,
      and acne scars, 108

308 / Subject Index

rhytids (*see* Rhytids, facial)
surgery
   aesthetic, 125
   plastic, liposhaver in, 184
Facelift
   biplane, with maximal skin underlining
     and vertical SMAS flap, results of,
     136
   incisions in, parallel hairline *vs.*
     perpendicular, 131
   SMAS, lateral and standard,
     comparison with extended SMAS
     and composite rhytidectomies, 138
   SMILE, 137
   smoking and, 266
Facial
   (*See also* Face)
   cervicofacial
     contours, value of liposuction in
      improvement of, 125
     liposuction, isolated, applied to
      treatment of aging, 127
   contour
     in craniofacial malformations,
      congenital, microsurgical correction
      of, 19
     new use for temporalis superficialis
      fascia in, 141
   craniofacial (*see* Craniofacial)
   dermoids, endoscopic plastic surgery
     for, in children, 42
   disfiguration, impact of social
     interaction skills training for
     patients with, 295
   hemifacial microsomia, mandibular
     asymmetry in, longitudinal analysis
     of, 21
   keratoses, widespread actinic, chemical
     peel *vs.* fluorouracil for, long-term
     efficacy and safety of, 45
   muscle function, coordinated lower,
     patterns of, 57
   paralysis after cervicofacial liposuction,
     125
   reanimation, and patterns of
     coordinated lower facial muscle
     function, 57
   skin, photoaged, histologic effects of
     high-energy pulsed carbon dioxide
     laser on, 102
Fascia
   lata, tensor, free flap, in abdominal wall
     reconstruction, 265
   temporalis superficialis, new use in
     facial contour, 141

temporoparietal and deep temporal
   fascia-tragal cartilage sandwich
   graft technique, modified, for repair
   of nasal septal perforations, 181
Fasciitis
   necrotizing, 294
Fasciocutaneous
   flap from hypothenar eminence of hand,
     anatomical basis for, 241
Fat
   in eyelid medial compartment, upper,
     surgical anatomy of, 154
   grafting, 184
   injection
     cheek augmentation by, large
      liponecrotic pseudocyst formation
      after, 198
     long-term follow-up, 195
   pad, nasolabial, pathogenesis and
     treatment of, 133
Fetus
   hyaluronic acid of wound fluid in (in
     rabbit), 274
Fibroplasia
   in wound healing, 272
Fibular
   free flap harvest, leg morbidity and
     function after, 259
Film
   dressing for full-thickness wounds (in
     pig), 283
Finger
   reconstruction, aesthetic refinements in
     toe-to-hand transfer for, 262
Fixation
   biodegradable positive, for endoscopic
     browlift, 149
   flap, endoscopic forehead-scalp, with
     K-wire, 152
Flap, 231
   closure, delayed bleeding after, effects of
     epinephrine infiltration on (in rat),
     284
   ear helical free, chondrocutaneous, for
     reconstruction of defects of nasal
     tip, columella and/or ala, 55
   fascia lata, tensor
     free, in abdominal wall
      reconstruction, 265
     myocutaneous, in reconstruction after
      ilioinguinal node dissection, 242
   fasciocutaneous, from hypothenar
     eminence of hand, anatomical basis
     for, 241
   fibular free, harvest, leg morbidity and
     function after, 259
   fixation, endoscopic forehead-scalp,
     with K-wire, 152

forearm, radial, donor site
    complications and morbidity, 263
free
  coverage of ischemic lower limb
      lesions after single-stage
      revascularization, 257
  failed, fate of lower extremities with,
      256
  reconstruction in massive upper
      extremity burns, 93
  success, and ischemia time, 251
galeo-pericranial, in forehead, 240
gracilis myocutaneous, in perineal
    hernia repair, 243
infrahyoid muscle, neurovascular, in
    tongue reconstruction, 54
latissimus dorsi
  donor site, seroma in, causes and
      prevention, 245
  donor site, seroma in, prevention of,
      246
  perfusion and function, in
      cardiomyoplasty, vascular delay
      improves (in dog), 238
  sliding shape-designed, 244
local, buried deepithelialized, in upper
    and lower lip augmentation, 143
lumbar periosteal turnover, in
    myelomeningocele closure, 37
musculocutaneous, reperfusion injury,
    E- and L-selectin adhesion
    molecules in (in pig), 232
neurocutaneous island, in upper limb
    coverage, 242
platysma, complete, for platysma bands,
    130
prefabricated
  allogeneically vascularized (in rabbit),
      235
  durability against bacterial challenge
      (in rat), 233
prefabrication
  free flap, for tracheal reconstruction
      (in goat), 236
  impact of tissue expansion on (in
      rabbit), 234
rectus abdominis, transverse
    myocutaneous (*see* TRAM flap)
TRAM (*see* TRAM flap)
YV-advancement, 247
Flexion
  elbow, results of functioning free muscle
      transplantation for, 264
Flexor
  digitorum profundus tendon gliding
      resistance through A2 pulley, 77
Fluid
  resuscitation

in necrotizing soft tissue infections,
    294
volume, reduced for second-degree
    burns with delayed initiation of
    ascorbic acid therapy (in guinea
    pig), 77
wound
  hyaluronic acid of, in adult and fetus
      (in rabbit), 274
  from leg ulcers, chronic, biochemical
      analysis of, 285
Fluorouracil
  vs. Jessner's solution and 35%
      trichloroacetic acid for widespread
      facial actinic keratoses, long-term
      efficacy and safety of, 45
Forearm
  flap, radial, donor site complications
      and morbidity, 263
  median and ulnar nerves in, tubular *vs.*
      conventional repair of, 73
Forehead
  galeo-pericranial flaps in, 240
  lift
    endoscopic, technique, 150
    transblepharoplasty, 152
  -scalp flap fixation with K-wire,
      endoscopic, 152
Fracture
  orbit, combined paresis and restriction
      of extraocular muscles after, 66
  radius, distal, scapholunate dissociation
      associated with, cast
      immobilization for, 76
Freezing
  storage, structural changes and cell
      viability of cultured epithelium
      after, 90
Fronto-orbital
  advancement in Apert's syndrome,
      extradural deadspace after, in
      infant, 14
Furosemide
  in pulmonary edema after tumescent
      liposuction, 189

G

Galea
  graft for lip augmentation revision, 145
Galeo-pericranial
  flaps in forehead, 240
Gene
  collagen α1, expression in cachexia,
      inhibition by tumor necrosis
      factor-α, and wound healing (in
      mice), 280

transfer, particle-mediated, with
transforming growth factor-β1
cDNAs enhances wound repair (in
rat), 276
Genioplasty
osseous, simultaneous with meloplasty,
119
Glucan
phosphate macrophage modulation,
effect on collagen biosynthesis (in
rodent), 278
Glutaraldehyde
-preserved allograft vein wrapping of
peripheral nerves, histologic effect
of (in rat), 72
Gluteal
thigh flap reconstruction in massive
upper extremity burns, 93
Goldenhaar's syndrome
microsurgical correction of facial
contour in, 20
Gore-Tex
implants, wide, in lip augmentation and
nasolabial groove correction, 142
Gracilis
flap
free, for recalcitrant chronic venous
ulcer, 261
myocutaneous, in perineal hernia
repair, 243
muscle transplant, functioning free, for
elbow flexion, results of, 264
Graft
allograft (*see* Allograft)
auricular composite, correction of
hypoplastic nasal ala with, 167
bone
alveolar, secondary, for cleft, 29
cranial, in mandibular condyle
reconstruction (in monkey), 1
dermofat, for correction of secondary
cleft lip deformities, 32
galea, for lip augmentation revision,
145
mini-slit graft hair transplantation using
Ultrapulse carbon dioxide laser
handpiece, 99
palate, hard, for postblepharoplasty
lower eyelid retraction, 161
sandwich, modified tragal
cartilage-temporoparietal and deep
temporal fascia, for repair of nasal
septal perforations, 181
skin, conchal bowel, in nasal tip
reconstruction, 51
subgalea, for lip augmentation revision,
145

vein, wrapping for recurrent
compression of median nerve, 71
Grafting
alveolar cleft, morbidity of iliac crest
harvest for, 30
fat, 184
of skin equivalents, living, produced
using collagens (in mice), 271
Granulation
tissue in wound healing, 272
Granulocyte
-macrophage colony-stimulating factor
in chronic leg ulcers, 279
Granuloma
after blepharoplasty, carbon dioxide
laser lower lid, 155
Growth
factor
angiogenic, and durability of
prefabricated flaps against bacterial
challenge (in rat), 233
transforming growth factor-β
isoforms, type I and type II
receptors for, expression subsequent
to TGF-β ligands during excisional
wound repair (in sheep), 282
transforming growth factor-β1
cDNAs, particle-mediated gene
transfer with, effect on wound
repair (in rat), 276
Gunshot
wounds to face, primary reconstruction
for, 65

H

Hair
transplantation
laser, 101
mini-slit graft, using Ultrapulse
carbon dioxide laser handpiece, 99
Hairline
elevation in endoscopic browlifts,
prevention of, 151
incisions, parallel, *vs.* perpendicular
incisions, in facelift, 131
Hand
hypothenar eminence of, anatomical
basis of fasciocutaneous flap from,
241
surgery, electrodiagnostic testing in, 67
toe joint transfer to, vascularized, 261
toe-to-hand transfer surgery, aesthetic
refinements in, 262
Handpiece
laser, Ultrapulse carbon dioxide, use in
mini-slit graft hair transplantation,
99

Head and neck
reconstruction, 51
microsurgical, selection of
appropriate recipient vessels in, 248
trauma, 61
Healing
surgical, impaired, and smoking (in
animals), 267
of tissue defects, use of negative
pressure to promote, 289
wound, 271
in cachexia, and tumor necrosis
factor-α inhibition of collagen α1
gene expression (in mice), 280
collagen biosynthesis in, effect of
macrophage stimulation on (in
rodent), 277
cutaneous, pulsed electromagnetic
fields in (in rat), 273
in diabetic ulcer patients, effects of
electrical stimulation on, 275
gene transfer with transforming
growth factor-β1 cDNAs enhances,
particle-mediated (in rat), 276
interferences, potential solutions for,
273
smoking and, 267
Health
-related quality of life before and after
aesthetic surgery, 97
status after breast reduction surgery,
216
Hearing
histories in children with and without
cleft palate, 29
Heating
microwave, in postmastectomy upper
limb lymphedema, 56
Hematoma
after fat injection, 196
after reduction of platysma bands, 130
small, after simultaneous osseous
genioplasty and meloplasty, 119
Hemifacial
microsomia, mandibular asymmetry in,
longitudinal analysis of, 21
Hemorrhage
in blepharoplasty, carbon dioxide laser
lower lid, 155
Hemostatic
process in wound healing, 272
Hernia
perineal, repair using gracilis
myocutaneous flap, 243
Herpetic
infections, facial, prevention after
chemical peel and dermabrasion,
111

Hirudo medicinalis
exploring use of, 248
Histoacryl Blue
lacerations repaired with, long-term
appearance of, 286
Histologic
alterations of adipose tissue after
liposuction, 194
effects
of barrier vein wrapping of peripheral
nerves (in rat), 72
of laser treatments, 585 nm pulsed
dye, 100
of laser treatments, high-energy
pulsed carbon dioxide, on
photoaged facial skin, 102
evaluation after conchal bowl skin
grafting in nasal tip reconstruction,
51
findings after Obagi's modified
trichloroacetic acid peel, 112
Histopathologic
changes in muscles affected by
distraction osteogenesis of
mandible (in dog), 25
Hospitalization
emotional and psychosocial factors in
burn patients during, 85
Hyaluronic acid
of wound fluid in adult and fetus (in
rabbit), 274
Hydrocolloid
dressings for full-thickness wounds (in
pig), 283
Hydroxyapatite
particulate, with crosslinked collagen, as
new cranial onlay and inlay
material (in rabbit), 2
Hyperbaric
oxygen therapy for burns, 83
Hyperpigmentation
late, after carbon dioxide laser lower lid
blepharoplasty, 155
Hypertonic
saline in burn resuscitation (in sheep),
78
Hypertrophic
scar (*see* Scar, hypertrophic)
Hypertrophy
masseteric, endoscope-assisted intraoral
approach for, 43
Hypoplastic
nasal ala correction using auricular
composite graft, 167
tuberous breast, extremely, surgical
correction of, 211

Hypothenar
 eminence of hand, anatomical basis of
  fasciocutaneous flap from, 241

I

Iliac
 crest harvest for alveolar cleft grafting,
  morbidity of, 30
Ilioinguinal
 node dissection, tensor fasciae lata
  myocutaneous flap reconstruction
  after, 242
Image
 analysis, quantification and distribution
  of nasal sebaceous glands using,
  170
Imaging
 magnetic resonance (*see* Magnetic
  resonance imaging)
Immobilization
 cast, in scapholunate dissociation
  associated with distal radius
  fractures, 76
Implant
 breast (*see* Breast, implant)
 polyethylene, porous, in reconstruction
  of microtic external ear, 62
 polytef, wide, in lip augmentation and
  nasolabial groove correction, 142
Incision
 labiocolumellar crease, in rhinoplasty,
  170
 parallel hairline *vs.* perpendicular, in
  facelift, 131
Infant
 Apert's syndrome in
  fronto-orbital advancement in,
   extradural deadspace after, 14
  prognosis for mental function in, 13
 septoplasty for obstructive sleep apnea
  in, after cleft lip repair, 31
 synostosis in, sagittal (*see* Synostosis,
  sagittal)
Infection
 after fat injection, 196
 flap failure due to, free, in lower
  extremities, 256
 herpetic, facial, prevention after
  chemical peel and dermabrasion,
  111
 after leech use, medicinal, 248
 necrotizing soft tissue, 294
 after reduction of platysma bands, 130
 after rhinoplasty with labiocolumellar
  crease incision, 171
 wound, after simultaneous osseous
  genioplasty and meloplasty, 119

Inflammatory
 conditions, 56
Infrahyoid
 muscle flap, neurovascular, in tongue
  reconstruction, 54
Infusion
 pump, tissue expansion for skin
  deformities using, 269
Inlay
 material, new cranial, ceramic
  containing crosslinked collagen as
  (in rabbit), 2
Insulin
 -induced lipohypertrophy treated by
  liposuction, 185
Interleukin
 -1RA levels and reperfusion injury in
  venous ulceration, 58
 -6 levels and reperfusion injury in
  venous ulceration, 58
Intestinal
 perforation after abdominal suction
  lipoplasty, 190, 191
Intradermal
 repair, polydioxanone *vs.* polyglactin
  910 in, 288
Intraoral
 approach, endoscope-assisted, for
  masseteric hypertrophy, 43
Intrasynovial
 tendon gliding resistance through A2
  pulley, 77
IQ
 in Apert's syndrome, 13
Iron
 burn injury and, 94
Ischemia
 lesions, lower limb, single-stage
  revascularization and free flap
  coverage for, 257
 -reperfusion injury in skeletal muscle,
  231
 time and free flap success, 251

J

Jejunal
 free-tissue transfer, prefabricated, for
  tracheal reconstruction (in rat), 237
Jessner's solution
 35% trichloroacetic acid and, *vs.*
  fluorouracil for widespread facial
  actinic keratoses, long-term efficacy
  and safety of, 45
Joint
 stiffness and instability after fibular free
  flap harvest, 260
 toe, vascularized, transfer to hand, 261

K

Kaplan Pendulaser 115
  periocular skin reshaping by, 156
Keratoses
  actinic, widespread facial, chemical peel
    vs. fluorouracil for, long-term
    efficacy and safety of, 45
Kirschner wire
  endoscopic forehead-scalp flap fixation
    with, 152
Klebsiella pneumoniae
  growth inside saline-filled implants, 208
Knee
  liposuction of, circumferential, 193
K-wire
  endoscopic forehead-scalp fixation with,
    152

L

Labial (*see* Lip)
Labiocolumellar
  crease incision in rhinoplasty, 170
Lacerations
  repaired with tissue adhesive, long-term
    appearance of, 286
Lactation
  preservation in two methods of breast
    reduction, 215
Lagophthalmos
  paralytic, surgical repair by medial
    tarsal suspension of lower lid, 159
Lambdoid
  stenosis and craniofacial asymmetry,
    long-term outcomes, 7
  synostosis, true, *vs.* positional molding,
    4
Laser
  carbon dioxide
    blepharoplasty, transconjunctival
      lower lid, complications of, 155
    handpiece, Ultrapulse, use in mini-slit
      graft hair transplantation, 99
    high-energy, for facial rhytids, 106
    high-energy, histologic effects on
      photoaged facial skin, 102
    periocular skin reshaping by, 156
    superpulsed, combined with
      cryotherapy, for facial rhytids, 105
    Ultrapulse, with CPG scanner, for
      full-face resurfacing for rhytids,
      photoaging, and acne scars, 108
    ultrapulsed, for skin resurfacing, 108
  dye
    flashlamp-pumped, for port-wine
      stains, 5-year assessment of, 36

    pulsed, 585 nm, are they all
      equivalent? 100
    hair transplantation, 101
    handpiece, Ultrapulse carbon dioxide,
      use in mini-slit graft hair
      transplantation, 99
    rhytidectomy, endoscopic, subperiosteal
      minimally invasive, 137
    skin resurfacing, 107
Latissimus
  dorsi
    flap, donor site, seroma in, causes
      and prevention, 245
    flap, donor site, seroma in, prevention
      of, 246
    flap, free, for venous ulcer,
      recalcitrant chronic, 261
    flap, free, in reconstruction after
      massive upper extremity burns, 93
    flap, musculocutaneous, reperfusion
      injury, E- and L-selectin adhesion
      molecules in (in pig), 232
    flap, sliding shape-designed, 244
    muscle transfer, free, endoscopic, 255
    muscle use in cardiomyoplasty,
      vascular delay improves muscle
      perfusion and function (in dog),
      238
Leatherneck
  skin after reduction of platysma bands,
    130
Leech
  medicinal, exploring use of, 248
Leg
  (*See also* Extremity, lower)
  lower, muscle transplant to, lack of
    significant postoperative contour
    change in, 258
  morbidity and function after fibular free
    flap harvest, 259
  ulcers
    chronic, granulocyte-macrophage
      colony-stimulating factor in, 279
    chronic, wound fluid from,
      biochemical analysis of, 285
    venous, reperfusion injury in, postural
      vasoregulation and mediators of,
      58
Lid (*see* Eyelid)
Lidocaine
  dose of 55mg/kg, tumescent anesthesia
    with, for liposuction, 198
  gel, 2%, in burn wound debridement
    pain, 89
Lift
  brow (*see* Browlift)

combined conventional and endoscopic
assisted, for facial rejuvenation,
134
face (*see* Facelift)
forehead
endoscopic, technique, 150
transblepharoplasty, 152
Limb (*see* Extremity)
Lip
augmentation
polytef implants in, wide, 142
revision, galea and subgalea graft for,
145
upper and lower, by buried,
deepithelialized local flaps, 143
cleft (*see* Cleft, lip)
incompetence as marker for progressive
bone resorption in Silastic chin
augmentation, 121
lower, unilateral, transient numbness,
after simultaneous osseous
genioplasty and meloplasty, 119
sculpture, 141
Lipectomy
suction-assisted (*see* Liposuction)
Lipohypertrophy
insulin-induced, liposuction for, 185
Liponecrotic
pseudocyst, large, after cheek
augmentation by fat injection, 198
Lipoplasty
in bulimic patient, 192
suction
(*See also* Liposuction)
abdominal, intestinal perforation and
peritonitis after, 191
intestinal perforation after, 190
Liposhaver
in facial plastic surgery, 184
Liposuction, 184
(*See also* Lipoplasty, suction)
anesthesia for, tumescent, with lidocaine
dose of 55mg/kg, 198
cervicofacial, isolated, applied to
treatment of aging, 127
circumferential, of knees, calves, and
ankles, 193
histologic alterations of adipose tissue
after, 194
for lipohypertrophy, insulin-induced,
185
mechanical properties of skin and, 195
photography for, standardization in,
187
tumescent, complicated by pulmonary
edema, 189
ultrasonic, for body sculpture, 188

value in improvement of cervicofacial
contours, 125
L-selectin
adhesion molecules in
musculocutaneous flap reperfusion
injury (in pig), 232
Lumbar
periosteal turnover flaps in
myelomeningocele closure, 37
Lymph node
ilioinguinal, dissection, tensor fasciae
lata myocutaneous flap
reconstruction after, 242
Lymphedema
postmastectomy upper limb, microwave
heating in, 56

M

McKissock reduction mammaplasty
silicone sheets in prevention of
hypertrophic scars after, 287
Macrophage
granulocyte-macrophage
colony-stimulating factor in chronic
leg ulcers, 279
stimulation, effect on collagen
biosynthesis in healing wound (in
rodent), 277
Magnetic resonance imaging
of carpal tunnel for median nerve
compression, 69
in combination with angiography,
diagnostic value in vascular
malformations, 34
fast, bilateral, of operated carpal tunnel,
68
of nasolabial fold changes, 132
of TRAM flap donor site, 228
Malarplasty
reduction, simple method of, 122
Malformations
(*See also* Deformities)
craniofacial, congenital, microsurgical
correction of facial contour in, 19
vascular, diagnostic value of MRI in
combination with angiography in,
34
Mammaplasty
augmentation, 199
characteristics of women with and
without, 199
implants for, textured or smooth,
3-year follow-up, 207
lack of association between
scleroderma and, 203
reduction, 213

bilateral, blood loss of scalpel *vs.*
cutting cautery in, 213
McKissock, silicone sheets in
prevention of hypertrophic scars
after, 287
methods, two, nipple sensitivity and
lactation in, 215
outpatient, safety of, 218
results of avoiding nipple-aerolar
amputation in cases of extreme
hypertrophy, 214
surgery, should it be rationed? 216
Managed care, 296
Mandible
asymmetry in hemifacial microsomia,
longitudinal analysis of, 21
condyle reconstruction, cranial bone
graft in (in monkey), 1
osteogenesis of, distraction,
histopathologic and biochemical
changes in muscles affected by (in
dog), 25
reconstruction with fibular free flap,
causes of, 260
Mandibular
nerve, marginal, transient weakness,
after simultaneous osseous
genioplasty and meloplasty, 119
Manganese
burn injury and, 94
Marketplace
new medical, 296
Masseter
muscle, histopathologic and biochemical
changes after distraction
osteogenesis of mandible (in dog),
25
Masseteric
hypertrophy, endoscope-assisted
intraoral approach for, 43
Mastectomy
lymphedema after, upper limb,
microwave heating in, 56
Mastopexy
breast implant removal combined with,
aesthetic outcome of, 206
Matrix
extracellular, in wound healing, 272
provisional, in wound healing, 272
Maxillary
morphology in patients with unilateral
complete cleft lip and palate, effect
of cleft lip repair on, 27
Mechanical
properties of skin and liposuction, 195
Median nerve
compression
MRI of carpal tunnel detecting, 69

recurrent, vein graft wrapping for, 71
in forearm, tubular *vs.* conventional
repair of, 73
Medical
marketplace, new, 296
Medicinal leech
exploring use of, 248
Melanoma
thin, recurrence of, effectiveness of
follow-up, 46
Meloplasty
genioplasty simultaneous with, osseous,
119
Meningococcal
septic shock, fulminant, treatment of
thromboembolic complications of,
293
Mental
function in Apert's syndrome, prognosis
for, 13
Metabolism
ornithine α-ketoglutarate, after enteral
administration in burn patients, 82
Microbial
growth inside saline-filled breast
implants, 208
Micrographic
surgery, Mohs, for dermatofibrosarcoma
protuberans
review of, 49
vs. wide surgical excision, 47
Microminerals
essential, and their response to burn
injury, 94
Microsomia
hemifacial, mandibular asymmetry in,
longitudinal analysis of, 21
Microsurgery, 231
facial contour in congenital craniofacial
malformations corrected by, 19
in head and neck reconstruction,
selection of appropriate recipient
vessels in, 248
smoking and, 266
Microtic
external ear reconstruction using porous
polyethylene implant, 62
Microvascular
free tissue transfers in elderly, 254
Microwave
heating in postmastectomy upper limb
lymphedema, 56
Mitek Mini GII Anchor System
for tendon reinsertion in medial
canthopexy, 158
Mohs micrographic surgery
for dermatofibrosarcoma protuberans
review of, 49

vs. wide surgical excision, 47
Morbidity
  of flap donor sites, radial forearm, 263
  of iliac crest harvest for alveolar cleft
    grafting, 30
  leg, after fibular free flap harvest, 259
Morphology
  maxillary, in patients with unilateral
    complete cleft lip and palate, effect
    of cleft lip repair on, 27
Motor
  nerve injury in composite rhytidectomy,
    139
MRI (*see* Magnetic resonance imaging)
Muscle(s)
  affected by distraction osteogenesis of
    mandible, histopathologic and
    biochemical changes in (in dog), 25
  digastric, contouring for rejuvenation of
    submental area of face, 198
  extraocular, combined paresis and
    restriction after orbital fracture, 66
  facial, lower, patterns of coordinated
    function, 57
  flap, neurovascular infrahyoid, in
    tongue reconstruction, 54
  individual, deletion alters walking-track
    parameters (in rat), 239
  latissimus dorsi
    free, endoscopic transfer, 255
    use in cardiomyoplasty, vascular delay
      improves muscle perfusion and
      function (in dog), 238
  rectus abdominis, vascular anatomy of
    tendinous intersections of, 222
  skeletal, ischemia-reperfusion injury in,
    231
  sling for prominent platysma bands,
    130
  transplant
    functioning free, for elbow flexion,
      results of, 264
    to lower leg, lack of significant
      postoperative contour change in,
      258
  underlying, wide and deep block
    excision for dermatofibrosarcoma
    protuberans including, 50
Musculocutaneous
  flap (*see* Myocutaneous, flap)
Myelomeningocele
  closure, lumbar periosteal turnover flaps
    in, 37
  repair with tissue expanders, 39
Myocutaneous
  flap
    gracilis, in perineal hernia repair, 243

rectus abdominis, transverse (*see*
  TRAM flap)
reperfusion injury, E- and L-selectin
  adhesion molecules in (in pig), 232
tensor fasciae lata, in reconstruction
  after ilioinguinal node dissection,
  242

N

Nasal
  ala
    hypoplastic, correction using
      auricular composite graft, 167
    reconstruction, chondrocutaneous ear
      helical free flap for, 55
    reductions in rhinoplasty, 174
  construction, total external and internal,
    in arhinia, 18
  CPAP for obstructive sleep apnea in
    children with craniofacial
    dysostosis, 16
  deviation, external bony, unilateral
    osteotomies for, 180
  packing, rhinoplasty, paraffinoma after,
    176
  sebaceous glands, quantification and
    distribution using image analysis,
    170
  septum
    perforations, repair with modified
      tragal cartilage-temporoparietal and
      deep temporal fascia sandwich
      graft, 181
    surgery for airway obstruction in
      rhinoplasty, 178
  surgery, aesthetic, 167
  tip
    cartilage concavities, suture correction
      of, 168
    reconstruction, conchal bowl skin
      grafting in, 51
    reconstruction, flap for,
      chondrocutaneous ear helical free,
      55
    surgery, cosmetic, and thick skin, 169
  valvular surgery for airway obstruction
    in rhinoplasty, 178
Nasofrontal
  angle, surgery of, 175
Nasolabial
  fat pad, pathogenesis and treatment of,
    133
  fold changes, MRI of, 132
  groove correction, wide polytef implants
    in, 142
Neck
  (*See also* Head and neck)

surgery, aesthetic, 125
Necrotizing
  soft tissue infections, 294
Negative pressure
  use to promote healing of tissue defects
    (*see* Vacuum, -assisted closure)
Neoplastic
  conditions, 45
Nerve
  injury, cold sensitivity after, long-term
    follow-up, 74
  mandibular, marginal, transient
    weakness, after simultaneous
    osseous genioplasty and meloplasty,
    119
  median (*see* Median nerve)
  motor, injury in composite
    rhytidectomy, 139
  peripheral
    injury, cold intolerance after, natural
      history and severity of symptoms,
      75
    vein wrapping of, barrier, histologic
      effect of (in rat), 72
  radial, entrapment, electrodiagnostic
    testing in, 67
  sural, endoscopic harvest, in children,
    250
  ulnar
    in forearm, tubular *vs.* conventional
      repair of, 73
    neuropathy, electrodiagnostic testing
      in, 67
Neurocutaneous
  island flaps in upper limb coverage, 242
Neuropathy
  peripheral, electrodiagnostic testing in,
    68
  ulnar nerve, electrodiagnostic testing in,
    67
Neurovascular
  flap, infrahyoid muscle, in tongue
    reconstruction, 54
Neutrophil
  -endothelial adhesion, CD18-dependent,
    in ischemia-reperfusion injury in
    skeletal muscle, 231
Nickel
  burn injury and, 94
Nipple
  -areolar amputation avoidance in
    reduction mammaplasty in cases of
    extreme hypertrophy, 214
  sensitivity and lactation in two methods
    of breast reduction, 215

Nose (*see* Nasal)
Numbness
  transient, in unilateral lower lip after
    simultaneous osseous genioplasty
    and meloplasty, 119

O

Obagi's modified trichloroacetic acid peel,
  112
Occlusive
  dressings for full-thickness wounds,
    comparison of three (in pig), 283
Office
  surgical facilities, accredited, patient
    safety in, 198
Onlay
  cranial bone allografts, cryopreserved,
    viability of (in sheep), 2
  material, new cranial, ceramic
    containing crosslinked collagen as
    (in rabbit), 2
OpSite
  for full-thickness wounds, comparative
    study (in pig), 283
Orbit
  fracture, combined paresis and
    restriction of extraocular muscles
    after, 66
Ornithine
  α-ketoglutarate metabolism after enteral
    administration in burn patients, 82
Osseous
  genioplasty simultaneous with
    meloplasty, 119
Ostectomy
  angle-splitting, for reducing width of
    lower face, 116
Osteogenesis
  distraction, of mandible, histopathologic
    and biochemical changes in muscles
    affected by (in dog), 25
Osteotomes
  four different types, comparison of, for
    lateral osteotomy, 177
Osteotomy
  lateral, comparison of four different
    types of osteotomes for, 177
  unilateral, for external bony deviation
    of nose, 180
Otoplasty
  endoscopic assisted, 42
Outpatient
  mammaplasty, reduction, safety of, 218
  surgery done under local anesthesia,
    reflex bradycardia in, 292
Oxygen
  therapy, hyperbaric, for burns, 83

P

Packing
  rhinoplasty nasal, paraffinoma after,
    176
Paecilomyces variotii
  growth inside saline-filled implants, 208
Pain
  burn
    procedural, intensity under conditions
      of varying physical control by
      patient, 89
    after wound debridement, topical 2%
      lidocaine gel for, 89
  donor site, after fibular free flap
    harvest, 260
Palate
  cleft (*see* Cleft, palate)
  hard
    closure, timing of, 27
    grafts, for postblepharoplasty lower
      eyelid retraction, 161
Palmaris
  longus tendon gliding resistance through
    A2 pulley, 77
Palsy
  Bell, time course of, 56
Paraffinoma
  after rhinoplasty nasal packing, 176
Paralysis
  facial, after cervicofacial liposuction,
    125
Paralytic
  lagophthalmos, surgical repair by
    medial tarsal suspension of lower
    lid, 159
Paresis
  combined paresis and restriction of
    extraocular muscles after orbital
    fracture, 66
Parotid
  leakage after rhytidectomy, management
    of, 140
Patient
  safety in accredited office surgical
    facilities, 198
Peel
  chemical
    blepharoplasty with,
      transconjunctival, 158
    Jessner's solution and 35%
      trichloroacetic acid in, *vs.*
      fluorouracil for widespread facial
      actinic keratoses, long-term efficacy
      and safety of, 45
    prevention of facial herpetic
      infections after, 111
  phenol, facial, 102

  trichloroacetic acid, Obagi's modified,
    112
Penile
  length in flaccid and erect states, and
    guidelines for penile augmentation,
    182
Perfusion
  latissimus dorsi, in cardiomyoplasty,
    vascular delay improves (in dog),
    238
Pericranial
  -galeo flaps in forehead, 240
Perineal
  hernia repair using gracilis
    myocutaneous flap, 243
Periocular
  skin reshaping by carbon dioxide laser,
    156
Periodontal
  evaluation, five-year, after secondary
    alveolar bone grafting, 29
Perioral
  area, chemical peel and dermabrasion
    of, prevention of facial herpetic
    infections after, 111
Periosteal
  turnover flaps, lumbar, in
    myelomeningocele closure, 37
Peripheral nerve
  injury, cold intolerance after, natural
    history and severity of symptoms,
    75
  vein wrapping of, barrier, histologic
    effect of (in rat), 72
Peritonitis
  after abdominal suction lipoplasty, 191
Pharyngeal
  wall augmentation, autogenous, for
    velopharyngeal dysfunction, 33
Phenol
  peel, facial, 102
Photoaging
  facial
    histologic effects of high-energy
      pulsed carbon dioxide laser for,
      102
    resurfacing for, full-face, with
      Ultrapulse carbon dioxide laser
      with CPG scanner, 108
Photodamaged skin
  appearance of, use of ultraviolet camera
    to enhance, 114
Photography
  standardization for body contour
    surgery and suction-assisted
    lipectomy, 187

Photometric
effects of 585 nm pulsed dye laser
treatments, 100
Physical
impairment of pediatric survivors of
burns of more than 80% total
body surface area, 87
Pi procedure
for correction of sagittal synostosis,
outcome analysis, 8, 9
Plagiocephaly
posterior
craniofacial asymmetry and,
long-term outcomes, 7
differential diagnosis of, 4
Plastic
surgery
endoscopic, pediatric, 42
facial, liposhaver in, 184
outpatient, under local anesthesia,
reflex bradycardia in, 292
smoking and, 266
Platelet
-activating factor levels and reperfusion
injury in venous ulceration, 58
Platysma
bands, management of, 130
Plexopathies
brachial, electrodiagnostic testing in, 68
Plications
two fusiform, for abdominoplasty, 183
Pocket
principle technique of ear replantation,
61
Polly beak
avoiding, 169
Polydioxanone
vs. polyglactin 910 in intradermal
repair, 288
Polyethylene
implant, porous, in reconstruction of
microtic external ear, 62
Polyglactin 910
vs. polydioxanone in intradermal repair,
288
Polytef
implants, wide, in lip augmentation and
nasolabial groove correction, 142
Polytetrafluoroethylene
expanded, in augmentation of lower
face, 147
Port-wine stains
treatment, 5-year assessment of, 36
Postauricular
hypertrophic scar after simultaneous
osseous genioplasty and meloplasty,
119

Postural
vasoregulation and mediators of
reperfusion injury in venous
ulceration, 58
Prefabricated
flap
allogeneically vascularized (in rabbit),
235
durability against bacterial challenge
(in rat), 233
jejunal free-tissue transfer for tracheal
reconstruction (in rat), 237
Prefabrication
flap
free, for tracheal reconstruction (in
goat), 236
impact of tissue expansion on (in
rabbit), 234
Premalignant
skin tumors, 45
Pressure
negative, use to promote healing of
tissue defects (*see* Vacuum, -assisted
closure)
ulcers, sacral, use of negative pressure
to promote healing, 289
Protein
provisions for thermally injured
children, 80
P-selectin
levels and reperfusion injury in venous
ulceration, 58
Pseudocyst
liponecrotic, large, after cheek
augmentation by fat injection, 198
parotid, after rhytidectomy, suction
drainage for, 140
Pseudomonas aeruginosa
growth inside saline-filled implants, 208
Psychological
well-being of facially disfigured people,
impact of social interaction skills
training on, 295
Psychosocial
factors in burn patients during
hospitalization, 85
Pulley
A2, gliding resistance of extrasynovial
and intrasynovial tendons through,
77
Pulmonary
edema complicating tumescent
liposuction, 189
Pump
infusion, tissue expansion for skin
deformities using, 269

Q

Quality of life
  health-related, before and after aesthetic
    surgery, 97
Quilting
  procedure in prevention of seroma in
    latissimus dorsi flap donor site, 246

R

Radial
  forearm flap donor site complications
    and morbidity, 263
  nerve entrapment, electrodiagnostic
    testing in, 67
Radiculopathy
  electrodiagnostic testing in, 68
Radiographic
  evaluation, five-year, after secondary
    alveolar bone grafting, 29
Radius
  fracture, distal, scapholunate
    dissociation associated with, cast
    immobilization for, 76
Reabsorption
  after fat injection, 196
Reanimation
  facial, and patterns of coordinated
    lower facial muscle function, 57
Reconstruction
  abdominal wall, tensor fascia lata free
    flap in, 265
  breast (see Breast, reconstruction)
  columella, chondrocutaneous ear helical
    free flap for, 55
  ear, microtic external, using porous
    polyethylene implant, 62
  facial, primary, for high-energy ballistic
    and avulsive injuries, 64
  finger, aesthetic refinements in
    toe-to-hand transfer for, 262
  flap
    free, in massive upper extremity
      burns, 93
    tensor fasciae lata myocutaneous,
      after ilioinguinal node dissection,
      242
  head and neck, 51
    microsurgical, selection of
      appropriate recipient vessels in, 248
  mandibular, with fibular free flap,
    causes of, 260
  mandibular condyle, cranial bone graft
    in (in monkey), 1
  nasal tip
    conchal bowl skin grafting in, 51

flap for, chondrocutaneous ear helical
    free, 55
  thumb, aesthetic refinements in
    toe-to-hand transfer for, 262
  tongue, neurovascular infrahyoid muscle
    flap in, 54
  trachea
    jejunal free-tissue transfer for,
      prefabricated (in rat), 237
    prefabrication of free flap for (in
      goat), 236
Rectus
  abdominis
    flap, free, for reconstruction in
      massive upper extremity burns, 93
    flap, free, for venous ulcer,
      recalcitrant chronic, 261
    flap, myocutaneous, transverse (see
      TRAM flap)
    muscle, vascular anatomy of
      tendinous intersections of, 222
  femoris
    flap, microneurovascular
      musculocutaneous free, for
      reconstruction in massive upper
      extremity burns, 93
    muscle transplant, functioning free,
      for elbow flexion, results of, 264
Reduction
  malarplasty, simple method of, 122
  mammaplasty (see Mammaplasty,
    reduction)
Re-epithelialization
  in wound healing, 272
Reflex
  bradycardia in outpatient surgery done
    under local anesthesia, 292
Rehabilitation
  of burn patients, critical pathways to
    enhance, 86
Rejuvenation
  facial
    implication of MRI dynamic analysis
      of changes in nasolabial fold in,
      132
    lift for, combined conventional and
      endoscopic assisted, 134
    submental area, digastric muscle
      contouring in, 198
    upper, transblepharoplasty, 152
Reperfusion
  injury
    musculocutaneous flap, E- and
      L-selectin adhesion molecules in (in
      pig), 232
    in skeletal muscle, 231

injury in venous ulceration, postural
vasoregulation and mediators of,
58
Replantation
digital, and smoking, 267
ear, without microsurgery, 61
Reshaping
periocular skin, by carbon dioxide laser,
156
Resident
level, teaching aesthetic surgery at, 98
Resource
costs of free *vs.* conventional TRAM
flap breast reconstruction, 223
Resurfacing
laser
full-face, with Ultrapulse carbon
dioxide laser with CPG scanner, for
rhytids, photoaging, and acne scars,
108
skin, 107
Resuscitation
burn (in sheep), 78
fluid
in necrotizing soft tissue infections,
294
volume for second-degree burns
reduced with delayed initiation of
ascorbic acid therapy (in guinea
pig), 77
Revascularization
single-stage, and free clap coverage for
ischemic lower limb lesions, 257
Rhinophyma
treatment, ultrasonic scalpel in, 173
Rhinoplasty
alar reductions in, 174
labiocolumellar crease incision in, 170
nasal packing, paraffinoma after, 176
primary, airway obstruction in, septal
and nasal valvular surgery in
correction of, 178
secondary, airway obstruction in, septal
and nasal valvular surgery in
correction of, 178
Rhytidectomy
composite
aesthetic and safety considerations in,
139
comparison with lateral and standard
SMAS facelifts, 138
intradermal repair after, polydioxanone
vs. polyglactin 910 in, 289
laser endoscopic, subperiosteal
minimally invasive, 137
parotid leakage after, management of,
140

SMAS, extended, comparison with
lateral and standard SMAS
facelifts, 138
Rhytids
facial
full-face resurfacing for, with
Ultrapulse carbon dioxide laser
with CPG scanner, 108
laser treatment of, superpulsed
carbon dioxide, 106
laser treatment of, superpulsed
carbon dioxide, combined with
cryotherapy, 105

S

Sacral
pressure ulcers, use of negative pressure
to promote healing, 289
Safety
patient, in accredited office surgical
facilities, 198
Sagittal
synostosis (*see* Synostosis, sagittal)
Saline
-filled breast implants, microbial growth
inside, 208
hypertonic, in burn resuscitation (in
sheep), 78
Scalp
-forehead flap fixation with K-wire,
endoscopic, 152
Scalpel
latissimus dorsi flap harvested by, and
seroma formation, 245
ultrasonic, in rhinophyma treatment,
173
vs. cutting cautery in bilateral reduction
mammaplasty, blood loss of, 213
Scanner
CPG, Ultrapulse carbon dioxide laser
with, for full-face resurfacing for
rhytids, photoaging, and acne scars,
108
Scapholunate
dissociation associated with distal
radius fractures, cast
immobilization for, 76
Scar, 271
acne
effects of dermabrasion on, 109
facial, full-face resurfacing with
Ultrapulse carbon dioxide laser
with CPG scanner for, 108
hypertrophic
breast, prevention with silicone
sheets, 287

postauricular, after simultaneous
osseous genioplasty and meloplasty,
119
submental, 119
revision, after reduction of platysma
bands, 130
from wound to scar, 272
Sclerosis
systemic, lack of association between
augmentation mammoplasty and,
203
Sculpture
body, 188
lip, 141
Sebaceous
glands, nasal, quantification and
distribution using image analysis,
170
Selectin
E-, adhesion molecules in
musculocutaneous flap reperfusion
injury (in pig), 232
L-, adhesion molecules in
musculocutaneous flap reperfusion
injury (in pig), 232
P-, levels, and reperfusion injury in
venous ulceration, 58
Selenium
burn injury and, 94
Self-esteem
after aesthetic surgery, 97
Septic
shock, fulminant meningococcal,
treatment of thromboembolic
complications of, 293
Septoplasty
for obstructive sleep apnea in infants
after cleft lip repair, 31
Septorhinoplasty
early secondary corrections after, 179
Septum
nasal
perforations, repair with modified
tragal cartilage-temporoparietal and
deep temporal fascia sandwich
graft, 181
surgery for airway obstruction in
rhinoplasty, 178
Seroma
after augmentation of lower face with
expanded polytetrafluoroethylene,
148
in latissimus dorsi flap donor site
causes and prevention, 245
prevention, 246
Serratus
flap

free, for recalcitrant chronic venous
ulcer, 261
reconstruction in massive upper
extremity burns, 93
Shock
septic, fulminant meningococcal,
treatment of thromboembolic
complications of, 293
Shotgun
wounds to face, primary reconstruction
for, 65
Silastic
chin augmentation, progressive bone
resorption in, labial incompetence
as marker for, 121
Silicone
breast implant (*see* Breast, implant,
silicone)
sheets in prevention of hypertrophic
breast scars, 287
tissue expanders in myelomeningocele
repair, 39
Skeletal
aesthetic surgery, 116
muscle, ischemia-reperfusion injury in,
231
Skin
aesthetic surgery on, 100
cancer, 45
conditions, ultraviolet camera to
enhance appearance of, 114
cryopreserved cadaver, for temporary
coverage of excised burn wounds,
92
deformities, continuous expansion for,
268
donor sites and deep partial-thickness
burns treated with cultured
epidermal allografts, 91
edema after burns, effect of
recombinant neutral endopeptidase
on (in guinea pig), 94
equivalents, living, produced with
collagens, grafting of (in mice), 271
expansion in burn patients, problems,
rules, and indications, 83
extender, clinical evaluation of, 270
facial, photoaged, histologic effects of
high-energy pulsed carbon dioxide
laser on, 102
graft, conchal bowl, in nasal tip
reconstruction, 51
irregularities after cervicofacial
liposuction, 125
leatherneck, after reduction of platysma
bands, 130
mechanical properties of, and
liposuction, 195

photodamaged, appearance of, use of
ultraviolet camera to enhance, 114
replacement, biosynthetic temporary, for
burns, 92
reshaping, periocular, by carbon dioxide
laser, 156
resurfacing, laser, 107
thick, and cosmetic surgery of nasal tip,
169
tumors, premalignant and malignant, 45
underlining, maximal, and vertical
SMAS flap, results of biplane
facelifts with, 136
wound healing, pulsed electromagnetic
fields in (in rat), 273
Skoog breast reduction technique
modified, nipple sensitivity and lactation
in, 215
Skull
surgery, posterior, in craniosynostosis,
15
Sleep
apnea, obstructive
craniofacial dysostosis and, nasal
CPAP for, 16
septoplasty for, after cleft lip repair in
infant, 31
SMAS
facelift, lateral and standard,
comparison with extended SMAS
and composite rhytidectomies, 138
flap, vertical, results of biplane facelifts
with, 136
rhytidectomy, extended, comparison
with lateral and standard SMAS
facelifts, 138
SMILE facelift, 137
Smoking
effect on plastic surgery and
microsurgery, 266
Social
interaction skills training for facially
disfigured people, impact of, 295
Soft tissue
defects, use of negative pressure to
promote healing of, 289
infections, necrotizing, 294
Stahl's ear
operation for, 36
Stains
port-wine, treatment, 5-year assessment
of, 36
Staphylococcus epidermidis
growth inside saline-filled implants, 208
Stenosis
lambdoid, and craniofacial asymmetry,
long-term outcomes, 7

Subgalea
graft for lip augmentation revision, 145
Submandibular
gland prolapse after simultaneous
osseous genioplasty and meloplasty,
119
Submental
area of face, rejuvenation of, digastric
muscle contouring for, 198
scar, hypertrophic, after simultaneous
osseous genioplasty and meloplasty,
119
Submucosal
aponeurotic system (*see* SMAS)
Subperiosteal
minimally invasive laser endoscopic
rhytidectomy, 137
Suction
-assisted lipectomy (*see* Liposuction)
drainage for parotid leakage after
rhytidectomy, 140
lipoplasty (*see* Lipoplasty, suction)
Sural
nerve harvest, endoscopic, in children,
250
Surgery
cosmetic, nasal tip, and thick skin, 169
microsurgery (*see* Microsurgery)
outpatient, done under local anesthesia,
reflex bradycardia in, 292
Surgical
facilities, accredited office, patient safety
in, 198
healing, impaired, and smoking (in
animals), 267
Suture
correction of nasal tip cartilage
concavities, 168
material, polydioxanone *vs.* polyglactin
910, in intradermal repair, 288
Synostectomy
vs. complex cranioplasty for sagittal
synostosis, 9
Synostosis
lambdoid, true, *vs.* positional molding,
4
sagittal
correction of, late, 10
pi procedure for, outcome analysis, 8
synostectomy *vs.* complex
cranioplasty for, 9

T

Tarsal
strip, lateral, for postblepharoplasty
lower eyelid retraction, 161

suspension, medial, lower lid, for
paralytic lagophthalmos, 159
Teaching
aesthetic surgery at resident level, 98
Temporal
fascia, modified tragal
cartilage-temporoparietal and deep
temporal fascia sandwich graft
technique for repair of nasal septal
perforations, 181
Temporalis
superficialis fascia, new use in facial
contour, 141
Temporoparietal
fascia, modified tragal
cartilage-temporoparietal and deep
temporal fascia sandwich graft
technique for repair of nasal septal
perforations, 181
Tendinous
intersections of rectus abdominis
muscle, vascular anatomy of, 222
Tendon
extrasynovial and intrasynovial, gliding
resistance through A2 pulley, 77
reinsertion in medial canthopexy, new
anchoring device for, 158
Tensor
fascia lata flap
free, in abdominal wall
reconstruction, 265
myocutaneous, in reconstruction after
ilioinguinal node dissection, 242
Thermal
injury (*see* Burns)
Thigh
flap, gluteal, in reconstruction in
massive upper extremity burns, 93
Thoracic
outlet syndrome, electrodiagnostic
testing in, 68
Thromboembolic
complications of fulminant
meningococcal septic shock,
treatment of, 293
Thrombosis
arterial, causing free flap failure in
lower extremities, 256
venous, causing free flap failure in
lower extremities, 256
Thumb
reconstruction, aesthetic refinements in
toe-to-hand transfer for, 262
Tissue
adhesive, long-term appearance of
lacerations repaired with, 286
adipose, postliposuction histologic
alterations of, 194

autologous, breast reconstruction with,
spontaneous return of sensibility in
breasts after, 229
defects, healing of, use of negative
pressure to promote, 289
expansion, 231
continuous, for skin deformities, 268
external device for, 270
impact on flap prefabrication (in
rabbit), 234
in myelomeningocele repair, 39
pediatric, 42
pediatric, risk factors for
complications in, 268
granulation, in wound healing, 272
soft, necrotizing infections of, 294
transfer, free
in children, 252
jejunal, prefabricated, for tracheal
reconstruction (in rat), 237
microvascular, in elderly, 254
smoking and, 267
in venous ulcer, recalcitrant chronic,
260
Toe
big, weakness after fibular free flap
harvest, 260
joint transfer to hand, vascularized, 261
-to-hand transfer surgery, aesthetic
refinements in, 262
Tongue
reconstruction, neurovascular infrahyoid
muscle flap in, 54
Torticollis
release, endoscopic, in children, 42
Trachea
reconstruction
jejunal free-tissue transfer for,
prefabricated (in rat), 237
prefabrication of free flap for (in
goat), 236
Tragal cartilage
-temporoparietal and deep temporal
fascia sandwich graft technique,
modified, for repair of nasal septal
perforations, 181
Training
social interaction skills, for facially
disfigured people, impact of, 295
TRAM flap
breast reconstruction
abdominal wall recovery after, 226
abdominal wall sequelae after, 227
bilateral, for post
implantectomy/capsulectomy breast
deformity, 224
free and conventional, comparison of
resource costs of, 223

donor site, MRI of, 228
Transblepharoplasty
  forehead lift and upper face
    rejuvenation, 152
Transconjunctival
  blepharoplasty
    with chemoexfoliation, 158
    lower lid, carbon dioxide laser,
      complications of, 155
Transfer
  latissimus dorsi muscle, endoscopic free,
    255
  tissue, free (*see* Tissue, transfer, free)
  toe joint, vascularized, to hand, 261
  toe-to-hand, aesthetic refinements in,
    262
Transforming growth factor
  -β isoforms, type I and type II receptors
    for, expression subsequent to
    TGF-β ligands during excisional
    wound repair (in sheep), 282
  -β1 cDNAs, particle-mediated gene
    transfer with, effect on wound
    repair (in rat), 276
Transplantation
  hair
    laser, 101
    mini-slit graft, using Ultrapulse
      carbon dioxide laser handpiece, 99
  muscle
    functioning free, for elbow flexion,
      results of, 264
    to lower leg, lack of significant
      postoperative contour change in,
      258
Trauma, 61
  extremity, upper, 67
  face, high-energy ballistic and avulsive,
    64
  head and neck, 61
  orbital fracture due to, combined
    paresis and restriction of
    extraocular muscles after, 66
Trichloroacetic acid
  35%, and Jessner's solution, *vs.*
    fluorouracil for widespread facial
    actinic keratoses, long-term efficacy
    and safety of, 45
  peel
    blepharoplasty with,
      transconjunctival, 158
    Obagi's modified, 112
Trunk
  surgery, aesthetic, 182
Tube
  ventilation, and hearing loss in children
    with cleft palate, 29

Tuberous
  breast
    deformity, classification and
      treatment, 209
    hypoplastic, extremely, surgical
      correction of, 211
Tubular
  vs. conventional repair of median and
    ulnar nerves in forearm, 73
Tumescent
  anesthesia with lidocaine dose of
    55mg/kg for liposuction, 198
  dermasanding with cryospraying, 110
  liposuction complicated by pulmonary
    edema, 189
Tumor
  modeling, growth characteristics of
    dermatofibrosarcoma protuberans
    based on, 49
  necrosis factor-α inhibits collagen α1
    gene expression and wound healing
    in cachexia (in mice), 280
  skin, premalignant and malignant, 45

U

Ulcer
  diabetic, effects of electrical stimulation
    on wound healing in patients with,
    275
  leg, chronic
    granulocyte-macrophage
      colony-stimulating factor in, 279
    wound fluid from, biochemical
      analysis of, 285
  pressure, sacral, use of negative pressure
    to promote healing, 289
  venous
    chronic recalcitrant, free tissue
      transfer in, 260
    reperfusion injury in, postural
      vasoregulation and mediators of,
      58
Ulnar
  nerve
    in forearm, tubular *vs.* conventional
      repair of, 73
    neuropathy, electrodiagnostic testing
      in, 67
UltraCision Harmonic Scalpel
  in rhinophyma treatment, 173
Ultrapulse carbon dioxide laser
  with CPG scanner for full-face
    resurfacing for rhytids, photoaging,
    and acne scars, 108
  handpiece, use in mini-slit graft hair
    transplantation, 99

Ultrasonic
   liposuction for body sculpture, 188
   scalpel in rhinophyma treatment, 173
Ultraviolet
   camera use to enhance appearance of
      photodamage and other skin
      conditions, 114

V

Vacuum
   -assisted closure
      animal studies and basic foundation,
         290
      clinical experience, 291
      clinical trial using, 289
Valvular
   surgery, nasal, for airway obstruction in
      rhinoplasty, 178
Vascular
   anatomy of tendinous intersections of
      rectus abdominis muscle, 222
   delay improves latissimus dorsi muscle
      perfusion and function for use in
      cardiomyoplasty (in dog), 238
   lesions, endoscopic excision of, in
      children, 42
   malformations, diagnostic value of MRI
      in combination with angiography
      in, 34
Vascularized
   prefabricated flaps, allogeneically (in
      rabbit), 235
   toe joint transfer to hand, 261
Vasoconstriction
   arteriolar, CD18-dependent, in
      ischemia-reperfusion injury in
      skeletal muscle, 231
Vasoregulation
   postural, and mediators of reperfusion
      injury in venous ulceration, 58
Vein
   graft wrapping for recurrent
      compression of median nerve, 71
   thrombosis causing free flap failure in
      lower extremities, 256
   ulcer
      chronic recalcitrant, free tissue
         transfer in, 260
      reperfusion injury in, postural
         vasoregulation and mediators of,
         58
   wrapping, barrier, of peripheral nerves,
      histologic effect of (in rat), 72
Velopharyngeal
   dysfunction, surgical management of,
      33

Ventilation
   tube and hearing loss in children with
      cleft palate, 29
Vessels
   (*See also* Vascular)
   appropriate recipient, selection in
      microsurgical head and neck
      reconstruction, 248
Veterans
   World War II, severely wounded, late
      follow-up of, 296

W

Walking
   -track parameters, deletion of individual
      muscles alters (in rat), 239
Washing
   self-washing effect on procedural burn
      pain intensity, 89
Waterhouse-Friderichsen syndrome, 293
Wattles
   small, after cervicofacial liposuction,
      125
Wire
   K-wire, endoscopic forehead-scalp flap
      fixation with, 152
World War II veterans
   severely wounded, late follow-up of,
      296
Wound
   burn
      debridement pain, topical 2%
         lidocaine gel in, 89
      excised, Dermagraft-transitional
         covering of, 92
      excisional, repair, type I and type II
         receptors for transforming growth
         factor-β isoforms are expressed
         subsequent to TGF-β ligands
         during (in sheep), 282
   fluid
      hyaluronic acid of, in adult and fetus
         (in rabbit), 274
      from leg ulcers, chronic, biochemical
         analysis of, 285
   full-thickness, comparative study of
      three occlusive dressings for (in
      pig), 283
   healing (*see* Healing, wound)
   infection after simultaneous osseous
      genioplasty and meloplasty, 119
   from wound to scar, 272
Wounded World War II veterans
   severely, late follow-up of, 296
Wrapping
   vein

barrier, of peripheral nerves,
    histologic effect of (in rat), 72
graft, for recurrent compression of
    median nerve, 71

Y

YV-advancement, 247

Z

Zinc
  burn injury and, 94

Z-plasty
  for platysma bands, 130
  principle, theoretical consideration of
    extensions of, 247
Zygoma
  prominent, simple method reduction,
    122

Author Index

A

Abbott AH, 14
Ågren MS, 283
Allmann KH, 69
Alster TS, 106
Amadio PC, 77
Amarante MTJ, 132
Amato D, 91
Anderson RL, 161
Aniceto C, 279
Antonacci R, 66
Antonyshyn OM, 158
Antrobus SD, 148
Apfelberg DB, 108
Arámbula-Alvarez H, 91
Argamaso R, 7
Argenta LC, 290, 291
Arnaud E, 11, 13
Arndt KA, 100
Aronsson A, 109
Asato H, 239
Asko-Seljavaara S, 93, 227
Aston SJ, 138

B

Baena-Montilla P, 236
Bajec J, 55
Baker LL, 275
Baker SS, 155
Baker TJ, 102
Baker TM, 102
Banis JC Jr, 237
Barak A, 185
Batchelor AGG, 254
Bays RA, 1
Bazán A, 2
Becker DG, 184
Bekkelund SI, 68
Bell JL, 243
Benacquista T, 256
Bengtson BP, 218
Ben-Izhak O, 154
Benn SI, 276
Bertelli JA, 242
Berton M, 88
Birely B, 64
Blakeney P, 87
Bolgiani A, 273
Bonanad E, 236
Boop FA, 8, 9
Borg DH, 34
Bosshardt TL, 294

Botti G, 169
Boyd B, 259
Brannen AL, 83
Brenda E, 183
Brenner E, 245
Bresnick S, 2
Briggs JC, 46
Broadley KN, 276
Broen PA, 29
Brogan WF, 29
Bruns TB, 286
Buchman SR, 37
Buck M, 280
Budo JA, 188
Buncke G, 266
Burstein FD, 42
Button B, 78

C

Cacou C, 57
Camirand A, 131
Campion D, 67
Canady JW, 214
Cannon B, 296
Capek L, 250
Capozzi A, 98, 293
Carlson GW, 265
Carlstrom J, 29
Carpaneda CA, 194
Carroll SM, 238
Carver N, 264
Castroviejo-Bolibar M, 159
Cavadas PC, 236
Celiköz B, 39
Chadduck WM, 8, 9
Chajchir A, 195
Chambers R, 275
Chang LD, 266
Chang P, 214
Chen H-C, 261, 262
Chen SH-T, 261
Cherry GW, 58
Chiarello SE, 110
Cho BC, 255
Chojkier M, 280
Cholon A, 2
Chuang DC-C, 262, 264
Chumas PD, 11
Chun JT, 243
Churukian K, 237
Ciletti SJ, 10
Cinalli G, 11, 13
Clardy RB, 178

Clark N, 64
Clarke HM, 250
Clarren SK, 4
Coates N, 189
Coert JH, 77
Cohen SR, 42
Coleman DJ, 207
Colen LB, 240
Collins ED, 74
Conrad K, 142
Constantian MB, 178
Cook LS, 199
Cooter RD, 254
Coudray-Lucas C, 82
Covington DS, 79
Cox SE, 45
Crespo LD, 61
Cruz-Korchin NI, 287
Cunningham JJ, 80
Cutting CB, 31

D

da Costa RM, 279
Dagum AB, 158
Dahlin L, 73
Dalal AV, 242
Daling JR, 199
Daniel RK, 150
DeBiasse MA, 94
de Benito J, 145
de Chalain TMB, 248
de Damborenea A, 159
Deguchi M, 116
de la Cruz L, 165
de la Fuente A, 134
de la Plaza R, 165
Demling RH, 94
DeMuth SK, 275
Deuber MA, 252
Dijkstra R, 215
Diniz VM, 141
Dodson TB, 1
Donelan M, 84
Doucet J, 131
Dover JS, 100
Dufresne RG, 173
Dzubow LM, 51

E

Echinard C, 83
Elejabeitia J, 2
Elias AC, 121
Elias RL, 121

Elmaraghy MW, 70
Enacar A, 27
Eriksson M, 270
Eriksson T, 109
Ersek RA, 149, 193
Espinoza LR, 201
Evans GRD, 223
Exner K, 209

F

Fan J, 270
Fanous N, 180
Fatah MFT, 246
Feakins R, 176
Feldberg L, 207
Fernández-Sanza I, 145
Fernández-Vega A, 159
Fiala TGS, 37
Figueroa AA, 21
Fisher E, 25
Fisher SE, 263
Fitzpatrick R, 97, 216
Fitzpatrick RE, 101
Flageul G, 127
Flock S, 36
Fontana AM, 175
Franulic A, 85
Franzén L, 283
Friedland JA, 157
Friedman RM, 268
Fukuta K, 240
Fulton JE Jr, 114

G

Gabriel SE, 200
Gamliel Z, 94
Gan J-L, 56
Gang RK, 55
Garg S, 106
Gault DT, 42
Germain L, 271
Gherardini G, 187
Giannakopoulos PN, 71
Gilbert SE, 158, 174
Gilbert SEA, 75
Gilliland MD, 189
Gloster HM Jr, 47
Goffin V, 195
Gold LI, 282
Goldin JH, 15
Gonsalez S, 16
González X, 85
Goode RL, 105
Goodrich JT, 7

Gordon DJ, 46
Gosain AK, 132
Graham KE, 42
Grana D, 273
Greenfield BE, 57
Griffin ME, 107
Grong K, 191
Gruss JS, 4
Gu YQ, 76
Guha SC, 78
Guidi MC, 268
Gunji H, 36
Gunter JP, 148
Gürlek A, 251
Gürsu KG, 27, 50
Guyuron B, 288

H

Hage JJ, 247
Hamas RS, 151
Hansbrough JF, 92
Hansen MT, 243
Haramoto U, 167
Harashina T, 248
Harris KR, 47
Har-Shai Y, 185
Hata K, 90
Haycox CL, 49
Haynes M, 83
Hayward R, 16
He C, 58
Heilman SJ, 238
Henderson VJ, 294
Henry F, 195
Hergrueter CA, 234
Hertl MC, 208
Hibino Y, 90
Hirai T, 235
Ho C, 99
Hochberg MC, 203
Hockley AD, 15
Hoffman LA, 190
Holder IA, 94
Honda T, 43
Horch RE, 69
Horie K, 90
Houglum K, 280
Hovius SER, 34
Howell RL, 265
Huang MHS, 4, 42
Huang V, 222
Hughes K, 235
Hunt NP, 57
Hurst LN, 70, 213
Hurwitz PJ, 292
Hussain A, 181
Hwang YJ, 122

Hyde JS, 132

I

Isik S, 62
Ichinose H, 112
Iio Y, 116
Illouz Y-G, 127
Imwalle AR, 94
Ingram AE Jr, 268
Inoue T, 248
Irwin MS, 75
Isenberg JS, 258
Ivy EJ, 138

J

Jackson BA, 100
Jacobsen WM, 157
Jacobsson S, 109
Jenkinson C, 97, 216
Jeon JY, 122
Jesus FM, 279
Johns DF, 27
Johnson JB, 112
Josephson GD, 31

K

Kaila S, 213
Kaplan I, 156
Kappel RM, 215
Kapucu MR, 27
Karp NS, 256
Kasabian AK, 256
Kealey GP, 92
Kerrigan CL, 232
Khan JI, 176
Kim M, 237
Kim SK, 152
Kind GM, 226
Kinsky MP, 78
Klassen A, 97, 216
Ko CY, 229, 233
Kobayashi K, 116
Kobayashi S, 167
Koman LA, 72
Kostakolu N, 50
Kostianovsky AS, 143
Krieger LM, 296
Kroll SS, 223, 251
Kruft S, 209
Kuo H-R, 170
Kuran I, 177
Kuzon WM, 219
Kwasny O, 289

L

Landon BN, 204
Langton SR, 285
Larrabee WF Jr, 147
Lask G, 99, 107
Laubenberger J, 69
Lawrence N, 45
Leblanc P, 136
Le Bricon T, 82
Lee JH, 255
Lee MS, 122
Levi Y, 154
Levine J, 31
Li S-l, 56
Lieberman M, 190
Linares HA, 272
Linder S, 293
Linder SA, 98
Lioret N, 82
Liou EJ-W, 21
Longaker MT, 19
López Valle CAL, 271
Lorenc ZP, 138
Love EJ, 277
Lowe NJ, 107
Lowery JC, 219
Lue TF, 182
Lundborg G, 73

M

MacDonald MR, 142
Mackinnon SE, 74
Mahdi S, 220
Maitz PKM, 234
Majocco AM, 54
Maladry D, 136
Malata CM, 207, 254
Manders EK, 235
Manson PN, 64
Marques A, 183
Marsh JL, 33
Marshall D, 224
Maruyama Y, 244
Matarasso A, 121, 187
Matsuda H, 77
Mauriello JA Jr, 66
Maxwell D, 89
McAninch JW, 182
McCarthy JG, 25
McComb HK, 29
McDermott RE, 192
McGeorge DD, 220
McKinney P, 130, 140

McLario DJ, 286
Medsger TA Jr, 203
Mele JA, 293
Mele JA III, 98
Mellgren SI, 68
Memore L, 277
Mertz PM, 283
Meyer R, 18
Michelson LN, 170
Miller PJ, 184
Mitsionis GI, 71
Mitz V, 136
Mole B, 125
Moller KT, 29
Moloney DM, 46
Monstrey S, 257
Montgomery PQ, 176
Moore M, 87
Moore MH, 14
Moore P, 87, 88
Morykwas MJ, 290, 291
Mostafavi R, 66
Mozingo DW, 92
Mrkonjic L, 289
Müllner T, 289
Muraszko KM, 37
Murray PR, 208
Murthy P, 181
Mustoe TA, 226
Muti E, 175, 211
Muuronen E, 93

N

Nasri S, 105
Neely AN, 94
Neligan P, 259
Netscher DT, 205
Neu BR, 168
Newman JP, 105
Nguyen D, 284
Nguyen Q, 99
Ninkovic M, 245
Nordström REA, 270
Novak CB, 74
Nunes PHF, 268

O

Obagi ZE, 112
O'Brien J, 89
O'Daniel TG, 33
Odland PB, 49
O'Fallon WM, 200
Ogilvie M, 292
Ohmori K, 167
Olbricht SM, 49

Omokawa S, 241
Ono I, 36
Organ CH Jr, 294
Orgill DP, 61
Orringer JS, 229
Orten SS, 36
Ovrebo KK, 191
Özcan G, 50
Özcan H, 177

P

Paans PR, 34
Pakkanen M, 149
Parks DH, 79
Partridge J, 295
Patel BCK, 161
Patel SG, 242
Patiño O, 273
Patipa M, 161
Peck GC Jr, 170
Pensler JM, 10
Pereira MD, 183
Perkins SW, 111
Perlmutter DL, 203
Pfeffle RC, 1
Phil D, 58
Pierre-Jerome C, 68
Pina DP, 139
Polley JW, 21
Portera CA, 277
Potparić Z, 240
Pozner JN, 137
Prelack K, 80
Pribaz JJ, 61, 234

Q

Qi WW, 56

R

Rademaker AW, 226
Ramasastry SS, 255
Ramirez OM, 137, 152
Reece GP, 223
Remmert SM, 54
Renier D, 13
Rey RM Jr, 284
Reynolds JL, 239
Rice JC, 201
Richard R, 86
Richards AM, 32
Richardson D, 263
Rigau J, 156
Ringler SL, 218

Rivas-Torres MT, 91
Robert R, 88
Robinson E, 295
Roenigk RK, 47
Rohrer TE, 51
Rohrich RJ, 27, 151, 268
Rosén B, 73
Rouabhia M, 271
Routh AC, 231
Rowsell AR, 27
Rozelle A, 173
Ruch DS, 72
Rudman RA, 30
Rumsey N, 295
Ryu J, 241

S

Salisbury AV, 149, 193
Sando K, 274
Santamaría AB, 134
Sanz J, 2
Sasaki K, 43
Savant DN, 242
Sawai T, 274
Sawaizumi M, 244
Schendel S, 2
Schingo VA Jr, 252
Schuler J, 260
Schusterman MA, 251
Schwabegger A, 245
Sengezer M, 39, 62
Serletti JM, 252
Serure AS, 187
Sgouros S, 15
Shaaban AF, 214
Sharma S, 205
Shaw WW, 229, 233
Shelton-Brown EI, 290
Sheridan R, 84
Sheridan RL, 80
Sherris DA, 147
Shewmake K, 8, 9
Shi D, 76
Shimazaki S, 77
Short KK, 218
Shpitzer T, 259
Siebert JW, 19, 282
Simon HK, 286
Sklarew EC, 111
Slezak S, 266
Smith JW, 140
Smoot EC III, 284
Sommer KD, 54
Sotereanos DG, 71

Sparkes G, 89
Spinner RM, 72
Spiro SA, 119, 170, 224
Spyrou GE, 246
Stacey MC, 285
Staffenberg DA, 25
Staley M, 86
Stephenson LL, 231
Still J, 83
Storm van Leeuwen JB, 215
Stotland MA, 232
Stremel RW, 238
Stucker FJ, 56
Stuzin JM, 102
Sung JJ, 282
Suominen S, 227, 228
Sutherland S, 89
Svahn JK, 204
Szalay L, 179

T

Takamatsu A, 248
Takeuchi M, 43
Talmor M, 190
Tan AES, 29
Tanaka H, 77
Tang J-B, 76, 241
Tateshita T, 36
Tenenbaum SA, 201
Terenghi G, 75
TerKonda S, 157
Tervahartiala P, 228
Thompson D, 16
Thornby J, 205
Ting J, 155
Tirkanits B, 150
Titley OG, 246
Tomita T, 10
Trelles MA, 155, 156
Trengove NJ, 285
Trepsat F, 133
Trucco M, 85
Tsekouras A, 220
Tukiainen E, 93
Türegün M, 39, 62

U

Uchiyama S, 77
Ullmann Y, 154, 185
Urbanchek MS, 239

Usta A, 177
Usui N, 274

V

Van Landuyt K, 257
Van Look, 195
Vargas VEB, 268
Vastine VL, 204
Vaughan C, 288
Vaughan ED, 263
Vegter F, 247
Vermassen F, 257
Vindenes H, 191
Voigt LF, 199
von Heimburg D, 209
von Smitten K, 227, 228

W

Wainwright DJ, 79
Waner M, 36
Waterhouse N, 32
Wei F-C, 261, 262, 264
Weinberg MJ, 158
Weinberger MS, 184
Weinzweig N, 260
Wessells H, 182
Whetzel TP, 222
Whitsitt JS, 276
Wider TM, 119, 170
Wilkins EG, 219
Willard SG, 192
Williams JK, 265
Witheiler DD, 45
Withey SJ, 32
Witt PD, 33
Wolfe SA, 119, 170
Woodhouse LM, 192
Woods JE, 200

Y

Yin SS, 56
Young VL, 208

Z

Zamboni WA, 231
Zhu X, 84
Zienowicz RJ, 173
Zuckerbraun BS, 140
Zuker RM, 250